RADIOLOGY
AND INJURY
IN SPORT

RADIOLOGY
AND INJURY
IN SPORT

Jack W. Bowerman, M.D.
Associate Professor of Radiology
Joint Appointments in Emergency
Medicine and Orthopedic Surgery
Director of Skeletal Radiology
Department of Radiology and Radiological Science
Johns Hopkins Medical Institutions
Baltimore, Maryland

APPLETON-CENTURY-CROFTS/New York

Library of Congress Cataloging in Publication Data

Bowerman, Jack W   1938-
    Radiology and injury in sport.

    Includes bibliographies and index.
    1.   Sports—Accidents and injuries—Diagnosis.
2.   Diagnosis, Radioscopic.   I.   Title. [DNLM:
1.   Athletic injuries—Radiography.   QT260 B786r]
RD97.B67   617′.1027   77-2287
ISBN 0-8385-8250-8

Credits

Baseball (p. 147) is courtesy of the Baltimore Orioles, photograph by Jay Spencer.
Basketball (p. 160) is taken from a photograph by Jocelyn Hinsen.
Football (p. 178) is courtesy of the Baltimore Colts, with permission of Ernie Accorsi.
Gymnastics (p. 200) is reprinted courtesy of Frank Yapps.
Squash (p. 205) is reprinted courtesy of George Mars from a Theodore Lane print done in 1827.
Hockey (p. 208) is reprinted courtesy of the Chicago Black Hawks.
Horseback Riding (p. 214) is courtesy of the Maryland Horsebreeder's Association; credit to Marzani.
Lacrosse (p. 218) is from a print by George Catlin; courtesy of the Lacrosse Hall of Fame, Skeeter Chadwick, Curator, Johns Hopkins University.
Boxing (p. 172), *Cricket* (p. 176), *Fencing* (p. 177), *Hang-Gliding* (p. 207), *Soccer* (p. 238), and *Track and Field* (p. 256) are all reprinted courtesy of the *Baltimore Sun-papers*.

Prentice-Hall International, Inc., London
Prentice-Hall of Australia, Pty. Ltd., Sydney
Prentice-Hall of India Private Limited, New Delhi
Prentice-Hall of Japan, Inc., Tokyo
Prentice-Hall of Southeast Asia (Pte.) Ltd., Singapore
Whitehall Books Ltd., Wellington, New Zealand

PRINTED IN THE UNITED STATES OF AMERICA

ACKNOWLEDGMENTS

Many people have contributed in some measure to this effort. Martin W. Donner has provided constant leadership and the direct opportunity for my work in skeletal radiology. Robert A. Robinson and Lee H. Riley have encouraged, welcomed, and instructed me in the orthopedic department. Behind the scenes Russell H. Morgan has always provided personal counsel and his own model of excellence. Ronald O. Murray, Harold G. Jacobson, and B. "Gil" Brogdon have made unique and enthusiastic contributions to my studies and to this work. My co-workers and teachers Bob W. Gayler, Fred J. Hodges III, and John P. Dorst have always offered advice and support.

Special thanks is due to those people who loaned precious case material. Edmond McDonnell and Kenneth Spence have been particularly generous in this regard. Other material has been provided by many colleagues presently or formerly at Johns Hopkins including Jeremy Altman, Klemens Barth, Richard Ferguson, David Filtzer, Charles Fisher, Olga Baghdassarian Gatewood, Bill Gatewood, Donald Harrington, Fred J. Hodges III, James Hughes, A.J. Kumar, Maxwell Lai, James Milgram, Charles Morreels, Ole Ottesen, Pedro Purcell, Lee Riley, and Robert White. Case material has also been generously provided by Frank Cawley, Overton Himmelwright, Harold G. Jacobson, Thomas Meaney, Ronald O. Murray, Lee Rogers, and K. Tan. William Stripp has cooperated in providing copies of selected cases from the Royal National Orthopaedic Hospital in London. Susan Baker kindly reviewed sections of the manuscript and made valuable suggestions that led to information from scholars in the field of trauma.

Information and photographic material has been provided by Bob Brown of the public relations office of the Baltimore Orioles and Ernie Accorsi of the Baltimore Colts. Technologists Deborah Braun, John Freeland, George Flickinger, and Jeff Sneeringer have contributed useful radiographs. Perspective on injury in several areas of sport has been offered by Charlie Jeffrey, Abie Grossfeld, Muriel Grossfeld, R.D. Meyer, and Leroy Brandimore.

At our art department Ranice Crosby spearheaded a team including Amalie Dunker, Margorie Gregerman, and Gary Lees. They produced all the drawings in the book and did so in a painstaking manner. Ms. Crosby was particularly helpful in preparing all the illustrations. The original photographs of the radiographs were prepared by Henri Hessels and Willie Ragsdale.

My secretary, Kristy Shea, prepared the entire manuscript faithfully and diligently. Other parts of the initial stages of the manuscript were typed by Monica Masanielo, Dorothy Magner, and Scottie Dohme.

Finally, the publishers deserve their own lines of praise. Doreen Berne and Steven Abramson have been patient editors and deserve credit and gratitude for their work in this project. Rodelinde Albrecht, as art director, designed the cover.

PREFACE

The following material is grouped according to sites of injury and activity. Part I includes information on the x-ray examination of injured body areas. Its aim is to provide a guide for radiologic assistance in the evaluation and treatment of the injured person. It includes comments on pitfalls in the diagnosis and it provides advice to aid in a comprehensive evaluation of the x-ray evidence following injury. Part II includes a description of the activity and hazards in sport. Wherever possible, injuries are documented by abstracts of case reports and articles illustrating features of injury in sport. The sports included are listed in alphabetical order. Part III is a section of radiographs used to show examples of injury. In nearly every example, an amateur or professional athlete was injured in his or her sport. The plan of x-ray presentation is similar to that used in a recent important radiology text on skeletal disorders. The radiographs are presented as a series of unknown problems so that the reader can actively assess his or her diagnostic skills before the denouement of each example.

In the chapters to follow I will refer at times to anteroposterior and posteroanterior radiographic views. In an anteroposterior view, the diagnostic x-rays enter the anterior part of the body or extremity and exit via the posterior wall, to be recorded on the film placed behind the person or body part. The reverse is true in a posteroanterior view.

CONTENTS

INTRODUCTION

The number of injuries that occur in sport and recreation in the world each year is vast. In the United States, in one year alone approximately 700 deaths occur in bicycling, compared to 4500 deaths due to tuberculosis.[1,2] Medical, economic, and psychosocial aspects of the injuries and fatalities in sport are of considerable importance. The era in which only the mortality associated with sport was recorded is now giving way to a period of closer scrutiny in which the morbidity of sport is being evaluated as well. The extent and significance of injury has great variability from patient to patient. In certain patients an injury is a single chance event with no untoward sequelae and no psychologic or financial complications. However, in the serious amateur and in the professional athlete every injury is viewed as a career-threatening event. The treatment and prevention of these injuries is predicated on adequate diagnosis and recognition of the injury. This can be accomplished with knowledge of the particular patterns of injury after trauma, particularly after sports injury. Physicians and trainers interested in trauma must constantly remember to be complete in their evaluation of the patient's problem. From a radiographic standpoint, this requires care in choosing useful views and, more importantly, skill and thoroughness in evaluating them. The busy practitioner must be able to concentrate on the problem at hand and consider alternative diagnostic techniques including arthrography, xeroradiography, and radioisotopic procedures.

It may take days, weeks, or months to establish an accurate picture of an injury. The initial x-ray examination is not the only item to consider. Some subtle fractures will only be detected by subsequent radiographic study. Too often the novice in radiology or orthopedics attempts to decide resolutely on the basis of a single inadequate examination. He or she may not pursue an elusive diagnosis out of false confidence and unrecognized ignorance. The pattern in some training programs in radiology has been to ignore many aspects of skeletal and visceral trauma in favor of other medical pursuits that tend to occupy the talents of the senior workers, while the junior members are assigned to the front lines of the emergency rooms and accident wards.

Certain other issues must be considered. Is the injured athlete likely to suffer injuries different from those in nonathletes with trauma? Stress fractures, skeletal hypertrophy and other overuse phenomena are the obvious candidates for a positive answer. Athletic activity of some type, including prolonged walking and dancing, must lead to these findings. Many other injuries in sport, including epiphyseal and avulsion injuries, can be reproduced in the nonathlete after falls, motor vehicle collisions, and the like. It is the circumstances of injury, the risk taking involved, and the continued exposure to risk that produce interesting characteristics of the injury in sport.

What in the athlete contributes to injury in sport? Infrequently, in studies of injury, personal and social factors have been considered. Previous aggressive behavior and the use of alcohol and drugs have been associated with some reports of injury in sport. Motivational and personal factors must play a tremendous role in creating the entire distribution of injuries in and away from sport. Research efforts are needed to emphasize these contributions and possibly lead to modification of the conditions at hand. One type of modification employed in injury control involves changes in both the design and use of protective equipment. Boxers, for example, might be required to use protective headgear. Motorcyclists or snowmobile operators might be required to use helmets equipped with visors to protect the face. A second type of modification is restriction of activity shown to be harmful if done excessively, for example, limiting javelin throwing and baseball pitching in the adolescent athlete. This adaptation is ideal in that it permits continued involvement in sport yet tempers the activity as a result of the contributions of sports medicine.

A word of caution is needed for the serious student of injury regarding the pertinent literature. The study of prior publications on sports injury includes the review of varied work. Some papers give an exact time period of studies so that the injuries observed in a defined period of time are reported and compared to those in other athletes or age-matched controls not involved in that sport. Some papers give only anecdotal experiences in which one or two examples of a certain injury are recalled without a complete study involving extensive numbers of subjects and controls. Such anecdotal reports have some value, however, in pinpointing possible areas for more extensive study. The long-term effects of athletic activity on the mental, physical, social, and economic aspects of human life are additional factors to consider.

Haddon discussed the principles of research in the effects of sports on health from a broad standpoint in 1966.[3] He noted that basic data on the incidence and prevalence of sports injuries have not yet been obtained. He emphasized that the factors of exposure—that is, the nature and amount of participation—must be defined and measured as precisely as possible. He considers several variables worthy of consideration and evaluation: the rules of sport (objectives, circumstances of play, equipment, etc); the participants (age, sex, physical and mental attributes, etc.); the immediate sport environment (coaches, influence of spectators, weather conditions, etc); medical variables (regular screening for injury or evaluation of the injured); late effects of sports injuries (possible long-term medical benefits or liabilities); and, lastly, the time and place of sports activity in relation to the possibilities of seasonal or geographic variation of injury in sport.

The role the radiologist can play in this entire picture of sports injury depends on his or her understanding of the patterns of injury and other variables. The enlightened radiologist can effect change in the medical variables cited by Haddon. As an example, the regular screening of radiographic examinations of football and baseball players has become a part of yearly physical examinations. A comprehensive knowledge of the contributions made in the study of trauma assists in this difficult task.

References

1. Editorial: Cycling fatalities on the rise. Stat Bull Metropol Life Ins Co 48:4–6, 1967
2. Editorial. Current status of tuberculosis in the United States. Stat Bull Metropol Life Ins Co 55:9–11, 1974
3. Haddon W Jr: Principles in research on the effects of sports on health. JAMA 197:885–888, 1966

HISTORICAL

Prehistoric records of the activities of man include the petrographs of the Old Stone Age. Drawings in caves such as those at Lascaux and at Altamira depict the animals known to early man as objects of hunting.[2,5] In the Lascaux cave in France the human figure is portrayed in a drawing of a man either injured or dead adjacent to a wounded bison.[2,3] One theory holds that the man was gored by the bison, probably in the hunt.[3] This then suggests that these art treasures, between 30,000 and 100,000 years old, are the earliest records of injury in what are considered by today's standards to be sporting events.

The early records of sport are part of the history of the ancient peoples of the world. The early Greek, Roman, Egyptian, Chinese, and Central American cultures contributed to this history. The games of ancient Greece were important as a unifying force for the members of the different countries and states of Greece. The Olympic Games was the feature event, beginning in the shadowy past and undergoing reemphasis by Lycurgus the Lawgiver in 776 BC.[6] That year is counted as the first Olympiad, according to McGregor, and the second occurred in 772 BC.[6] In their earliest form the games lasted only one day and consisted simply of running events. Later other events were added to include wrestling, boxing, racing, and chariot races covering a five-day period.

The word *athlete* stems from a Greek word of two forms.[4] One form was used to indicate a contest and another to refer to a contest prize. Homer used the word to describe the contest of the ten-year struggle of the Trojan War. In the Odyssey the word *athlete* is used in a jibe. This appears at a point when Odysseus has reached the land of the Phaeacians after being shipwrecked. Excusing himself from an invitation to try his skill at sports Odysseus finds one of the young Phaeacians appraising his disinterest in games with a passage ending "thou art no athlete." Odysseus is stung by this taunt and hurls a diskos—a heavy stone—far beyond the established marks.

Gardiner, in *Athletics of the Ancient World,* recounts some of the early history of sport.[4] The tombs of Beni-Hassan (circa 1991–1778 BC), located along the Nile between the ancient cities of Thebes and Gizeh, depict the early

Egyptian sports. Among them is one wall showing 220 groups of wrestlers in various poses of action. According to Gardiner, wrestling is the oldest of sports. Running, boxing, polo, and an early form of soccer are mentioned as other activities of these ancient peoples. The Tartars, Gardiner believes, must have played polo centuries before that game came to China in 600 AD. Boxing is mentioned by the Marquis of Chin in a campaign in 631 BC: he dreamed that he was boxing with the Viscount Chu. The inhabitants of a town in China called Lin-tzu are known to have played a form of soccer in the third century BC. Gardiner cites an account of this game by Giles in which bamboo goals were used. The goals were joined by a silk cord over which the ball was kicked. The ball was round and was formed of eight pointed strips of leather stuffed with hair.

The stories of individual heroes, political ramifications of sport, and early athletic injuries are included in Gardiner's work.[4] Leonidas of Rhodes is an overwhelming choice as a heroic runner. In 164 BC he won the stade race, the diaulos, and the long race at Olympia, garnering the title of Triple Victor or Triastes. He repeated this performance in four successive Olympiads. The statesmanship of Mark Antony was called upon by a priest in 41 BC in Ephesus. The priest, representing a synod of sacred Victors or professional athletes, appealed to Antony to maintain the rights of athletes and to grant them the privileges of exemption from military service and other favors. Antony wrote a letter on their behalf to the Greek community in granting this petition. The early casualties of sport include two deaths in field events described by Gardiner. Hyacinthus was accidentally killed by a diskos thrown by Apollo, and another youth accidentally killed a boy with a javelin. The boy had crossed the range while the youth was throwing the javelin.

The appeal of ancient ballgames is described by Masterson.[7] The earliest known examples included catching, juggling, hitting, kicking, throwing, and chasing balls. Masterson cites a reference by Galen (130–201 AD) that mentions a game with tackling in his *Exercise with the Small Ball*. The ballgames of the ancient Olmecs, Mayans, and Aztecs are also cited. Pottery figures from British Honduras depict the masks, mitts, and thigh protectors of Mayans active in the game Pok-ta-Pok, a forerunner of soccer. Players were required to kick or pass a ball using only their legs, hips, or buttocks. Stones were used for goal areas. Collisions, contusions, and exhaustion were apparently commonplace. The ancient Chinese, too, participated in forms of sport that resemble football, soccer, and polo. Injuries must have been similar to those of today's horsemen and athletes participating in football, soccer, and rugby.

Since these earlier times man has continued the pursuit of sport. Along with this participation the medical supervision and evaluation of athletes has increased to an elaborate point in the later years of the twentieth century. The first United States medical delegation to the modern Olympic Games was a group of three physicians and a nurse sent to the 1924 games in Paris. The present-day contingent of 16 medical people includes five physicians, several trainers, two nurses, and one dentist.[1] They serve a United States team that includes 500 athletes.

References

1. Anderson JB (Chief Physician, United States Olympic Team, Summer 1976): Personal communication
2. Bataille G: Lascaux, The Birth of Art. Wainhouse A (trans), Lausanne, Switzerland, Skira, 1955
3. Casteret N, Williams MO: Lascaux cave, cradle of world art. Nat Geogr Mag 94:771–794, 1948
4. Gardiner EN: Athletics of the Ancient World, Oxford, Clarenden, 1930
5. Leroi-Gourhan A: Treasures of Prehistoric Art. Guterman N (trans), New York, Abrams, 1967
6. MacGregor M: The Story of Greece. Edinburgh, Nelson, 1960, pp 84–96
7. Masterson D: The early history of ball games. Med Biol Illus 15:259–265, 1965

This is a book on trauma and sport. It is written in support of athletic endeavor with no intention of masking the emotional and physical value of sport by emphasizing its misfortune. Most of all, this book is written in the hope that athletes will benefit from better medical care through its use.

PART I
RADIOGRAPHIC EVALUATION OF
SITES OF INJURY

The radiographic evaluation of injury to various body sites is recorded briefly in this section. Primary and secondary clues of injury are outlined. These must be recognized on the radiograph so that accurate diagnosis is established. In several instances radiographic positions are shown for those not totally familiar with standard and special views.

SOFT TISSUES

The majority of injuries in sport are musculotendinous and often will have no significant radiographic abnormalities. However, certain soft tissue injuries do have x-ray manifestations that can be of considerable help toward accurate diagnosis.

Avulsion Injuries

Sudden violent contraction of muscle groups can lead to avulsion of bony fragments at origin and insertion sites.[8] The subject has been reviewed by Bavendam and Nedelman[2] and is discussed by Zatzkin.[17] Following injury, one must anticipate such possibilities and study the margins of bones at each suspected site of injury. Several locations in the lower back and pelvis are common among avulsion type injuries. A useful checklist begins with the lumbar spine and then progresses more distally to various pelvic muscle origin and insertion points. In the lumbar region, muscle avulsions may occur with fragmentation of the transverse processes of the lumbar vertebrae, this being the site of origin of the psoas muscle. The gluteal muscles may avulse their origin at the iliac crest. Moving distally along the lateral pelvic margins, the anterior superior iliac spine marks the origin of the sartorius muscle and the anterior inferior iliac spine marks that of the rectus femoris. Either location may be an avulsion point. The ischial tuberosity is the site of avulsion injuries of the hamstring muscle origins. Just below the pelvis, either trochanter can be displaced as an avulsion fragment following injury to the gluteal insertion at the greater trochanter or following injury to the iliopsoas muscle insertion at the lesser trochanter. Figure 1 shows these important check points.

Figure 2 shows an avulsion injury site in a young athlete. Use the checklist from Figure 1 to evaluate this x-ray. The patient is a 14-year-old boy who fell while running in a gymnasium and complained of severe pain at the right hip.

Upper Extremity

The soft tissues of the upper extremity may show clues on radiographs that indicate specific joint, soft tissue, or bone injury.

Weston has described the x-ray findings of biceps brachii rupture.[16] A telltale hump of soft tissue appears in the lower or midarm level anterior or anterolateral to the middle of the humerus. Fat planes may be displaced (Fig. 3).

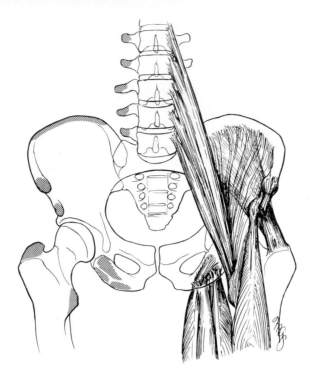

Fig. 1. The check points for evaluation of the more common avulsion injuries in the lumbar spine, pelvis, and hip are shown as shaded areas in this drawing. Both the origin and the insertion sites of the iliopsoas and gluteus medius muscles are shown. In addition the origins of the sartorius, rectus femoris, and hamstring group are shown.

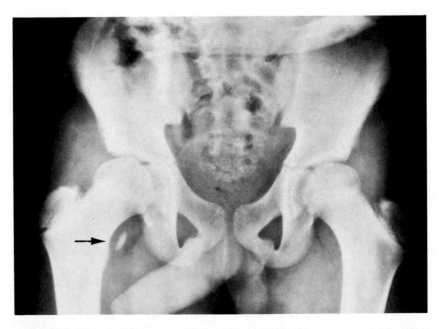

Fig. 2. The right lesser trochanter is displaced, indicating an avulsion injury of the insertion of the iliopsoas muscle.

4

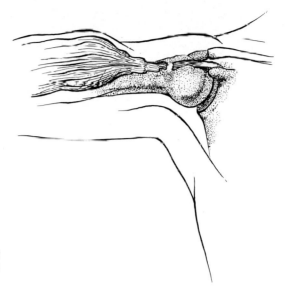

Fig. 3. The soft tissue deformity that accompanies a rupture of the long head of the biceps brachii muscle.

Fat pad displacements have been most extensively described at the elbow.[4,12] Norell points out that on a lateral view of the elbow the anterior fat pad may be seen normally.[12] The fat pad posterior to the humerus is hidden in normal circumstances by the posterior extensions of the epicondyles of the humerus. Elbow effusions, of traumatic and nontraumatic causes, will displace the posterior fat pad so that it is visible at the posterior edge of the humerus on the lateral view[12] (Figs. 4, 5). Again, careful attention to the bone–soft tissue interface on available x-rays contributes to an adequate examination.

Just proximal to the wrist, a pronator muscle fat pad sign has been described adjacent to the distal radius.[10] This sign is useful in situations wherein a distal radius fracture is suspected but is not readily seen at first glance. The fat pad is visible on normal lateral views of the wrist. It separates the pronator quadratus muscle and the tendons of the flexor digitorum profundus. Injury or disease in the radius or volar soft tissues will bow, blur, or obliterate the fat pad. The examiner should check this radiolucent fat stripe adjacent to the pronator muscle, especially in comparison to the same soft tissue area in views of an uninjured forearm. This may be rewarding and lead to the only sign of injury (Figs. 6, 7).

Lower Extremity

The soft tissues of the lower extremities also offer several useful areas in studying an x-ray following injury. Any patient with hip pain warrants careful examination of the soft tissues medial and lateral to the hip and within the pelvis at the obturator internus area. At the knee joint, the most common soft tissue abnormality is effusion shown by water density enlargement of the su-

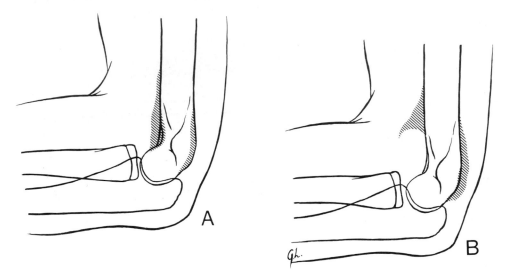

Fig. 4A. An anterior fat pad is often visible in a normal elbow. The posterior fat pad is hidden within the confines of the olecranon fossa and is not visible in a normal lateral view. **B.** The elbow with effusion often shows displacement of the anterior and posterior fat pads.

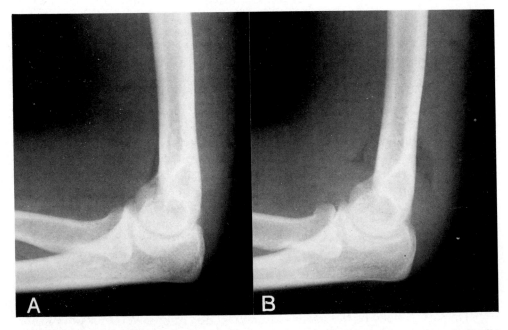

Fig. 5A. Normal lateral elbow view. **B.** Abnormal view. Both the anterior and posterior fat pads are present and displaced in the injured elbow. A subtle fracture of the radial head was detected on this and other elbow views.

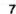

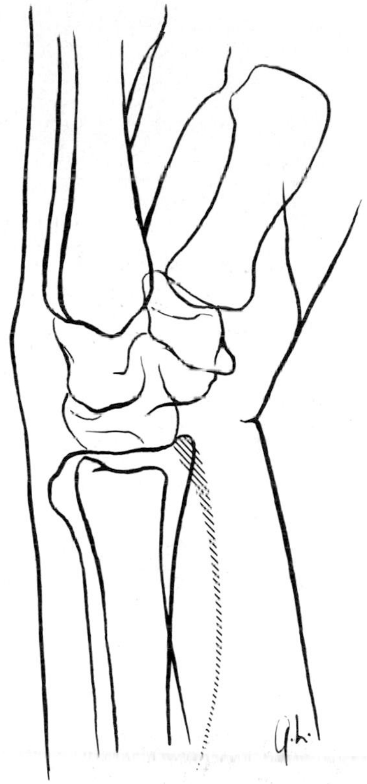

Fig. 6. Swelling along the volar margin of the radius displaces the pronator muscle fat pad. This may be a clue to a subtle radial fracture.

prapatellar joint space and again by displacement of the adjacent fat stripes in that area.

The lateral knee radiograph is most helpful in deciding for or against knee effusion, although small effusions may escape detection on x-ray examinations. In the normal knee, there is usually some lucency due to fatty tissue superior to the patella, anterior to the femur, and posterior to the quadriceps tendon as it begins to envelope the patella (Figs. 8, 9). In the joint with effusion, be it post-traumatic or associated with inflammatory disease, the normal suprapatellar and retroquadriceps tendon fatty area is replaced by water density that matches the density of the thigh musculature (Figs. 10, 11). The same fatty area on radiographs obtained in the crosstable lateral position is occasionally the site of a fat–fluid level. This occurs following knee fracture in which blood layers in the suprapatellar portion of the knee joint beneath a supernatant layer of fat within the anteriormost portion of this suprapatellar pouch. Berk and others have described this sign.[3,9] The patient's leg is radiographed when it is horizontal in position with the knee held in extension or moderate flexion. When the crosstable view is obtained, the central ray of the x-ray tube travels on a horizontal path. Thus, the fat–fluid interface will be shown parallel to the floor (Fig. 12).

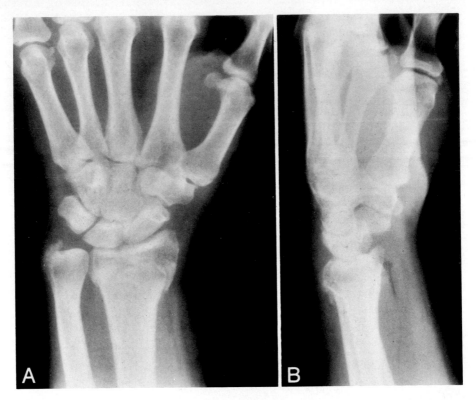

Fig. 7. A displaced pronator fat pad in a patient with a fracture of the radius. The ulnar styloid process also has been fractured. **A.** The posteroanterior view shows the fracture sites clearly. **B.** The lateral view shows the displaced fat pad.

Fig. 8. (See facing page, top) This normal lateral view of a teen-ager's knee shows several important landmarks. Area A represents the area of the normal fat pad occupying the margin of the suprapatellar portion of the knee joint. Obliteration of this area occurs in abnormal knees that contain an effusion. Area B marks the line of the residual epiphyseal cartilage in the distal femur. This should be of rather uniform thickness and show no displacement of its margins. Area C denotes the normal smooth articular margins of the femoral condyles. Osteochondral fractures and the fragmentation of osteochondritis dissecans alter these smooth margins. Area D indicates the apophysis of the tibial tubercle and the site of insertion of the quadriceps tendon. This area may appear markedly fragmented and still be within normal limits. The diagnosis of Osgood-Schlatter's disease rests on swelling of the quadriceps tendon insertion showing on the x-ray examination and not on fragmentation of this portion of the tibia.

Fig. 9. (See facing page, bottom) Diagrammatic representation of the structures in the normal lateral radiograph of the knee. The lettered areas correspond to those discussed in the legend to Figure 8.

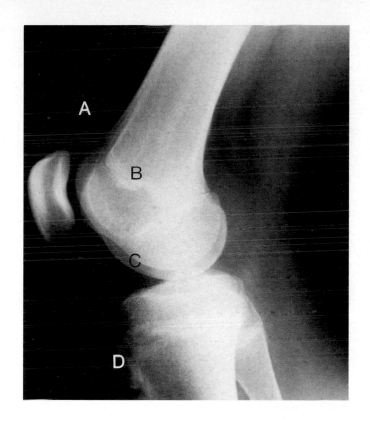

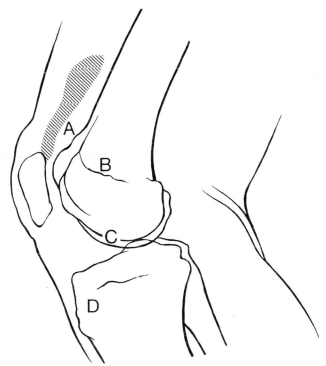

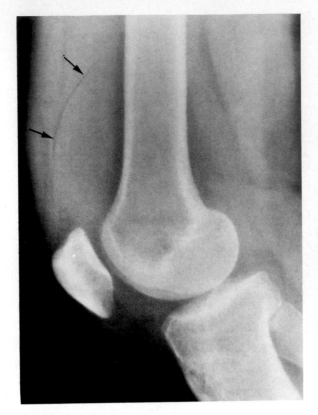

Fig. 10. The enlarged area of water density superior to the patella and anterior to the femur represents an extensive joint effusion. Normally this zone contains deposits of fat outlining the suprapatellar portion of the joint cavity and delimiting the posterior margin of part of the quadriceps tendon. Large effusions, such as this one, after joint injury are easily detected on physical and x-ray examination.

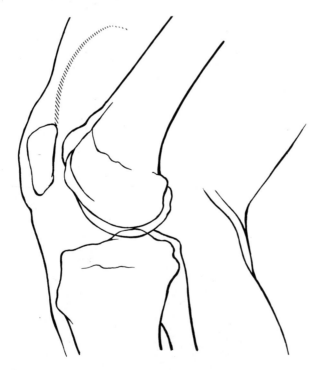

Fig. 11. The lateral view is helpful in showing an effusion at the suprapatellar area. The shaded curvilinear area represents the fatty outline of this portion of the joint. The fatty border is displaced and bowed by an effusion.

10

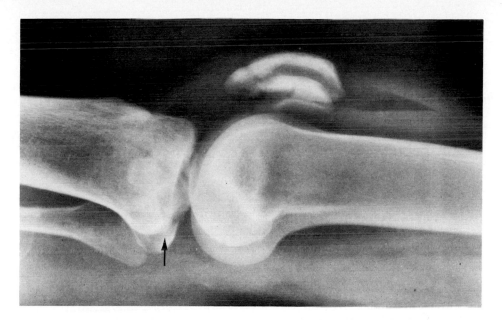

Fig. 12. A severe knee injury led to this radiograph of a young man. A horizontal x-ray beam was employed as his leg was held straight on the x-ray table. A fat–fluid level is present proximal to the patella, indicating a fracture with marrow release and hemorrhage. The patella has a double outline, indicating a vertical fracture splitting the patella into medial and lateral fragments. In addition, the cortical margins of the tibial plateau are disrupted, indicating a tibial fracture (arrow).

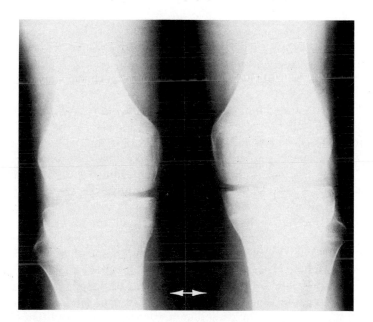

Fig. 13. This comparison anteroposterior view of normal knees is useful in showing the symmetry of the soft tissues of each upper medial calf (arrows). Occasionally this zone will show marked swelling in patients with Baker's cysts that distort the popliteal fossa and upper calf. Remember to check these zones in assessing frontal views and do not confine your search for abnormality to the cartilage space between the femur and tibia.

Occasionally, the anteroposterior view of the knee will show soft tissue density below the level of the joint line and medial to the tibia. This can occur in patients with synovial cysts that extend medially and posteriorly beyond the normal paratibial soft tissue confines[5] (Figs. 13, 14).

Patients with these findings usually have knee swelling due to effusion. The effusion is often caused by an injury to the knee but can follow arthritis of rheumatoid, post-traumatic, and other types. As the fluid increases within the joint, the synovial space expands directly or indirectly through bursal communications in the popliteal space. The resultant synovial cysts may be confined to the popliteal space, as they usually are, or may extend to the medial-posterior portion of the upper calf. The synovial enlargement rarely extends into the soft tissues of the posterior thigh. Symptoms of pain and swelling in the calf may predominate in these patients, masking the underlying knee disease or injury and leading to a misdiagnosis of thrombophlebitis. Arthrography has been useful in showing the gross anatomy of these popliteal and calf cysts in addition to demonstrating meniscus tears following injury[5] (Figs. 15, 16).

Avulsion injuries of soft tissue and bone can involve the knee. Smillie records examples of avulsions of the iliotibial band in which small fragments of bone can be detected at the lateral articular edge of the proximal tibia[14] (Figs. 17, 18).

A common site of athletic injury is the Achilles tendon. The early work by McMaster[11] showing the tremendous tensile strength of normal tendons is worth reviewing. He demonstrated that femoral or calcaneus fractures occurred before the Achilles tendon ruptured in an Achilles tendon loading experiment using rabbit limbs. Only tendons with prior injury or disease ruptured in circumstances of sudden excessive loading. Thus, one is led to believe that the athlete who suddenly feels he has been hit in the lower leg, only to realize that no possible offender is nearby, has ruptured a tendon that was compromised by some earlier insult.

Sir Harry Platt and others have called attention to the use of soft tissue radiographs in the lateral projection of the Achilles tendon in cases of suspected rupture.[13] The normal lateral ankle radiograph shows a radiolucent triangle of fatty tissue bounded by the posterior tibial musculature anteriorly, the smooth margins of the Achilles tendon posteriorly, and the margin of the calcaneus inferiorly (Figs. 19, 20). Following rupture, the smooth margin of the Achilles tendon will usually be totally altered at the rupture site (Fig. 21). This occurs as edema and hemorrhage ensue in the tendon and within the relatively fatty radiolucent triangle through which pass the arteries and veins to and from tendon segments. The lateral radiograph will then show water density filling in the radiolucent triangle (Fig. 22). Furthermore, if one is careful to note which edge of the triangle is obliterated one can be led to suspect injury not only in the Achilles tendon but also in the posterior tibialis tendon or in the ankle joint. In the latter instance, the radiolucent triangle will be obliterated by water density that extends out from the ankle joint and thus alters the angle of the triangle made by the posterior tibial and calcaneal margins. This form of radiologic geometry can be most helpful in ankle sprains with significant effusion.

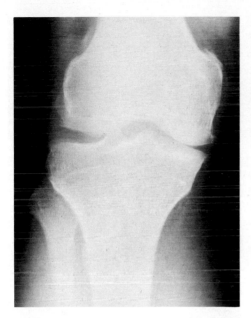

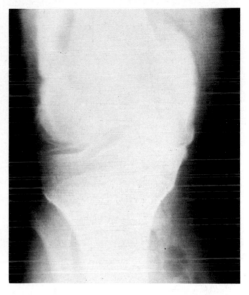

Fig. 14. A 30-year-old man has swelling of the upper medial calf on physical and x-ray examination. He was examined because of knee and upper calf pain and swelling after a football injury.

Fig. 15. Air and contrast material, placed in the knee at arthrography, outline portions of a post-traumatic synovial cyst in the upper medial portion of the calf. Note that this cyst corresponds to the area of suspected soft tissue swelling on the plain radiograph of the knee (Fig. 14).

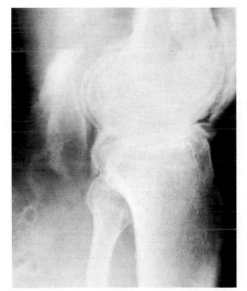

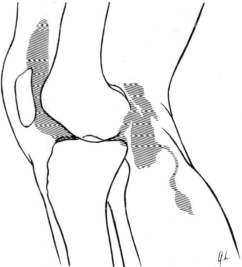

Fig. 16 Left. The lateral arthrographic view shows the posterior position of the popliteal and upper calf synovial cysts. The bursal connections at the posterior margins of the femoral condyles are through the semimembranosus and gastrocnemius bursae. **Right.** The shaded areas represent the synovial space and its posterior extension through the popliteal bursae in this outline drawing of a complex synovial cyst.

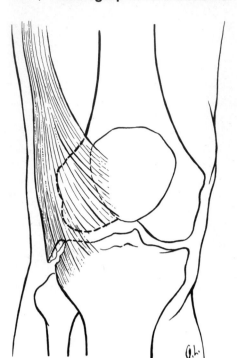

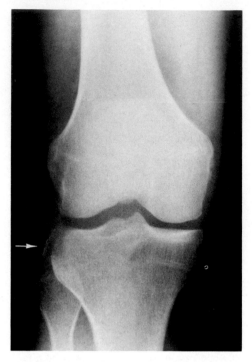

Fig. 17. The iliotibial band is shown in diagram with an avulsion fracture at the lateral margin of the tibia.

Fig. 18. An avulsion injury of the insertion site of the iliotibial band produced a partially displaced bone fragment in this anteroposterior view.

Ossification may occur in tendon sites such as the patellar tendon or Achilles tendon following hemorrhage in partial tendon tears. Similarly, soft tissue ossification may follow joint dislocation. Often, heterotopic bone formation occurs in soft tissues following blunt trauma to a limb[7] (Fig. 23). Although we refer to this condition as *myositis ossificans traumatica,* it is a misnomer in that muscle inflammation per se is not found histologically. Furthermore, the ossification usually is not found solely within muscle, but is found in fascial planes as well. Because the reactive fibromuscular proliferation can mimic sarcoma in certain fields on microscopic examination, it behooves us to gain an overall view both in histologic and clinical terms regarding such an abnormality. Histologically, an outer shell of organized bone often characterizes myositis ossificans.[1] Osteosarcoma, on the other hand, lacks a peripheral shell of relatively well-developed bone. The usual course of events is trauma, eg, to the thigh in a so-called charley horse, followed by hemorrhage in the soft tissues.[15] In the next 2 to 5 weeks, ill-defined densities of calcification and ossification may occur.[6] A hallmark of such early ossification is its ill-defined margin and almost ghostlike quality on the x-ray (Fig. 24). Excision or surgical exploration of such developing bone at this stage is likely to complicate matters in two ways. In the first instance, a biopsy may well lead to the microscopic examina-

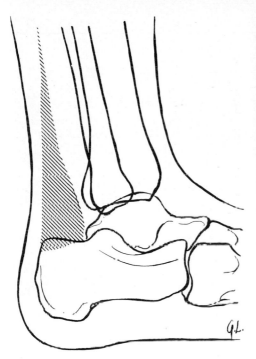

Fig. 19. A drawing of the posterior triangle of the ankle. The shaded area denotes the fatty space anterior to the Achilles tendon.

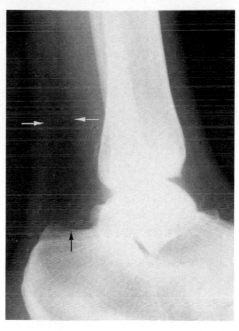

Fig. 20. The posterior triangle of normal fat is shown on the lateral view of the ankle (arrows). A fine avulsion fracture of the posterior tibial cortex has not altered the margins of the triangle.

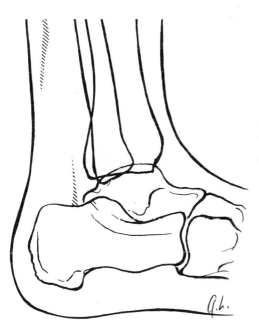

Fig. 21. The radiolucent triangle is obliterated by hemorrhage and edema in this example of rupture of the Achilles tendon.

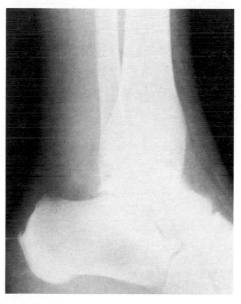

Fig. 22. Shadows of water density fill in the area of the posterior triangle of the ankle after rupture of the Achilles tendon and its blood supply.

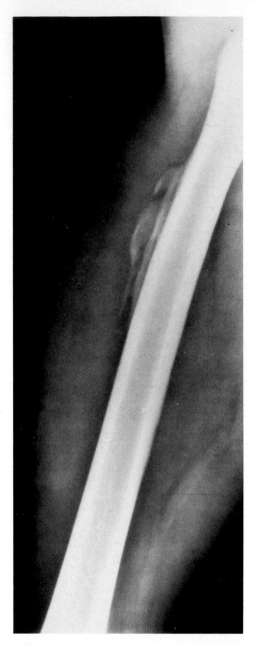

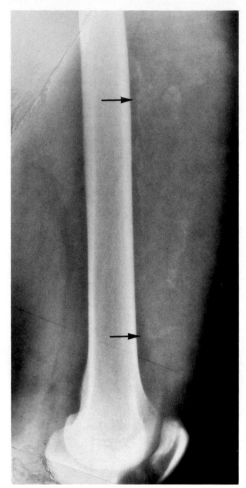

Fig. 24. An 18-year-old was struck on the thigh during a football game. Swelling, pain, and induration developed immediately and in the first few days after injury. This x-ray view shows a 20 cm-long zone of cloudlike mineralization (arrows) anterior to the femur in the first weeks following injury. Note that the edges of the lesion are mineralized rather than its center. This peripheral mineralization supports the diagnosis of myositis ossificans.

Fig. 23. A 16-year-old boy was struck in the thigh during a football game. The above view of the femur shows ossification along the anterolateral margin of the upper shaft. The circumscribed nature of the bone and its rather uniform density suggest that the injury occurred several weeks prior to this x-ray examination. The original x-rays showed small areas of trabeculation within the lesion, indicating the early maturation of the added bone.

tion of confusing reactive tissue at this point. Second, the surgical dissection alone may stimulate additional tissue reaction, leading to a more exuberant local ossification. In 1 to 2 months the newly formed bone gains a cortical outline and recognizable trabeculae on radiographic examination, and at this point it can be considered relatively mature and resectable, if necessary. On occasion, excision is indeed necessary as the bony mass may cause poor function of overlying soft tissues and muscle planes or may simply be painful enough to warrant surgery.

References

1. Ackerman LV: Extra-osseous localized non-neoplastic bone and cartilage formation (so-called myositis ossificans). Clinical and pathologic confusion with malignant neoplasms. J Bone Joint Surg 40A:279–298, 1958
2. Bavendam FA, Nedelman SH: Some considerations in roentgenology of fractures and dislocations. Semin Roentgenol 1:407–436, 1966
3. Berk RN: Liquid fat in the knee joint after trauma. N Engl J Med 277:1411–1412, 1967
4. Bledsoe RC, Izenstark JL: Displacement of fat pads in disease and injury of the elbow. Radiol 73:717–724, 1959
5. Bowerman JW, Muhletaler C: Arthrography of rheumatoid synovial cysts of the knee and wrist. J Can Assoc Radiol 24:24–32, 1973
6. Coley WB: Myositis ossificans traumatica. Ann Surg 57:305–337, 1913
7. Jackson DW, Feagin JA: Quadriceps contusion in young athletes. J Bone Joint Surg 55:95–105, 1973
8. Kessler FB, Driscoll R: Bilateral anterior superior iliac spine avulsions. J Trauma 3:129–131, 1963
9. Kling DH: Fat in traumatic effusions of knee joint. Am J Surg 6:71–74, 1929
10. MacEwan DW: Changes due to trauma in the fat pad overlying the pronator quadratus muscle: a radiologic sign. Radiology 82:879–886, 1964
11. McMaster PE: Tendon and muscle ruptures. J Bone Joint Surg 15:705–722, 1933
12. Norell HG: Roentgenologic visualization of the extra capsular fat. Acta Radiol 42:205–210, 1954
13. Platt H: Observations on some tendon ruptures. Br Med J 1:611–615, 1931
14. Smillie IS: Injuries of the Knee Joint, 4th ed. Essex, Longman, 1971
15. Thorndike A: Myositis ossificans traumatica. J Bone Joint Surg 22:315–323, 1940
16. Weston WJ: The soft tissue signs with rupture of the long head of biceps. Br J Radiol 42:539–540, 1969
17. Zatzkin HR: The Roentgen Diagnosis of Trauma. Chicago, Year Book, 1965

SKULL

An analysis of skull radiographs must be orderly as in other examinations, although a compulsive sequential scrutiny of area by area usually rapidly breaks down through impatience with visual scanning techniques. One must always revert to orderly analysis when clinical findings are present. The standard views usually include frontal and lateral views and a view of the vault of the skull, without overlapping facial bones, known as the Townes view. For purposes of x-ray interpretation, the skull is composed of three main examination areas: the craniocervical junction, the calvarium and its contents, and the facial bones (Figs. 25, 26). These three areas will be discussed individually.

Craniocervical Junction

Subluxation and dislocation of C1–C2 or C1 at the craniocervical junction may be apparent on radiographs of the skull. The normal relationships of C1 and C2 to the foramen magnum are shown on the lateral view in Figure 26. The prespinal soft tissues may be widened here following hemorrhage and may be most apparent on the lateral view of the skull. Normally the soft tissues anterior to the upper cervical spine are not wider than a vertebral body's anteroposterior dimensions, and the normal soft tissue shadow is narrowest anterior to the upper cervical spine. Such observations are made on the lateral radiographs of the skull.

Calvarium and Its Contents

The second examination area of each skull x-ray is the calvarium and its contents. The use of a bright light to illuminate the scalp margins may aid in the detection of soft tissue swelling and localization of the injury site. The examiner should then look for abnormal radiolucent lines as well as radiodense lines, because both can occur following skull fracture. This is a difficult task because we often forget that depressed skull fractures produce overlapping bony margins which appear as radiodensity (Fig. 27). The density is produced by two thicknesses of skull in a focal area. The more common radiolucent frac-

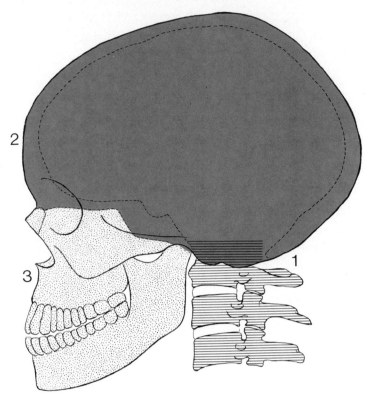

Fig. 25. The lateral view of the skull provides three main areas for evaluation: (1) the head–neck junction, (2) the calvarium with its contents including the base of the skull, and (3) the facial structures.

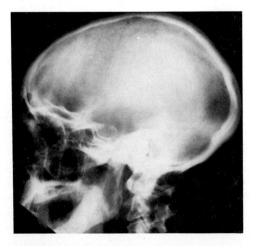

Fig. 26. The lateral radiograph, as in this normal skull, provides much of the information in a skull examination. Remember to inspect all three areas shown in Figure 25.

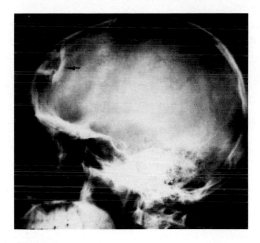

Fig. 27. Abnormal radiodensities are present at the frontal bone on this lateral view. The densities represent a depressed skull fracture caused by a blunt object. Overlapping bits of bone produce the density and remind us to look for these findings in addition to radiolucency in patients with possible fracture.

ture lines are often sharply angled or straight, unlike the gentle arcs and branching of vascular markings in the skull (Figs. 28, 29). Usually fracture lines appear as radiolucent lines that are more lucent than the vascular grooves in the skull.[1] Remember that vascular markings in the skull occupy only part of the thickness of bone, whereas fractures are rifts or ravines through the entire thickness of bone. Fractures at bony junctions in the skull are diastatic fractures, that is, they produce diastasis of skull bones through suture lines. Skull suture lines are still present in teenagers and young adults and usually measure less than 3 mm.

Beware the fracture line that extends across the parietal distribution of the middle meningeal artery. This fracture can produce epidural hemorrhage within hours. Similarly, one must consider the dural sinuses at the sagittal suture and lambdoidal suture as potential bleedings sites. Venous bleeding or thrombosis can also occur there. Rarely, the meninges may herniate into a fracture preventing healing and gradually eroding the margins of the fracture[13] (Figs. 30, 31).

A negative standard skull examination does not exclude a basilar skull fracture, which is the most difficult of all skull fractures to detect. Bleeding from the ear or within the ear may indicate that a basilar fracture is present. Battle's sign may be present. This sign consists of subcutaneous hemorrhage at the mastoid region and bleeding in the ear.[5] Facial nerve injury and deafness can occur via fracture in the temporal region (Fig. 32). Basal views of the skull are helpful in detecting basilar fractures, and tomograms of the temporal bone may be needed to demonstrate this abnormality.

A sign of skull fracture that may be overlooked is pneumocephalus. Such collections of air tracking along the meningeal margins need not be large. Pneumocephalus is usually secondary to a fracture that involves the sinuses or skull base (Fig. 33).

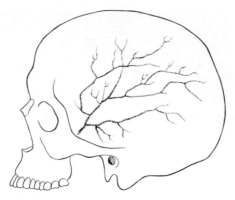

Fig. 28. The arterial markings on the normal skull are part of the meningeal vascular system. The lines produced are graceful arcs with branches and do not generally resemble the straight and curvilinear lines of a fracture.

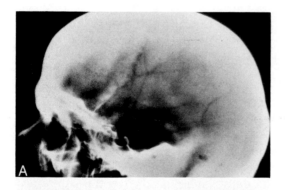

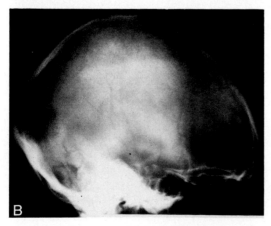

Fig. 29. Two examples of the branching patterns produced by arterial grooves in the inner table of the skull are shown here. **A.** In this dried skull preparation there are three main arterial branches centered in and about the parietal area. **B.** Among several larger vascular grooves a slightly curved radiolucent line crosses the temporal area above the sella turcica. This groove is caused by a segment of the superficial temporal artery, a branch of the external carotid system. Occasionally this vascular groove is mistaken for a fracture line.

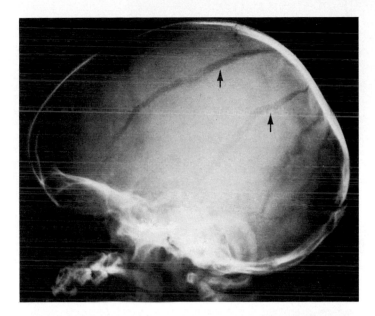

Fig. 30. A child fell from a height and injured her head in September 1966. Two prominent fractures cross the parietal area in this lateral view.

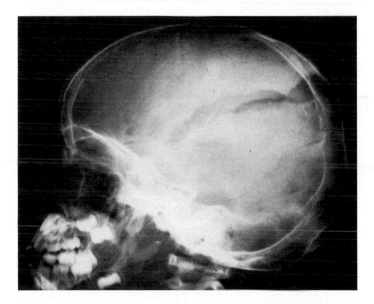

Fig. 31. Follow-up radiographs in October 1967 showed that one fracture line had healed, yet the other had widened considerably. This represents a leptomeningeal cyst that has eroded the skull as the cyst protrudes through a dural tear. This uncommon complication of fracture may also be associated with herniation of the brain into the fracture site. Dural grafting and repair is usually required.

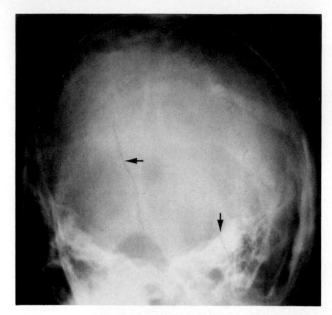

Fig. 32. A 20-year-old man fell from his motorcycle and later complained of hearing loss. A Townes view of the skull shows a long fracture extending into the foramen magnum and a vertical fracture across the temporal bone. Temporal bone fractures are seldom seen on plain skull views and often require tomography for accurate delineation.

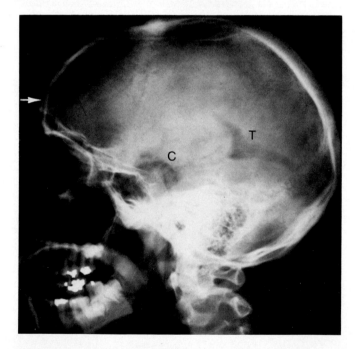

Fig. 33. Fractures are present in the frontal area (arrow) of another man injured in a fall from his motorcycle. The radiolucent fracture lines are rather straight and fine and are darker or more radiolucent than ordinary vascular grooves. In addition, there are no branching patterns present and the fracture lines are located in an area usually devoid of prominent vascular markings. Another secondary sign of fracture is shown on this view. Pneumocephalus is present and is seen as abnormal patches of radiolucency in the parasellar cisterns (C) and in the trigone portion of the cerebral ventricle (T). The fractures of the frontal area involved the frontal sinus and air tracked beneath the brain and into the ventricle via a cerebral laceration or through the fourth ventricular foramina.

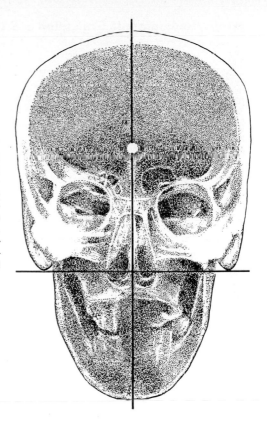

Fig. 34. The midline localization of the calcified pineal gland can be checked in a number of ways. One method uses the mastoid tips as lateral landmarks for a line segment. This line is then bisected by a perpendicular line that should be within 1 to 2 mm of the midpoint of the calcified pineal gland. Other methods use different lateral landmarks including the cochlea and other temporal bone points. Asymmetry of the mastoid tips may compromise the method illustrated.

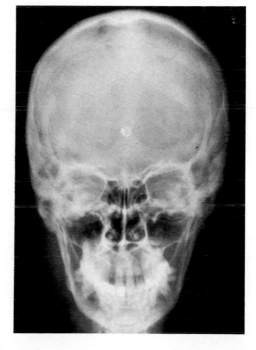

Fig. 35. The pineal gland is densely calcified in this patient. Its midline location can be calculated by the method shown in Figure 34 or by using the superior semicircular canals or the cochlea.

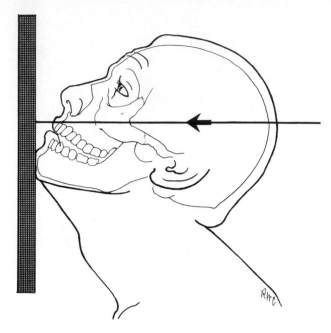

Fig. 36. In the Waters view the central ray (solid line) is perpendicular to the film. The chin is placed against the cassette (shaded area) while the central ray exits at the tip of the nose. The orbitomeatal line forms an angle of 40° with the plane of the film. (See Figure 41 for an x-ray in the Waters projection.)

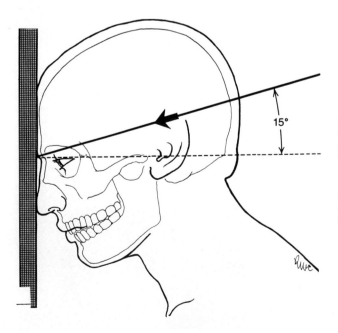

15°

Fig. 37. In the modified Caldwell view, another basic frontal display of facial bone anatomy, the central ray (solid line) is directed through the nasion at a 15° caudad angle. The brow and nose are against the cassette. The dotted line represents the orbitomeatal line.

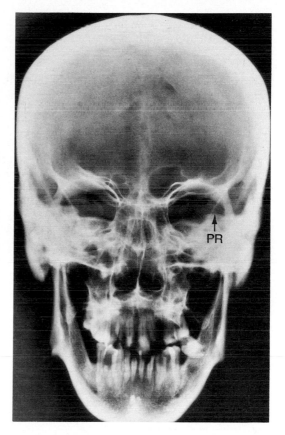

Fig. 38. This frontal view of the dried skull is similar to the Caldwell view used to assess facial injury or skull abnormality. The petrous ridges (PR) overlap the lower portions of the orbits. This position can be used to advantage to evaluate the petrous bones. If the area of inquiry is the orbital margin, then the chin can be elevated slightly to give a clear view of the entire orbital margins and project the petrous bones over the maxillae.

In the central portion of the brain, on frontal and lateral radiographs, the only radiographic indicator of a large hematoma affecting a shift of cerebral structures is a displacement of the calcified pineal gland. This interesting structure can calcify as early as 6 years of age and is usually calcified in 60% of adults,[9] so it should be used when present. How to use it is yet another problem and several methods have been proposed. One method is to construct a horizontal line on a frontal view from mastoid tip to mastoid tip making certain that rotation of the skull is not an interfering factor. A perpendicular line constructed to the midline of this horizontal line should then fall within 1 to 2 mm of the calcified pineal gland (Figs. 34, 35).

Facial Bones

The facial bones are the third large area for radiographic examination within the skull. To most people they represent a confusing array of overlapping and finely contoured structures. Again, one needs a plan of attack for their examination. Campbell suggests a sensible and easily remembered plan for frontal views of the face[4] (Figs. 36–38). Such views include the Waters

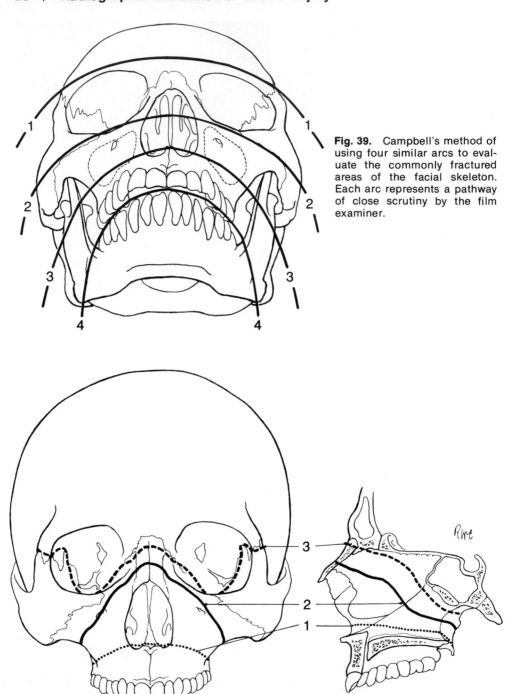

Fig. 39. Campbell's method of using four similar arcs to evaluate the commonly fractured areas of the facial skeleton. Each arc represents a pathway of close scrutiny by the film examiner.

Fig. 40. LeFort's classic lines of facial fracture after severe skull injury (Adapted from Rowe and Killey: Fractures of the Facial Skeleton, 2nd ed, 1968, Courtesy of E. S. Livingstone). Line 3 is a craniofacial separation. Lines 1 and 2 are lesser fractures through the maxilla.

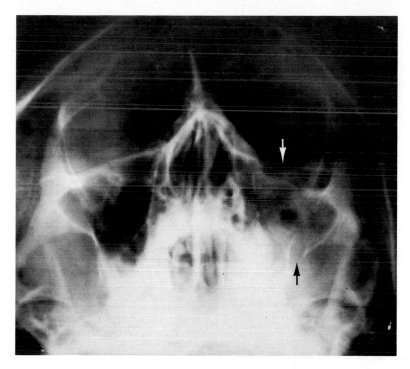

Fig. 41. In this Waters view, obtained after blunt trauma to the patient's left cheek, there are fractures of the left orbital floor and lateral maxillary antral wall (arrows). The chin is elevated in this projection and the temporal bones are projected over the rami of the mandible. The zygoma and zygomatic frontal junctions were also fractured on the left.

view (chin up) and the Caldwell view (a standard frontal view of the skull). The plan is this: visually construct, or in fact literally construct with a wax marking pencil, four similar arcs that represent portions of concentric circles. Each arc will take the viewer through frequently damaged areas within the face and serve as a reminder that each has been examined. Figure 39 demonstrates this method. In addition, one should be familiar with the classic lines of facial fractures described by LeFort[4,10] (Fig. 40). In fact, the LeFort classification parallels the lines suggested by Campbell, and one can easily apply the label LeFort 1 fracture to the lower maxillary line (3) in Figure 39, the label LeFort 2 to the next higher line (2) and so on, leading up to the craniofacial separation of a LeFort 3. In sports, only injuries involving high-speed collisions with racing vehicles, snowmobiles, and the like would result in the severe degrees of facial injury included in the LeFort cleavage planes. Incidentally, boxing is reported to contribute very little in the way of facial fractures apart from nasal cartilage and nasal bone injury.[2]

Blyth and Arnold,[3] Gonzalez,[7] Gurdjian et al,[8] and Schneider[11] have reported examples of severe and fatal injuries in football, with the majority involving damage to the head and neck. Gonzales, in his report on fatal injuries in sport in New York City, showed a surprising number of deaths from head

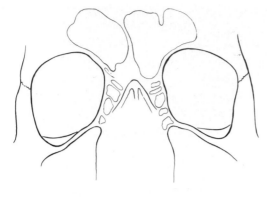

Fig. 42. The normal orbital margins feature a complex but smooth overlay of the anterior medial and inferior bony walls. To use this view to evaluate subsequent cases of injury, pay particular attention to the normal air space in the maxillary and ethmoid sinuses. Edema and soft tissue injury will often obscure the medial and inferior orbital margins after trauma.

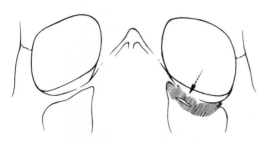

Fig. 43. The blow-out fracture of the orbital floor follows blunt trauma to the eye. Soft tissue bulges inferiorly from the orbital margins and alters the upper maxillary sinus margin. Occasionally bone fragments of the broken floor may be detected (arrows).

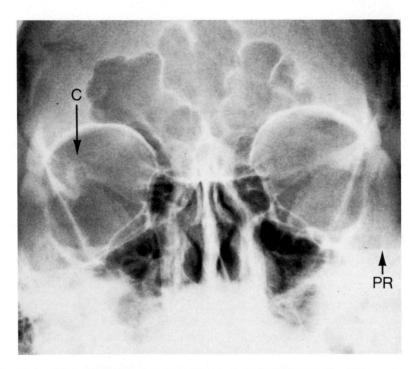

Fig. 44. The orbital margins are normal bilaterally in this frontal view. The petrous ridges (PR) have been positioned so that they are projected through the maxillary antra. An orbital calcification (C) is present on the patient's right side and probably represents an old hemorrhage in the periorbital tissue.

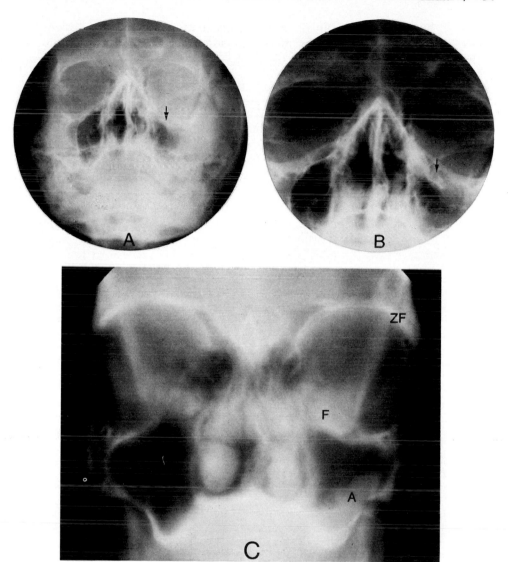

Fig. 45. Facial bone views were obtained in a 50-year-old man after a fist fight. **A.** The Waters view shows soft-tissue swelling at the left zygoma and at the lateral margin of the left maxillary antrum. The left orbital floor and lateral antral wall are indistinct, unlike the right counterparts of those structures. **B.** A coned down view of the orbital floors shows a bone fragment displaced downward (arrows in A and B) into the maxillary antrum. **C.** Tomography (arrows in A and B) shows clearly the fracture sites at the left orbital floor (F), lateral antral wall (A), and zygomatic frontal junction (ZF). Soft tissue swelling is present at the orbital blow-out fracture and at the lateral and inferior margins of the left maxillary antrum. The right side is normal. The normal nasal turbinates and the crista galli are also shown.

injury in baseball as a result of thrown balls, batted balls, and collisions with other players or barriers.[7] This study was done before the batting helmet was introduced as a safety measure in baseball.

Blow Out Fractures

Finally, in addition to anticipation of the above injuries to the skull, the examiner should be familiar with blow out fractures of the orbit.[6,12] Such fractures usually occur following a direct blow to the eye from a fist, elbow, knee, or blunt object (Fig. 41). The thin inferior and medial margins of the orbit are most often damaged. The novice at x-ray diagnosis is apt to have difficulty in detecting orbital floor fractures because of the slightly confusing appearance of the normal lower orbit margin. Here there are two overlapping contours: the anterior inferior rim of the orbit (the anterior rim that we can easily palpate on our own faces), and the more deeply seated posterior lowermost bony margin of the orbit (Figs. 42, 43). In the case of fracture of the orbital floor, a third line may be present indicating a loose bony fragment (Figs. 44, 45). This fragment may hinge medially or laterally and is usually associated with a downward bulge of periorbital soft tissue. At times only this soft tissue bulge will be apparent. Tomography of the facial bones is often of value in showing the extent of facial fractures and in determining the presence of a fracture in doubtful cases[6] (Fig. 45).

References

1. Allen WE, Kier EL, Rothman SLG: Pitfalls in the evaluation of skull trauma. Radiol Clin North Am 11:479–503, 1973
2. Blonstein JL: Medical care of the boxer. In Bass AL, Blonstein JL, James RD, Williams JGP (eds): Medical Aspects of Boxing. London, Pergamon, 1965, p 35
3. Blyth CS, Arnold DC: The Forty-Second Annual Survey of Football Fatalities 1931–1973. Prepared for: American Football Coaches Association National Collegiate Athletic Association and The National Federation of State High School Athletic Associations. February 26, 1974
4. Campbell W: Fractures of the middle third of the face. In Lodge T (ed): Recent Advances in Radiology. Boston, Little, Brown, 1964, pp 239–251
5. Dorland's Illustrated Medical Dictionary, 25th ed. Philadelphia, Saunders, 1974, p 1414
6. Fueger GF, Milauskas AT, Britton W: The roentgenologic evaluation of orbital blow-out injuries. Am J Roentgenol 97:614–617, 1966
7. Gonzales TA: Fatal injuries in competitive sports. JAMA 146:1506–1511, 1951
8. Gurdjian ES, Lissner HR, Patrick MS: Protection of the head and neck in sports. JAMA 182:509–512, 1962
9. Ozonoff MB, Burrows EH: Intracranial calcification. In Radiology of the Skull and Brain. Newton TH, Potts DG (eds) St. Louis, Mosby, 1971, p 824
10. Rowe NL, Killey HC: Fractures of the Facial Skeleton, 2nd ed. Edinburgh, Livingstone, 1968
11. Schneider RC: Serious and fatal neurosurgical football injuries. Clin Neurosurg 12:226–236, 1964

12. Smith B, Regan W: Blow-out fracture of the orbit. Am J Ophthalmol 44:733–739, 1957
13. Taveras JM, Ransohoff J: Leptomeningeal cysts of the brain following trauma with erosion of the skull. J Neurosurg 10:233–241, 1953

CERVICAL SPINE

Standard Views

The initial period of x-ray examination of the cervical spine can be a critical one. Expert guidance of the patient and paramedical personnel is necessary to obtain adequate views in a safe manner. The usual sequence of views employed at Johns Hopkins begins with anteroposterior and lateral views of the neck. Both of these views are obtained with the patient supine. The lateral view is made with a crosstable exposure so that the patient is not moved. The film is stood on end alongside the patient's neck as he lies facing the ceiling (Figs. 46, 47). The standard anteroposterior and lateral views of the cervical

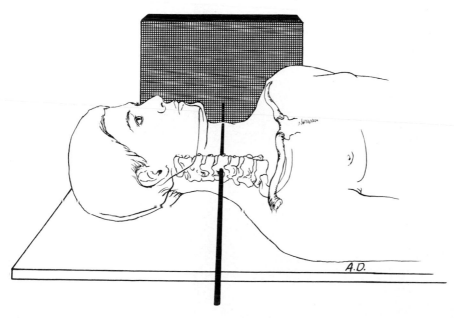

Fig. 46. The film is placed along the shoulder lateral to the neck so that C1 through C7 are included. The shoulders should be lowered. The central ray (solid line) is perpendicular to the film.

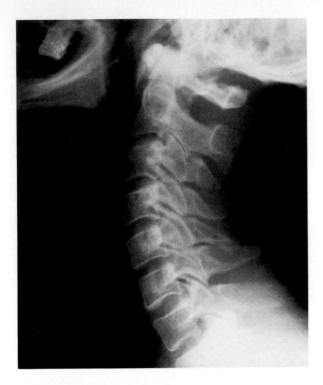

Fig. 47. This is a normal cervical spine lateral view. The patient's neck is slightly rotated judging by the margins of the facet joints that do not overlap evenly. Note the main areas that must be checked as indicated in the text.

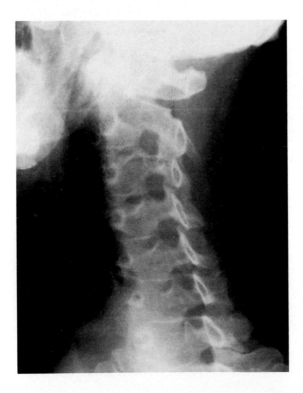

Fig. 48. The normal overlapping of facet joints in a shinglelike manner is shown in this oblique view. The end-on images of the lamina between the facets appear as a chain of ovals that overlap like shingles on a roof.

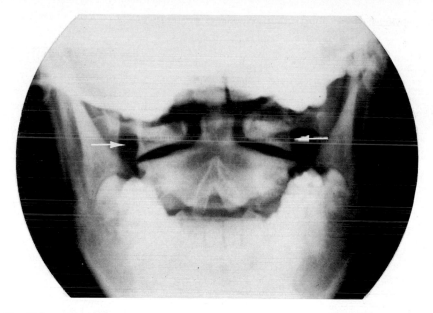

Fig. 49. This normal odontoid view was made by positioning the patient so that his mouth was open. Each side of the body of C1 articulates exactly with a facet of C2 (arrows). The lateral margins of the articulation match evenly as the neck is viewed from the front without rotation of patient. The spaces between the odontoid peg and each side of C1 are symmetrical.

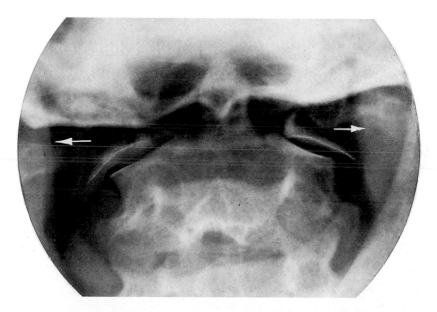

Fig. 50. This open mouth odontoid view was obtained in a 57-year-old man. His truck slid on a wet road surface and rolled over. He struck the top of his head on the windshield and experienced severe neck pain. Both sides of the vertebral ring of C1 are displaced laterally and do not articulate normally with the facets of C2. This type of injury requires two fracture sites in the ring of C1 to permit such displacement. G. Jefferson described this type of injury (see Br J Surg 7:407–422, 1920) and since then it has been popularly called a Jefferson fracture.

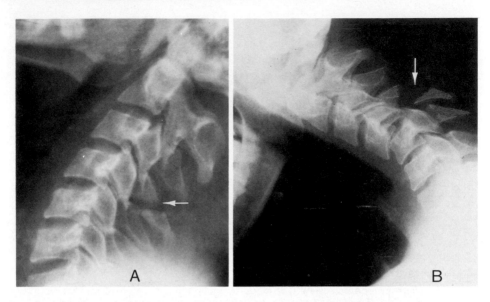

Fig. 51A. The initial lateral view in this patient involved in an auto accident shows an oblique fracture at the fourth spinous process. The alignment of the vertebral bodies is normal. **B.** The view in flexion shows dislocation of C4 and C5 and separation of the fracture fragments in the C4 spinous process. This dramatic example indicates the need for flexion views to show the full extent of ligament rupture and the need for the utmost care in obtaining those views.

spine may not suffice, however, to show injury in the neck. If symptoms and signs are present and these views are normal, then oblique and odontoid views are in order (Figs. 48–50). These views also can and should be made without moving the patient's neck. The odontoid view is exposed by directing the central ray vertically down through the patient's mouth to the film placed beneath the patient. Finally, if these also are unremarkable, then flexion and extension views should be obtained, taking care to insure that the patient alone moves his neck with a physician in attendance (Fig. 51). If the patient is unconscious or unable to respond appropriately, then flexion and extension views should be avoided and the neck protected by a brace or traction.

Special Studies

Tomograms or laminagrams can be especially helpful in showing the subtle fracture in the vertebral appendages and at the important C1–C2 area (Figs. 52, 53). Myelography can be performed using air or radiopaque contrast material in order to show cord compression by a hematoma or bone fragment or to pinpoint cervical nerve root avulsions.[5,9,13] A careful and active evaluation is stressed pending the physical findings and diagnostic signs from the plain radiographs rather than a conservative "head in the sand" or "ostrich" approach. The latter is typified by an ill-fated early assumption that nothing can be done surgically in the acute situation to help the patient. Several reports

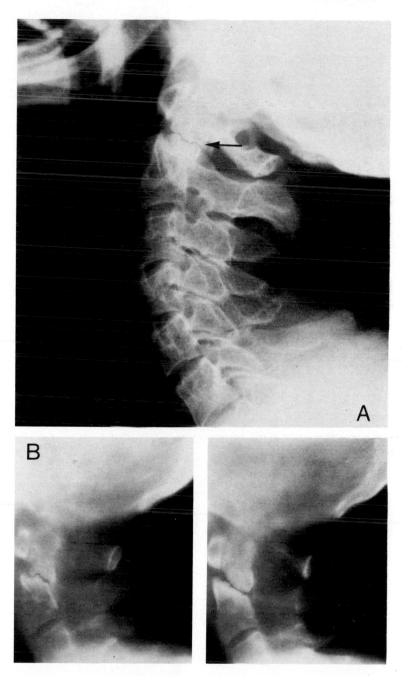

Fig. 52A. This view was obtained after a diving injury in which the patient's head was forced backward. A fracture is present at the base of the odontoid process and the entire odontoid peg is displaced posteriorly. **B.** Two parts of a series of tomographic lateral views of the C1–C2 area show the oblique fracture line through the base of the odontoid process. This young man was diving in shallow water when he injured his neck.

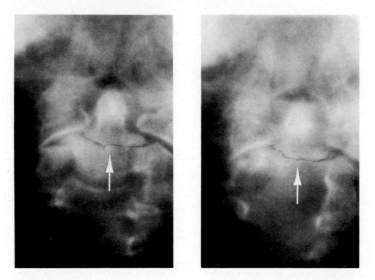

Fig. 53. Two views of a series of anteroposterior tomographic views of a different patient's C1–C2 area following injury show a horizontal fracture in C2 undermining the base of the odontoid process.

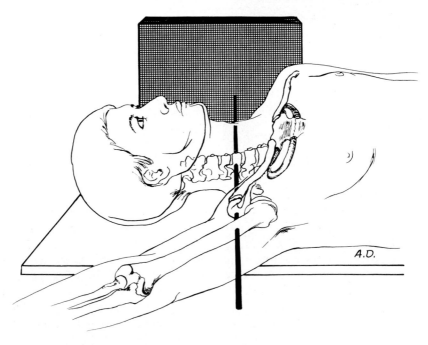

Fig. 54. The "swimmer's" position is useful for obtaining a view of the cervicothoracic junction. Note the arm positions resembling those of a swimmer. The central ray (solid line) is again perpendicular to the film.

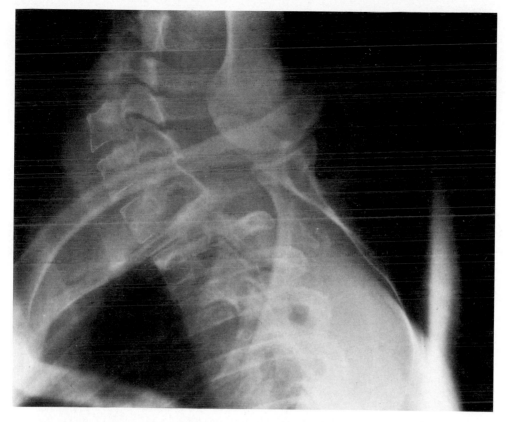

Fig. 55. In this "swimmer's" view the lower cervical and upper thoracic vertebral bodies are visible.

deal with the syndrome of acute cord compression and surgical efforts to relieve hematomata.[2,4,7,8,11]

Interpretation of Lateral View

How does one go about evaluating radiographs of the cervical spine? We do not assume that adequate views have been obtained. The first step is to make certain that we do have adequate films. A frequent problem is that the patient's shoulders obscure the C6–C7–T1 area on the lateral view. Fractures and fracture–dislocations at these levels can be missed all too easily. A repeat lateral view with the shoulders repositioned may be necessary. Alternatively, if the patient's arms are mobile, one arm can be elevated and one lowered, so that the patient assumes a pose resembling the arm positions of a freestyle swimmer (Fig. 54). This so-called swimmer's lateral view can display the neck–thorax junction to advantage (Fig. 55).

The most frequent mistakes of interpretation are those of omission in which attention has been limited to too small a portion of the cervical spine,

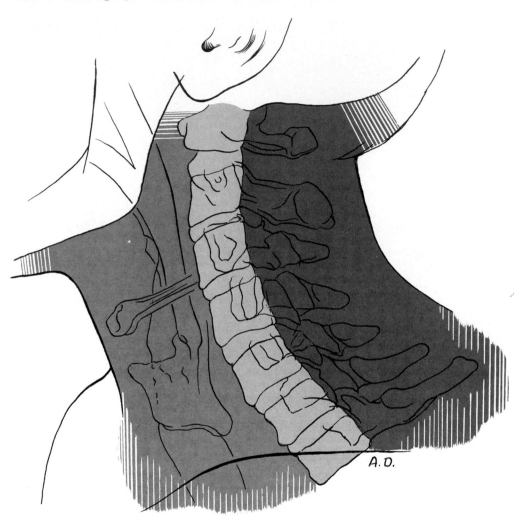

A.D.

Fig. 56. The three zones of inspection on the lateral view of the cervical spine. Remember to study all three areas in each patient.

eg, to the vertebral bodies only, neglecting the soft tissues, the disc spaces, the facet joints, the junction of the skull and cervical spine, etc. The lateral radiograph of the cervical spine in neutral position serves as an important first step in film analysis. It is helpful to divide this view into three zones: anterior, middle, and posterior (Fig. 56).

Anteriorly, one looks at the airway and hypopharynx, which can be key indicators to edema, soft tissue hemorrhage, or free air in the anterior neck or at prespinal tissues (Figs. 57, 58). The prespinal soft tissue space is usually 0.5 to 1 cm wide at the upper cervical region. The normal lower prespinal soft tissue seldom exceeds the anteroposterior dimension of a vertebral body at C5, C6, or C7.

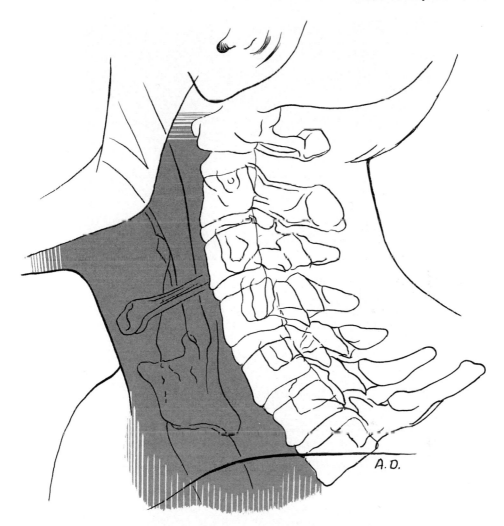

Fig. 57. The anterior zone of the lateral view of the cervical spine.

Occasionally, on close inspection of the soft tissue space one may see a radiolucent line that runs vertically along the anterior margin of the cervical vertebrae just 1 to 2 mm anterior to the spine. This is the prevertebral fat stripe that represents fat between the anterior longitudinal spinal ligament and the esophagus. Spinal injury can displace this fat stripe anteriorly. The observation of a local alteration of the fat stripe may be the only indication of injury.[12]

In the middle zone of the lateral view, the vertebral bodies and disc spaces offer the greatest return in terms of injury areas discovered per minute of examination (Fig. 59). Vertebral compression fractures are detected by observation of the anterior portions of the vertebral bodies and comparison of their margins at multiple levels. The margins are usually regular and show a smooth

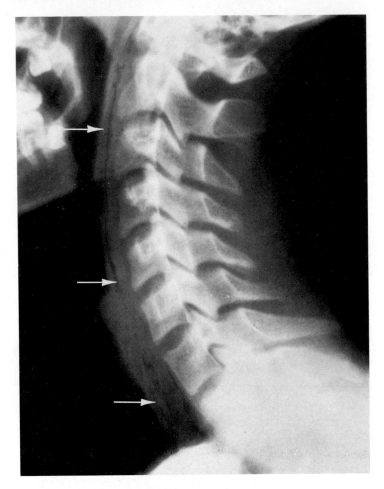

Fig. 58. A man fell from a scaffold and sustained blunt trauma to the chest and neck. He complained of mild neck pain. The lateral radiograph of the cervical spine showed air within the soft tissues (arrows) anterior to the vertebral bodies. The air was traced distally in the mediastinum as well. A barium swallow was negative and the interstitial emphysema resolved in several days. A small tear in one of his air-containing structures must have sealed quickly.

cortex. Compression fractures produce collapse of the anterior portion of the body (Fig. 60). Subluxation and dislocations are detected by noting the relationships of the posterior vertebral margins at each level (Fig. 61). A line drawn so that it passes through each posterior vertebral margin should create a regular unbroken line (Fig. 61A). Subluxed or dislocated vertebrae will alter this unbroken line. At the disc space gas sometimes appears in the anterior disc margins in patients who have had acute neck injury without dislocation.[6] An acute rupture of an intervertebral disc will usually show collapse of the disc space, readily noted by comparison of disc thicknesses at multiple levels.

The posterior third of the lateral view contains the apophyseal or facet

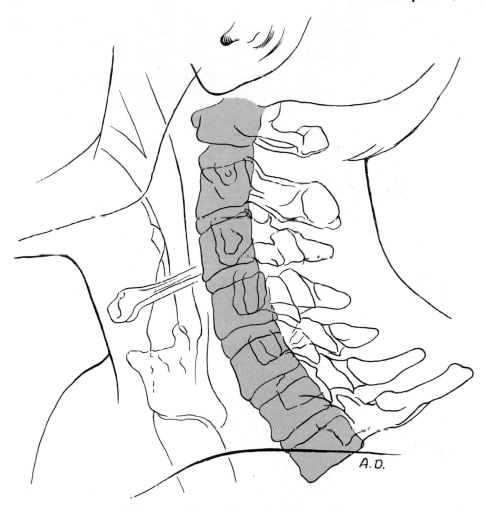

Fig. 59. The middle zone of the lateral view is a key area in a key examination. The vertebral bodies and disc spaces offer the greatest return in terms of injury areas discovered per minute of examination.

joints, spinous processes, and posterior soft tissues (Fig. 62). Here one should study the relationships of the normal apophyseal joints and posterior vertebral appendages to detect injury (Fig. 63). On oblique views each facet joint shows two articular processes. One process extends downward from the vertebral body above and the second extends upward from the vertebral body below the level of the facet joint. Each process surface faces either downward and anteriorly or upward and posteriorly (Fig. 63B). Occasionally, in subluxations of facet joints, an articular process will slip forward on its mate beneath and produce a "perched" appearance on the oblique view. The term "perched" refers to the position of one facet perched on top of the facet immediately beneath it, unlike the normal situation in which each facet sits above but behind the adja-

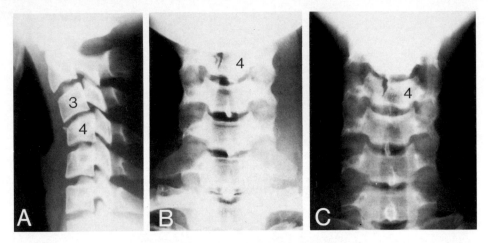

Fig. 60A. A 17-year-old girl was riding a spirited horse. Without warning she was thrown forward over the head of the horse landing on her helmeted head. She experienced immediate neck pain. Radiographs showed a fracture of C4 of the compression type. The subluxation of C3 on C4 is a residual feature of the partial dislocation that must have occurred. The intervertebral disc at C3–C4 is compressed and probably ruptured. The patient suffered no neurologic disability. **B.** It is most valuable to correlate the findings on the lateral view with those on the anteroposterior or oblique views. The anteroposterior view in the same patient showed an abnormality in the C4 vertebral body. A vertical split is present in C4 with two vertical fracture lines. Because these lines overlaid part of the shadow of the airway and larynx they were not detected initially. **C.** At a subsequent out-patient visit this comparison AP view was made. The vertical split had partially resorbed and was easily detected.

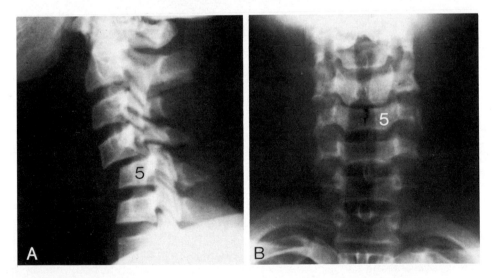

Fig. 61A. This cervical dislocation occurred in a 14-year-old gymnast who fell on his head during a running forward somersault. He fell because one of his feet caught in the springs of a mattress. He had been using the mattress to display his athletic skill at a city playground. The forward shift of the C4 vertebral body is obvious at the middle zone. The patient was rendered immediately and permanently quadriplegic. **B.** As the fourth cervical vertebral body is dislocated on C5 in this patient, as shown on the lateral view, a vertical fracture occurred in C5. The fracture site in C5 is shown through the overlying tracheal air column on the anteroposterior view.

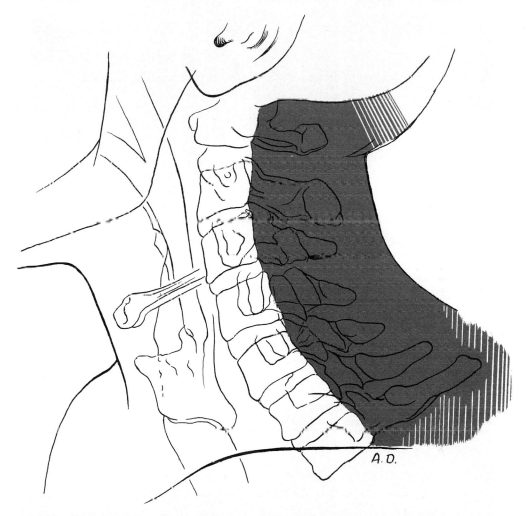

Fig. 62. The posterior zone of inspection of the lateral view of the cervical spine contains the apophyseal or facet joints, the spinous processes, and the posterior soft tissues.

cent inferior facet. Care must be taken to search for a fracture in a facet joint or neural arch whether or not a subluxation is detected (Fig. 64).

The lateral view shows each spinous process at the posterior margin of the spinal canal. The examiner should mentally connect the cortices of the anterior parts of the spinous processes (or actually employ a wax pencil to do so) so that a gentle regular line extends from posterior spinal canal limit to posterior spinal canal limit from C7 to C6 to C5 to C4, and so forth on upward to the skull. The same cortical margin in the spinous process of C1 will usually conform to this line, which should end at the posterior margin of the foramen magnum (Figs. 47, 66). In fracture–dislocations at C1–C2, C1 will often be displaced anteriorly with respect to C2. The spinous process of C1 will also be

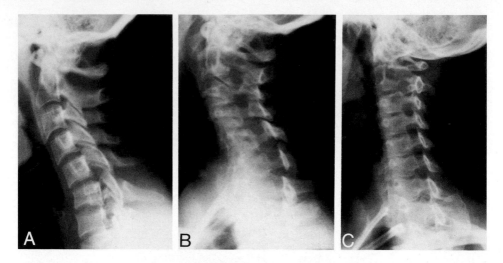

Fig. 63A. A 23-year-old equestrienne was thrown from her horse. She landed on her head, suffering a compression injury to the cervical spine. Several notable features are present on her radiographs. The intervertebral disc space is narrowed at C5–C6 following acute disc rupture. The lower facets of C5 are subluxed markedly on the upper facets of C6 at the zygoapophyseal joints. There is interspinous distance widening focally at the C5–C6 level, suggesting posterior rupture of interspinous ligaments. **B.** Following subluxation of facet joints in cervical spine trauma the oblique views are useful in showing the position of the displaced facet. Instead of the normal shinglelike arrangement in which an uppper facet drapes over a lower facet, the displaced facet perches upon the facet beneath it. In the same patient the facet of C5 is perched on C6 in this view. **C.** The normal relationships of the facet joints are shown in another patient by way of comparison.

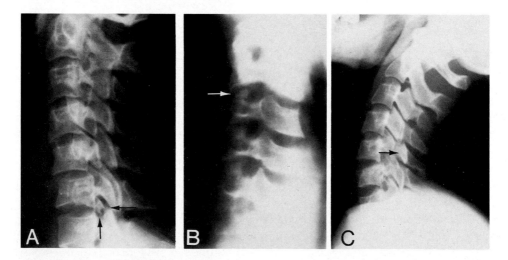

Fig. 64. Three examples of facet fractures are shown. It is often difficult to see the actual fracture line or the slightly displaced fragment of a facet. **A.** In the plain radiograph in a lateral view a fracture line and fragment is present at a C7 superior facet. **B.** In another patient a tomographic study showed a superior facet fracture that was not clearly shown on prior plain films. **C.** A fragment of a facet has been displaced posteriorly after a C5–C6 fracture dislocation in another patient. The fragment overlies the posterior limit of the spinal canal but is lateral to and outside the canal. The old fracture deformity of the C6 vertebral body is also evident.

48

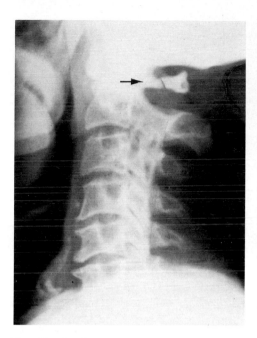

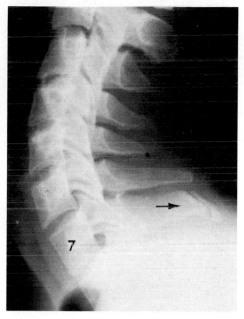

Fig. 65. In the patient with the Jefferson fracture (Fig. 50) the lateral view showed a fracture site in the neural arch of C1. This represents one of the two suspected fractures of the ring of C1. The second suspected site in the anterior part of the ring was not demonstrated.

Fig. 66. This lateral view of the cervical spine shows an old avulsion fracture of the posterior tip of the spinous process of C7. This represents the clay-shovelers type fracture. The patient, a young man in his early twenties, was playing golf when he injured his neck. He swung forcefully at the ball but hit the ground behind the ball and experienced immediate pain in the C7 area.

moved anteriorly, thus altering the regular appearance of the posterior "check line." Remember too that occasionally a congenitally short spinous process occurs at C1, and also that C1 may fuse with the occiput as a congenital anomaly. In these two instances the normal check line may be altered at the C1 level without indicating trauma.

The value of this posterior check line is that it provides the necessary evidence that can lead to a greater suspicion of C1–C2 dislocation and fracture. This suspicion then will lead to the appropriate use of supervised flexion and extension views and/or tomograms of C1–C2.

The outlines, extent, and relationships of the spinous processes remain to be examined in the posterior portion of the lateal view of the cervical spine (Fig. 65). Spinous process fractures can be subtle, especially if nondisplaced[3,10] (Fig. 66).

Nerve Root Injury

Do not forget that plain radiographs can be normal despite neurologic damage in the neck. This is especially true of patients who fall on what Bate-

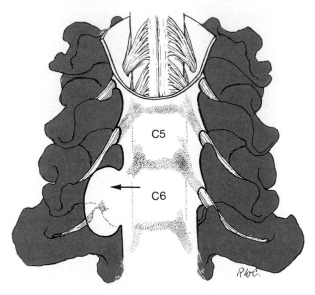

Fig. 67. This composite drawing illustrates the result of direct injury or traction injury to the cervical plexus. This injury, if severe, leads to avulsion of the nerve root and nerve root sleeve in the cervical spine. On one side the nerve roots emerge from normal root sleeves. On the opposite side a torn root sleeve (arrow) balloons about an avulsed nerve. The ballooning actually represents pooling of contrast material in this torn root sleeve at myelography.

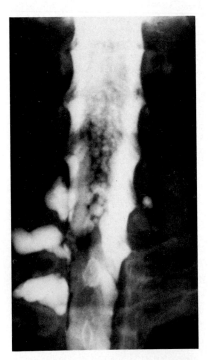

Fig. 68. This view was obtained at myelography in a patient who had been involved in an automobile accident. His chief symptom was inability to move the right arm. Contrast material tracks laterally into three abnormal collections at nerve root sleeves. This demonstrates widespread traumatic avulsion of the dura covering these nerve roots. In such cases the nerves are usually avulsed also. The normal nerve root shadows are present in the upper cervical spine but are absent in the three large areas of contrast material. Thus three major nerve roots and contributors to the brachial plexus have been torn and displaced. Such injuries are usually associated with permanent disability. Motorcycling injury has produced identical findings.

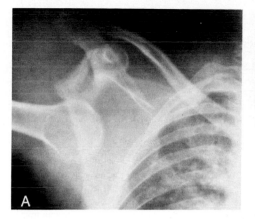

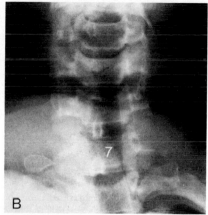

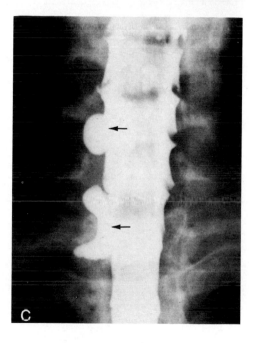

Fig. 69A. A motorcyclist was severely in-jured in a fall from his cycle. An anterior dis-location of the shoulder is present. Motor and sensory changes were present in his right arm and persisted after the shoulder dislocation was reduced. **B.** An anteropos-terior view of the cervical spine showed a fracture of the right transverse process of C7. **C.** At myelography nerve root and root sleeve avulsions were found at two levels on the patient's right side (see Figure 67).

man refers to as the acromionmastoid dimension.[1] Such a patient may have avulsed nerve roots of the brachial plexus. Think of the motorcyclist who is thrown from his cycle so that the side of his head hits the roadway (Fig. 67). Cervical myelography can then be of direct value in showing contrast material escape from the normal dural confines through the avulsed cervical nerve root sleeves[5,9,13] (Figs. 68, 69). In this regard, myelography may be of additional value in showing intramedullary hemorrhage or edema as well as bone frag-ments following acute injury.

References

1. Bateman JE: Nerve injuries about the shoulder in sports. J Bone Joint Surg 49A:767–773, 1967
2. Bohlman HH: The results of cervical spine trauma: general and specific. In: Instructional Course #17, American Academy of Orthopaedic Surgeons. January 30, 1972
3. Cancelmo JJ Jr: Clay shoveler's fracture. Am J Roentgenol 115:540–543, 1972
4. Garger WN, Fisher RG, Halfmann HW: Vertebrectomy and fusion for "tear drop fracture of the cervical spine." J Trauma 9:887–893, 1969
5. Rayle AA, Gay BB Jr, Meadors JL: The myelogram in avulsion of the brachial plexus. Radiol 65:65–72, 1955
6. Reymond RD, Wheeler PS, Perovic M, Block B: The lucent cleft, a new radiographic sign of cervical injury or disease. Clin Radiol 23:188–192, 1972
7. Schneider RC: A syndrome in acute cervical spine injuries for which early operation is indicated. J Neurosurg 8:360–367, 1951
8. ———— The syndrome of acute anterior spinal cord injury. J Neurosurg 12:95–122, 1955
9. Varley WT: The importance of cervical myelography in cervical and upper thoracic nerve root avulsion. Radiology 76:376–380, 1961
10. Venable JR, Flake RE, Kilian DJ: Stress fracture of the spinous process. JAMA 190:881–885, 1964
11. Verbiest H: Anterolateral operations for fractures and dislocations in the middle and lower parts of the cervical spine. J Bone Joint Surg 51A:1489–1530, 1969
12. Whalen JP, Woodruff CL: Cervical prevertebral fat stripe: a new aid in evaluating the cervical prevertebral soft tissue space. Am J Roentgenol 109:445–451, 1970
13. Yeoman PM: Cervical myelography in traction injuries of the brachial plexus. J Bone Joint Surg 50B:253–260, 1968

SHOULDER

Golding referred to the shoulder as the forgotten joint.[11] In sports this reference hardly holds true. From dislocations and fractures to soft tissue injury, this joint is in the forefront among injury sites.

Soft Tissue Injury

Soft tissue injury, particularly to the attachments of the rotator cuff, are not uncommon in athletes.[4] Bateman has experience with full thickness tears of the rotator cuff in baseball pitchers and shortstops, football quarterbacks, golfers, skiers, hockey and tennis players, curlers, riders, wrestlers, yachtsmen, canoeists, jujitsu enthusiasts, and bowlers.[5] Sudden vertical force from a blow directed along the humerus, headlong falls on the point of the shoulder, and throwing injuries account for the majority of these tears. An upward malposition of the humeral head may be found on x-ray examination following injury. Rotator cuff injury, however, usually occurs without malposition of the humeral head and therefore one shoud not rely on this upward shift of the humerus to indicate such an injury. Plain radiographs are usually normal after rotator cuff injury (Fig. 70). If there is an abnormality on the plain radiograph in the acute condition it consists of narrowing of the space between the acromion and the humeral head reflecting the shift of the humerus through the tear on anteroposterior radiographs.[17] Arthrography is very helpful if a cuff tear is suspected and can show abnormal migration of contrast material into the subacromial or subdeltoid soft tissue areas.[14-16,20,24,26] In the normal shoulder, contrast material is confined to the glenohumeral joint and its normal subcoracoid recesses (Figs. 71, 72). Once the diagnosis is established both operative and nonoperative treatment can be considered.

Injury to the Clavicle

Clavicular fractures usually occur at the midpoint of the clavicle. Seldom does radiography show the relationship of fracture ends in two planes. Only by bowing the patient over so that a worm's eye view of the fracture fragments

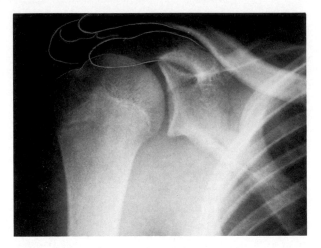

Fig. 70. In the normal shoulder, the humeral head is seated beneath the canopy of the acromion process. The margins of the glenohumeral articulation are parallel arcs and the cartilage space of that articulation is uniform and clearly shown. The residual cartilaginous growth plate in the proximal humerus in this young adolescent should not be confused with a fracture line. Lines have been added to this photograph so that structures evident on the original x-ray are appreciated.

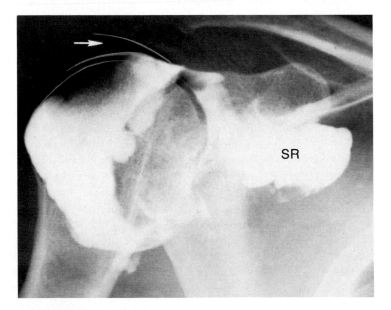

Fig. 71. Contrast material is confined in the glenohumeral cavity. The subcoracoid recess (SR) is a normal landmark in this normal shoulder arthrogram. Note the normal superolateral margins of the joint capsule preventing contrast from reaching the acromiohumeral space (arrow). This view was made with the humerus in internal rotation. Lines have been added to this photograph as in Figure 70.

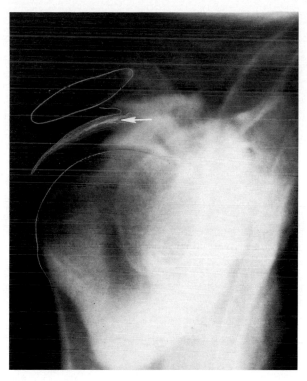

Fig. 72. This shoulder arthrogram was performed in a 48-year-old woman who fell many months earlier while playing tennis. As she fell she braced her fall with her right arm and injured her right shoulder. A rotator cuff tear shown here was not initially suspected. Other diagnoses were entertained to explain her continued shoulder pain and she underwent arteriography and acupuncture that were fruitless. The view illustrated shows an arc of contrast material in an abnormal location between the acromion and the superolateral part of the humerus. At surgery a superior rotator cuff tear was repaired and the patient recovered. Lines have been added to this photograph as in Figures 70 and 71.

can be obtained can we fully realize the extent of displacement (Fig. 73). This angled view or tangential view of the clavicle may show a fracture that is hidden in the anteroposterior view by exactly overlapping fragments (Fig. 74). Subclavian vessel or nerve injury may occur as a complication following fracture of the clavicle. Sir Robert Peel is said to have suffered a fatal hemorrhage from the subclavian vein following a fracture of the clavicle sustained in a fall from a horse.[18]

Both ends of the clavicle deserve as much attention as the frequently fractured midclavicular area. Medially, the clavicle can be dislocated anterior to the sternum and retrosternally. This injury is sometimes missed on physical examination and in the case of retrosternal dislocation can lead to compression of the great vessels, edema of the neck, and dyspnea. The x-ray diagnosis is facilitated by a chest x-ray in which the normal clavicular sternal articulation is shown adjacent to the abnormal side (Figs. 75, 76). Tangential lateral views of the sternum can be of value here.[19] If the central ray of the x-ray tube is

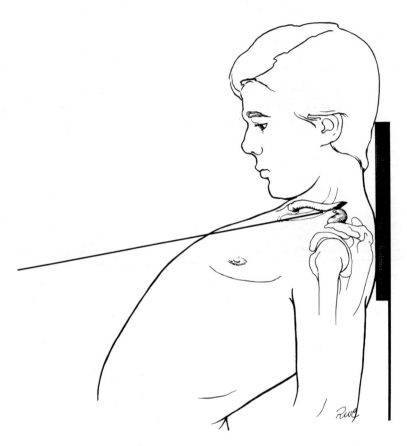

Fig. 73. By bowing the patient backward and angling the central ray (solid line) upward, a helpful view of the clavicular fracture site is obtained. This is useful in showing the degree of displacement of the fracture fragments. It may be the only view to show the fracture line.

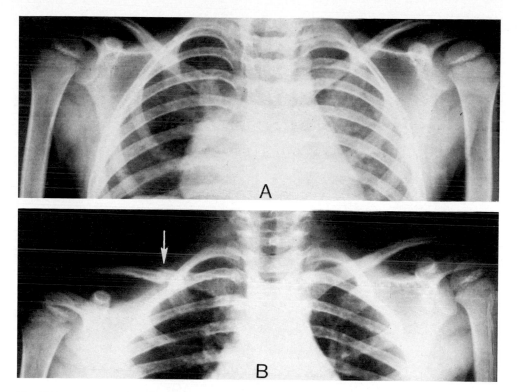

Fig. 74A. This view of the clavicles of a 3-year-old girl was obtained after she fell, injuring her right shoulder. No fracture line is noted. Because a fracture was strongly suspected from the physical examination alone a repeat angled view of the clavicle was obtained at the same time. **B.** This shows the suspected fracture (arrow) and indicates the extreme value of an axial or angled view of the clavicle. This view can also be used to show the degree of displacement in known fracture of the clavicle.

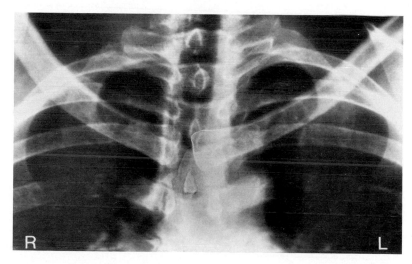

Fig. 75. A coned down view of the medial ends of the clavicles shows asymmetry of the sternoclavicular articulations. The left clavicle overlaps part of the sternum and is dislocated. The right clavicle articulates normally with the sternum. The dislocation was an anterior dislocation.

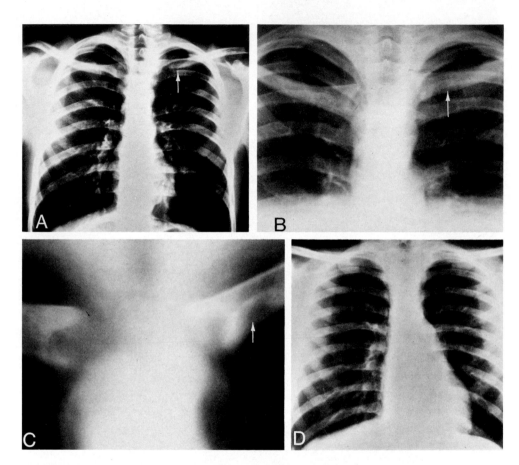

Fig. 76A. This chest x-ray was obtained after a 14-year-old batsman in baseball fell on the side of his shoulder as he narrowly avoided a pitched ball by diving to the ground. He complained of swelling and pain at the medial end of the left clavicle after the injury. The left clavicle is elevated at its dislocated sternoclavicular articulation. The clavicle was dislocated in an anterior superior direction. **B.** The upward displacement of the dislocated medial end of the left clavicle is shown better in this magnified view. **C.** In the course of evaluation of the patient and prior to the recognition of the dislocation, tomograms were made at the swollen left sternoclavicular joint because that area was indurated. This induration suggested the diagnosis of neoplasm to some of the physicians evaluating the patient. The medial ends of the clavicles are notched on the tomogram and are normal. The inferior edge of the left clavicle is also notched as is the right by the rhomboid fossae. The costoclavicular ligaments attach here. This is a normal landmark of the clavicle and is not to be mistaken as a pathologic lesion. **D.** At age 9 the same baseball player had been x-rayed for an upper respiratory infection. This normal chest x-ray shows the normal position of the medial ends of his clavicles at that time.

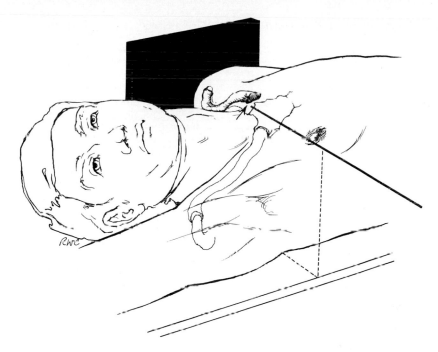

Fig. 77. The tangential view of the sternoclavicular joint is useful in showing the displacement of the clavicle in a patient with dislocation of the medial end of the clavicle. Comparison views obtained from both sides are a must. The central ray is angled along the opposite clavicle and is parallel to the table and perpendicular to the film.

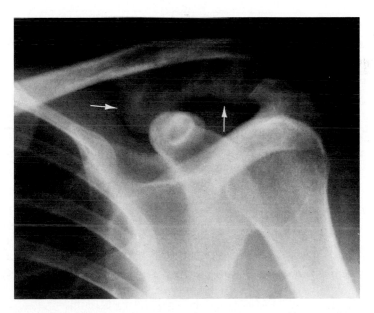

Fig. 78. Once there is rupture of the coracoclavicular and acromioclavicular ligaments, ossification may replace part of the normal ligaments (arrows). This result usually accompanies a severe separation of the acromioclavicular joint. Rarely, disease such as ankylosing spondylitis can lead to ossification of the coracoclavicular ligaments.

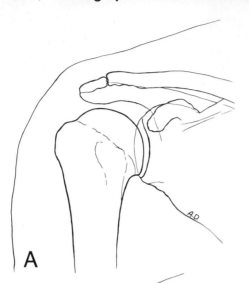

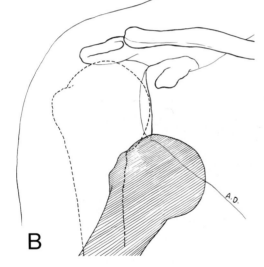

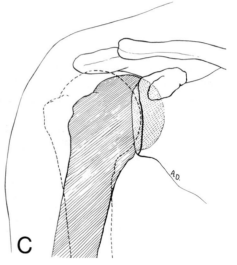

Fig. 79. The humeral head is shown in three positions: **A.** Normal. **B.** Anterior dislocation. **C.** Posterior dislocation. Note the resemblance of the position in posterior dislocation to that in the normal shoulder.

aligned with the clavicle, a comparison of the position of the medial end of the clavicle with the sternum can be made (Fig. 77). Both lateral views are needed for comparison. This combination provides a radiographic record of the sternoclavicular joint from the viewpoint of the clavicle. At the acromioclavicular and coracoclavicular joints various degrees of injury and displacement occur (Fig. 78). Comparison views of the normal and injured shoulders are useful if the patient holds weights of 10 to 15 pounds in each hand. The clavicle is elevated at its lateral end in abnormal radiographs in this injury and the distance between the coracoid process and the clavicle will be increased. The same ligamentous area between the coracoid process and the clavicle may show ossification after injury. The lateral end of the clavicle may be eroded or tapered following a fall or repeated falls on the shoulder.[13,27] Soft tissue calcification in injured tissue or hematomata can accompany this finding. Subclavian and axillary vessel injury are uncommon injuries in sports. However, hypertrophy of muscles can be a rare cause of venous thrombosis and venous insufficiency.[1,8] Occasionally, a violent or sudden movement of the shoulders produces rupture of the axillary artery or its branches.

The Dislocated Shoulder

Shoulder dislocation is a hazard of collisions and falls in many sports. At times, this injury is a difficult one to detect on x-ray examination. The usual dislocation is an anterior and inferior displacement of the humeral head in the subcoracoid or subglenoid positions[3] (Fig. 79). Less often, the humeral head moves posterior to the glenoid margins. Anteroposterior radiographs of the shoulder will readily show the downward and medial shift of the humerus in the anterior dislocation (Fig. 80). In the case of the posterior dislocation, however, the humeral head simply lies behind the glenoid margin, producing a picture that initially can be misinterpreted as normal (Figs. 81, 82). Careful examination of the relationships between the humeral articular surface and the glenoid articulation, however, will show incongruity of alignment in the posterior dislocation.[7,9,30]

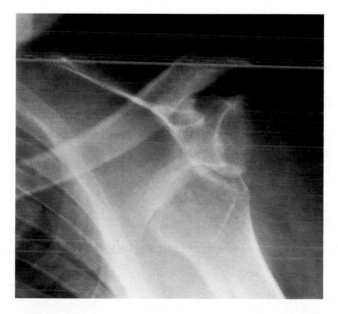

Fig. 80. This inferior position of the humeral head is diagnostic of an anterior dislocation of the shoulder. A wide variety of displacement positions exist. The humeral head may be shifted only slightly in an inferior medial direction in subluxations of the shoulder. Conversely, a humeral head (as in this example) may lie in a subglenoid or subcoracoid position in an overt anterior dislocation of the shoulder.

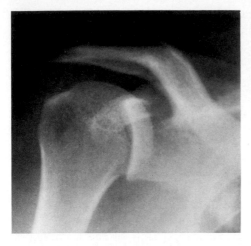

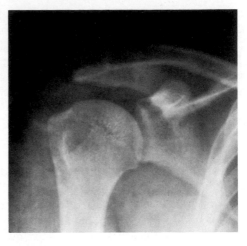

Fig. 81. To some readers this anteroposterior view of the shoulder will appear normal. The medial margin of the humeral head overlaps the glenoid in an abnormal relationship, indicating a posterior dislocation of the humerus. The dislocation cannot be an anterior one because anterior dislocations show an inferior displacement of the humeral head.

Fig. 82. The glenohumeral relationships are now normal after reduction of the posterior dislocation of the shoulder shown in Figure 81.

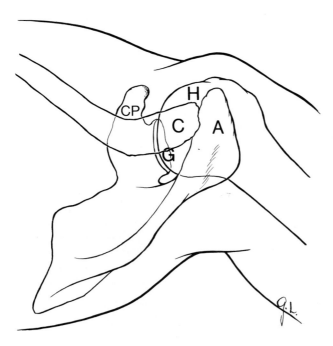

Fig. 83. The axillary view is a vital one in evaluating the shoulder. This worm's eye or bird's eye view displays the glenohumeral articulation to advantage. In this normal shoulder note how little depth the glenoid margin has and how small the glenoid process is compared to the area of the humeral head. (C, clavicle; CP, coracoid process; G, glenoid; H, humerus; A, acromion).

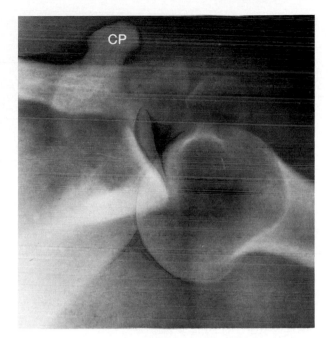

Fig. 84. The humeral head lies posterior to the major portion of the glenoid cavity, indicating a posterior dislocation of the shoulder. The coracoid process (CP) is intact and serves as an anterior landmark.

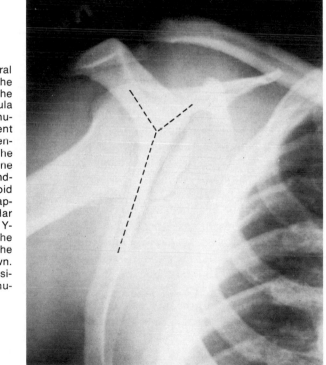

Fig. 85. By directing the central ray of the x-ray beam along the back as a tangent through the body of the scapula, the scapula is shown overlapping the humerus. This normal arrangement shows the humeral head centered at the glenoid area. The coracoid process and the spine of the scapula serve as landmarks to locate the glenoid area. With the body of the scapula, the coracoid and scapular spine form a triradiate or Y-shaped scapular profile. The humeral head should overlie the center of this Y figure as shown. In cases of dislocation the positions of the glenoid and the humeral head mismatch.

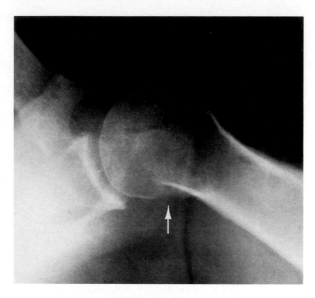

Fig. 86. Cortical fracture of the humerus often occurs after chronic dislocation of the shoulder. The irregular profile of the humeral head is shown in this axillary view. The glenoid margin is normal. The humeral head is in normal position with regard to the glenoid after reduction of a dislocation.

An extremely helpful radiographic view is the axillary view, which gives a bird's eye, or worm's eye view, if you prefer, of the shoulder (Fig. 83). The view is exposed by directing the central ray of the radiographic unit upward toward the axilla. The x-ray film is placed on top of the shoulder as an epaulette. If the patient has sufficient pain and limitation of motion to prevent access of the x-ray tube in the upright or supine position, then remember to use the patient's ability to bend his spine and assume a bowed or bending position to obtain this helpful exposure. With such a view, the anterior or posterior position of the humerus with respect to the relatively small glenoid rim is immediately apparent (Fig. 84). A tangential view of the scapula is another view that can be applied to the problem of shoulder dislocation (Fig. 85). The axillary view may be preferred not only for its clear exposition of the glenohumeral relationship, but also because the axillary view clearly shows the anterior and posterior margins of the glenoid and the coracoid process. The glenoid margin or the coracoid process may be fractured and shown only on the axillary view.[6] Armstrong indicated that the coracoid may be fractured in a recoil injury in target and game shooting and that brachial plexus injury is also possible after such recoil.[2]

Defects of the humeral articular margin are usually shown in the axillary view in the focal cortical impaction fracture that follows chronic dislocation.[23] This defect has been described by Hill and Sachs and has been given their eponymic designation[12] (Fig. 86). Several views of the humeral head may be required (including the axillary view) in order to best show the extent of the

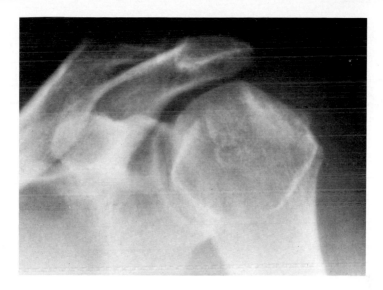

Fig. 87. This anteroposterior view in internal rotation also shows the notched appearance of the humeral head. The fracture occurs with the impact of the humerus on the glenoid margin.

cortical indentation by tangential projection (Fig. 87). Pseudodislocation is a term applied to inferior subluxation of the humeral head following hemarthrosis, effusion, or pyarthrosis.[21] Patients with hemophilia may show this sign following minimal trauma.

Other Injury

Scapular and soft tissue injury require radiographs that display these shoulder areas to best advantage. Tendon and bursal calcifications are best pinpointed by coned soft tissue views taken in internal and external rotation. The pattern of movement of the calcifications can be used to identify the location within the tendon sites.[29] Xeroradiography should be of value in improving radiographic detection of these soft tissue and tendon areas.

Finally, do not forget that in some athletes shoulder views may be the only chance to recognize rib, thoracic outlet, and pulmonary apex abnormalities. Stress fractures of the first rib do occur in baseball.[22] Violent throwing efforts have also been responsible for fractures of the proximal humerus or midshaft humerus in softball, baseball, and javelin throwing.[10,25,28]

References

1. Adams JT, Deweese JA: "Effort" thrombosis of the axillary and subclavian veins. J Trauma 11:923–930, 1971
2. Armstrong JR: Game shooting and injury. In Armstrong JR, Tucker WE (eds): Injury in Sport. London, Staples, 1964, pp 191–199

3. Bailey RW: Acute and recurrent dislocations of the shoulder. J Bone Joint Surg 49A:767–773, 1967
4. Bateman JE: Shoulder injuries in athletics. Clin Orthop 23:75–83, 1962
5. _____: Cuff tears in athletes. Orthop Clin North Am 4:721–745, 1973
6. Benton J, Nelson C: Avulsion of the coracoid process in an athlete. J Bone Joint Surg 53:356–358, 1971
7. Brown WH, Dennis JM, Davidson CN, Rubin PS, Fulton H: Posterior dislocation of the shoulder. Radiology 68:815–822, 1957
8. Estes JE: Thrombophlebitis. Springfield, Ill., Thomas, 1964, p 30
9. Figiel SJ, Figiel LS, Bardenstein MB, Blodgett WH: Posterior dislocation of the shoulder. Radiology 87:737–740, 1966
10. Gregersen HN: Fractures of the humerus from muscular violence. Acta Orthop Scand 42:506–512, 1971
11. Golding FC: The shoulder—the forgotten joint. Br J Radiol 35:149–158, 1962
12. Hill HA, Sachs MD: The grooved defect of the humeral head. Radiology 35:690–701, 1940
13. Jacobs P: Post-traumatic osteolysis of the outer end of the clavical. J Bone Joint Surg 76B:705, 1964
14. Kernwein GA, Roseberg B, Sneed WR Jr: Arthrographic studies of the shoulder joint. J Bone Joint Surg 39A:1267–1279, 1957
15. _____ Roentgenographic diagnosis of shoulder dysfunction. JAMA 194:1081–1085, 1965
16. Killoran PJ, Marcove RC, Freiberger RH: Shoulder arthrography. Am J Roentgenol 103:658–668, 1968
17. Kotzen LM: Roentgen diagnosis of rotator cuff tear. Am J Roentgenol 112:507–511, 1971
18. Lachman E: Anatomy as applied to clinical medicine. New Physician 2:115–117, 1962
19. Lee FA, Gwinn JL: Retrosternal dislocation of the clavicle. Radiology 110:631–634, 1974
20. Lipmann Kessel AW: Arthrography of the shoulder joint. Proc R Soc Med 43:418–420, 1950
21. Markham DE, Rowland J: The shoulder joint. Is it dislocated? Apparent dislocation of the shoulder joint. Clin Radiol 20:61–64, 1969
22. Meaney T: Personal communication.
23. Moseley HF: Recurrent dislocation of the shoulder. Postgrad Med 31:23–29, 1962
24. Neviaser JS: Arthrography of the Shoulders. The Diagnosis and Management of the Lesions Visualized. Springfield, Ill., Thomas, 1975
25. Peltokallio P, Peltokallio V, Vaalasti T: Fractures of the humerus from muscular violence in sport. J Sports Med Phys Fitness 8:21–25, 1968
26. Reeves B: Arthrography of the shoulder. J Bone Joint Surg 48B:424–435, 1966
27. Smart MJ: Traumatic osteolysis of the distal ends of the clavicles. J Can Assoc Radiol 23:264–266, 1972
28. Tullos HS, Erwin WD, Woods GW, Wukasch DC, Cooley DA, King JW: Unusual lesions of the pitching arm. Clin Orthop 88:169–182, 1972
29. ViGario GD, Keats TE: Localization of calcific deposits in the shoulder. Am J Roentgenol 108:806–811, 1970
30. Warrick CK: Posterior dislocation of the shoulder joint. Br J Radiol 38:758–761, 1965

ELBOW, FOREARM, WRIST, AND HAND

Elbow

Anteroposterior, lateral, and oblique views are the standard projections used to examine the elbow. Tomography is of occasional value in showing an intra-articular fragment of bone. The soft tissue signs of elbow injury have been discussed in the first chapter and will not be repeated. The normal bony landmarks are shown in Figures 88 and 89.

Prior to the attention centered on the elbow by the aches and pains of hundreds of Little League baseball players in this country,[1] reports of elbow injury occurred most commonly in tennis and golf.[6,7] The untoward effects of javelin throwing also produced an occasional report of injury.[23] Most elbow injuries produced in sport are of the avulsion type in which acute or chronic stress occurs at a ligament or tendon site. Bone fragments can be shown at the olecranon process and at the epicondyles following avulsion injury. Prominent spurs may occur at the epicondyles due to long-standing stress. The elbow of the adolescent is particularly apt to show signs and symptoms of undue exertion in sport.[3] Growth centers from the capitellum, trochlea, and epicondyles may be fragmented, displaced (even within the joint), enlarged, and prematurely fused following athletic activity. Careful comparison with the asymptomatic elbow in similar radiographic projections is necessary in evaluating the immature skeleton (Fig. 90). This last point bears restating. Comparison views should not be an optional tool but must be considered a vital part of an adequate examination. Fractures of the radial head and occult fractures of the distal humerus are often subtle. Repeat radiographs in one to two weeks will show such features to better advantage and may be the only views to show a definite fracture.

Forearm

Injuries from falls or from direct blows to the forearm produce the bulk of forearm skeletal injuries. The detection of injury here is usually straightforward. Certain pitfalls do exist, however. With a midforearm blow producing a fracture of the radius or ulna, remember, as in the case of the clavicle, to examine carefully each end of the forearm for associated subluxation–dislocation

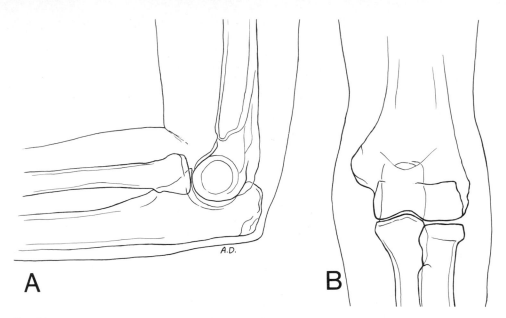

A   B

Fig. 88A. From the lateral viewpoint, the normal humerus has a distal articular portion that is positioned anterior to the plane of the shaft of the humerus. **B.** In the frontal view, the normal position of the medical epicondyle is not opposite the lateral epicondyle but at a more proximal point along the humerus.

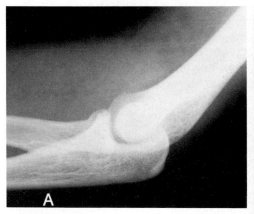

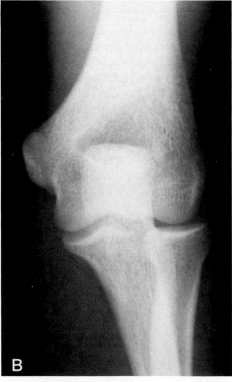

Fig. 89. The normal shapes and positions of the epicondylar, trochlear, capitellar, and radioulnar structures must be familiar to the examiner, who should know that the radial head articulates evenly with the capitellum on both these views. The smooth contours of the articular surfaces are important normal features. **A.** Lateral view. **B.** Anteroposterior view.

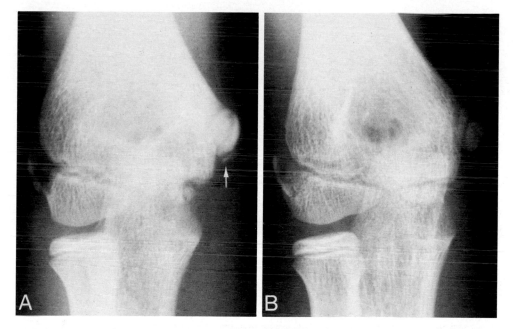

Fig. 90. An 11-year-old Little League pitcher complained of elbow pain. Comparison views of both elbows were obtained. Which elbow is abnormal and what findings do you anticipate in the elbow of a young baseballer? **A.** The right elbow is abnormal and shows a small bone fragment (arrow) at the distal edge of the ossification center for the medial epicondyle. This epicondylar area is the site of maximal stress in pitching and can fragment in the adolescent. Fragments can be displaced into the joint or lead to spur formation. The small fragment of bone in this case is next to a normal ossification center for the medial epicondyle. Four other ossification centers are shown in this adolescent elbow. **B.** The normal left elbow x-ray has been reversed so that it can be compared point by point with the abnormal right elbow.

or rotational abnormality. Dislocation of the proximal radius accompanies midulnar fracture in the Monteggia injury[21] (Figs. 91, 92). Midradius fracture is accompanied by distal ulnar subluxation in the Galeazzi fracture[5,21] (Fig. 93). Adequate lateral views of the elbow and wrist are needed to completely evaluate forearm injury in these circumstances. At the wrist, on a lateral radiograph, the distal ulna is normally lined up with and projected through the distal radius. In subluxation of the distal ulna, the ulna is usually displaced dorsally (Fig. 93B). Comparison views of the wrist may be necessary in order to evaluate distal ulnar subluxation. Rotational abnormalities of the ulna may complicate ulnar or radial fracture.[2] The helpful markers within the ulna that aid in the detection of rotation are the bicipital tubercle proximally and the ulnar styloid process distally. In a normal anteroposterior view the bicipital tubercle is in profile and is readily identified. Its absence in the anteroposterior view should raise the suspicion of proximal ulna rotation. The ulnar styloid process is located at the margin of the ulna on posteroanterior views of the wrist and distal forearm. This will be discussed below in the paragraphs that deal with the wrist.

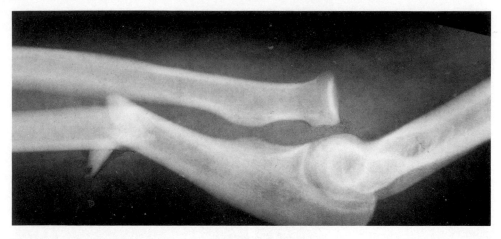

Fig. 91. A blow to the dorsum of the forearm is the mechanism of this Monteggia injury. The ulnar shaft fractures and the radius is separated from the ulna at their proximal interosseous connections. The normal radial head–capitellum articulation is lost, with the radius dislocated anteriorly at the elbow.

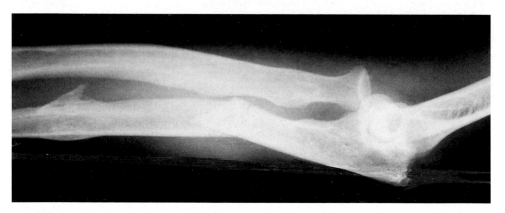

Fig. 92. The proximal radial dislocation is shown in this Monteggia injury featuring an old healed fracture of the midulnar shaft.

Wrist

The frequently encountered Colles' fracture of the distal radius may at first consideration offer little radiographic challenge. However, when one realizes that the entire radiocarpal and distal radioulnar joint relationships are disturbed in this injury the significance of the trauma is more fully appreciated. The normal relationships at the wrist of the radius, ulna, and carpal bones must be well understood (Figs. 94, 95). Distal radio-ulnar joint disruption is shown

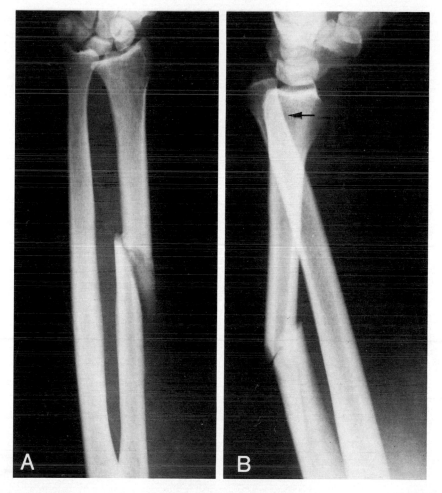

Fig. 93. A forceful impact to the ventral midforearm can produce radial fracture and disruption of the distal radioulnar joint. **A.** The ulna overlaps the radius abnormally at the wrist, indicating distal radioulnar separation. This is the counterpart of the Monteggia injury and is often referred to as the Galeazzi fracture. **B.** On the lateral view the distal ulna is displaced dorsally at the wrist.

as narrowing or widening of that joint on the posteroanterior view and as dorsal displacement of the distal ulna on the lateral view of the wrist. The radiocarpal joint alignment is normally best evaluated on the lateral view of the wrist. Here the distal articular margin of the radius is canted volarly so that an angle of approximately 35° is described by its distal margin and a perpendicular to the long axis of the radius at its volar end.[16] After a distal radius fracture of Colles' type, the articular margin of the radius usually is directed dorsally with loss of the normal angle just described. Occasionally the distal portion of the

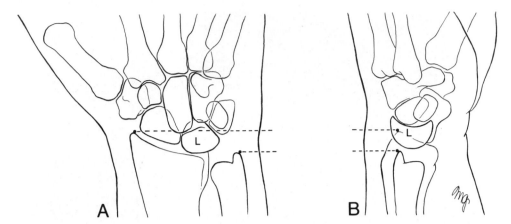

Fig. 94. The radial styloid process in the normal wrist is more distal than the ulnar styloid process in both these views. **A.** The frontal view. **B.** The lateral view. The articular surface of the distal radius is canted volarly on the lateral view. The lunate bone (L) is labeled as a reference for subsequent figures.

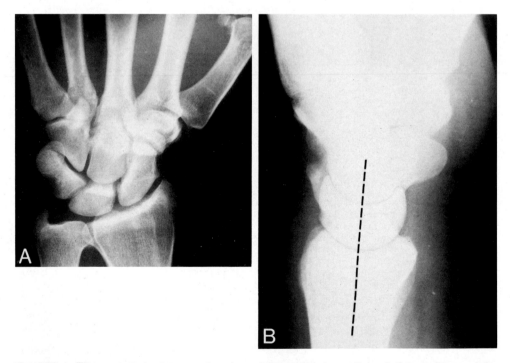

Fig. 95A. The normal posteroanterior view of the wrist shows the relative positions of the radial and ulnar styloid processes. The joint or cartilage spaces between carpal bones are rather uniform. **B.** In the lateral view the (demilune) shape of the lunate bone is evident. The longitudinal axis of the radius should extend through the midpoint of the lunate bone.

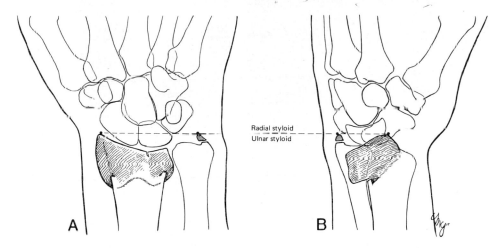

Radial styloid
Ulnar styloid

A

B

Fig. 96. An impacted radial fracture is shown. The ulnar styloid process is also fractured. The fragments of the radial fracture are telescoped so that the two styloid processes are at the same level. **A.** Posteroanterior view. **B.** Lateral view.

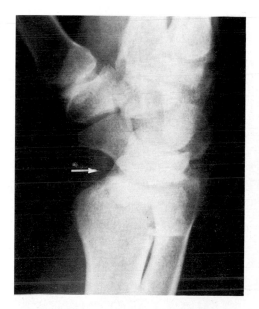

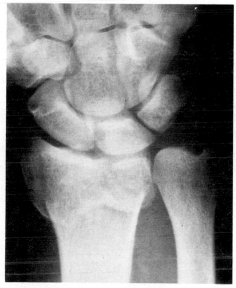

Fig. 97. This modified lateral view shows the dorsal displacement of the distal radial fracture fragment in a Colles fracture.

Fig. 98. The fracture lines in this injury of the distal radius involve the articular surface of the radius. This produces a variable degree of added morbidity and is not a typical Colles fracture.

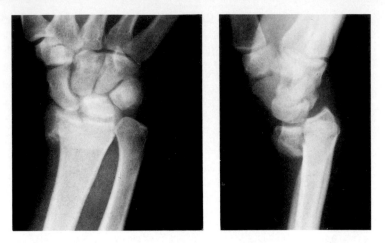

Fig. 99. In Barton's fracture an anterior and articular piece of the distal radius is separated from the main portion of the radius.

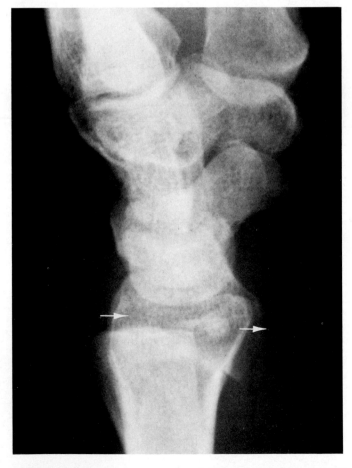

Fig. 100. A transverse fracture line crosses the distal radius in this injury. There is a slight volar shift (arrows) of the distal fragment, so that this is a variant of Smith's fracture.

radius is fragmented and impacted. The degree of impaction is detected by noting the relative positions of the ulnar and radial styloid processes. Normally the radial styloid process is 1 cm distal to the ulnar styloid process.[16] With impaction both styloid processes are at the same distal level (Figs. 96, 97). Other fracture variants exist at the wrist, including epiphyseal fractures[9,24,25] and fractures through the cartilaginous growth plate in adolescents or children (Figs. 98–101).

The conventional frontal radiographic view of the wrist is a posteroanterior view in which the ulnar styloid process is situated at the edge of the wrist and at the very outer margins of the ulna. When the wrist is rotated into a palm-up position and an anteroposterior view is exposed, one sees that the ulnar styloid process now occupies a central position with respect to the

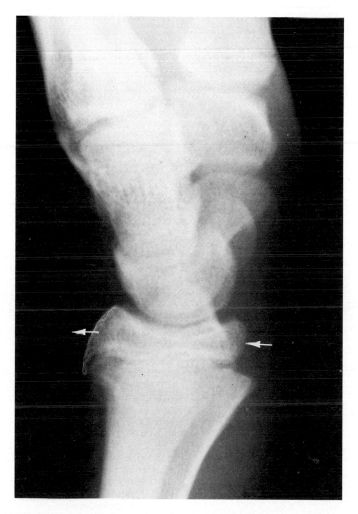

Fig. 101. The anterior margins of the distal radial epiphyseal growth plate are altered in a teenager following a fracture through the growth plate. The distal epiphysis of the radius is shifted slightly in a posterior direction (arrows).

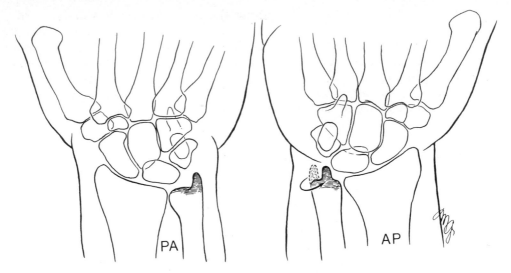

Fig. 102. The ulnar styloid shifts in the normal wrist during a position change of the wrist. The distal ulna rotates slightly in the normal wrist when the hand is shifted from the pronated position to a supinated position (or vice versa). This rotation is evident in the shift of the ulnar styloid process from its position in a posteroanterior view of the wrist to that in an anteroposterior view.

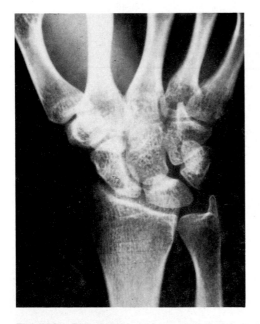

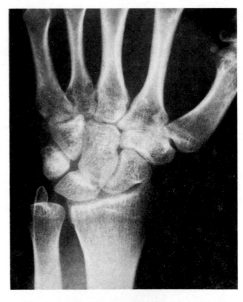

Fig. 103. The styloid process of the ulna is at the outer margin of the ulna in a posteroanterior view of a normal right wrist.

Fig. 104. Persistent wrist pain led to this view after a patient had fallen on the wrist. The ulnar styloid process is abnormally rotated along with the entire distal ulna in this posteroanterior view of the left wrist. The normal position for the styloid process of the ulna is at the outer margin of the ulna in the posteroanterior view. This indicates a rotational injury with partial disruption of the distal radioulnar joint.

76

longitudinal axis of the ulna. Hence in the normal person one can distinguish an anteroposterior view from a posteroanterior view by using the ulnar styloid as a guide (Fig. 102). The ulnar styloid can be positioned abnormally following disruption of the distal radioulnar joint.[2,13,14] In this unusual injury the ulna rotates and a posteroanterior view will give the appearance of an anteroposterior view (Figs. 103, 104).

Fractures of the carpal bones are not uncommon.[24] All carpal bones are potential fracture sites and the carpal navicular and lunate are among the commonest fracture sites. Usually the examiner remembers to scan the wrist for a fracture site but may not consider the possibility of a carpal bone dislocation. Lunate and perilunate dislocations are high on the list of overlooked injuries and may be the explanation for what is initially considered "a severe sprain." A lunate dislocation is present when the carpal lunate is displaced dorsally or ventrally (usually ventrally) so that it does not maintain its normal relationships with the radius and its carpal neighbors.[15] On the lateral radiograph of the normal wrist, the lunate lines up directly with the long axis of the radius (Figs. 94, 95). On the anteroposterior view the lunate has a quadrilateral shape (Figs. 94, 95). When the lunate is dislocated or subluxed this quadrilateral outline is lost and the bone resembles a triangle or slice of pie. The capitate and the third metacarpal may migrate proximally as the carpal and metacarpals are rearranged. A perilunate dislocation is one in which the lunate maintains its normal alignment with the radius and the distal row of carpal bones is displaced about the lunate.[15] In this dislocation one finds the distal carpal bones displaced dorsally and proximally or, less often, ventrally and proximally (Fig. 105). Combinations of these two main types of carpal dislocations do occur. The complete x-ray examination of the wrist thus will entail a careful check for fracture and dislocation (Figs. 106–109).

One may require multiple views of the wrist in several degrees of obliquity to show the fine fracture lines that occur in the carpal navicular bone, or in other carpal bones for that matter. Initially, the x-ray findings can be poorly defined and a positive diagnosis may only be established on repeat radiographs after the hand, wrist, and forearm are immobilized. Multiple views of the navicular bone or an elongated oblique view of the area of the anatomical snuff-box may be needed to show a navicular fracture (Fig. 110).

The carpal navicular, along with the femoral head and talus, is often supplied predominantly by a recurrent artery, ie, an artery that enters the distal portion of the bone and then proceeds to its proximal portion. Thus a fracture across the waist of the carpal navicular can interrupt the blood supply to the proximal fragment.[18] If a fracture is noticed, the examiner should carefully compare the densities of the two fragments to detect an increased radiographic density in the proximal fragment (Figs. 111–113). This density represents a reparative sclerosis following ischemia and does not indicate ischemia per se. Although this ischemic density denotes a severe local injury, revascularization may occur with the eventual return of normal density in the proximal fragment. Similar changes can occur in the lunate and in other bones elsewhere in the skeleton following fracture or dislocation.

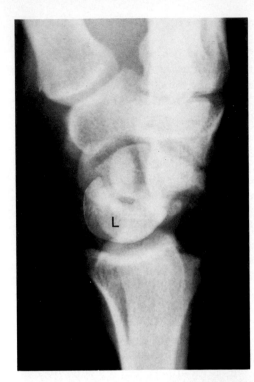

Fig. 105. The lunate bone (L) maintains a relatively normal relationship to the radius as the carpal bones shift around the navicular and lunate bones in this perilunate dislocation.

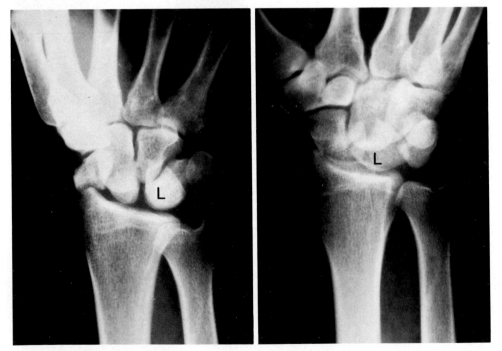

Fig. 106. Remember to search for a transnavicular (transscaphoid) fracture and a carpal dislocation in each injured wrist. Here both items are present with the carpal bones shifted in a partial perilunate position. The lunate bone is also shifted from its normal position so that a combination of a perilunate and lunate dislocation exists.

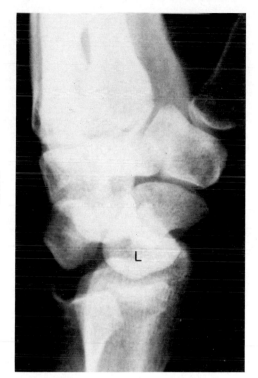

Fig. 107. The lateral view of the wrist shown in Figure 106 shows the partial displacement of the lunate bone and the perilunate shift of the capitate bone.

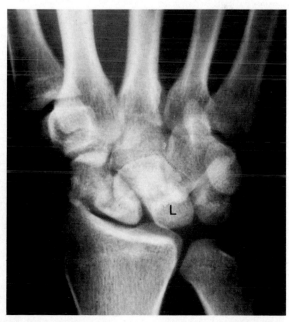

Fig. 108. The normal intercarpal joint spaces are lost in this marked rearrangement of the wrist. Fractures are present at multiple carpal bones (see surgical repair in Figure 109) and a perilunate dislocation is present. The patient was injured as his wrist was stepped on in a fight.

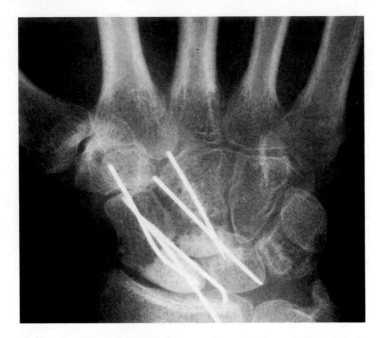

Fig. 109. At surgery the dislocated carpal bones shown in Figure 108 were reduced and fracture fragments were pinned with small Kirschner wires. Dense proximal fragments of aseptic necrosis are present at the navicular (scaphoid) and capitate bones.

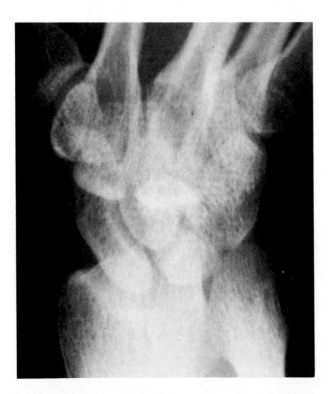

Fig. 110. This special view of the navicular or scaphoid bone is normal and is made such that there is elongation of that bone. The view is made with the hand palm down (pronated) and with the thumb at a right angle or nearly at a right angle with the hand. The x-ray tube is angled 35° toward the elbow and is pivoted so that the central ray is directed along the first metacarpal and the navicular bone. The value of the view is that it often accentuates a fracture line.

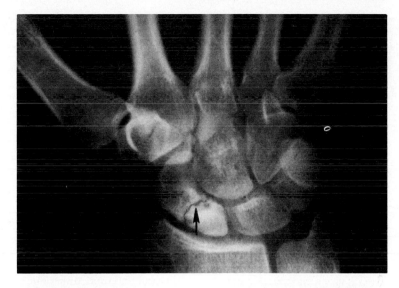

Fig. 111. The fracture line (arrow) across the waist of the carpal navicular is the most common type of fracture in that carpal bone. The increased density of the proximal fragment in this particular example suggests the presence of aseptic necrosis.

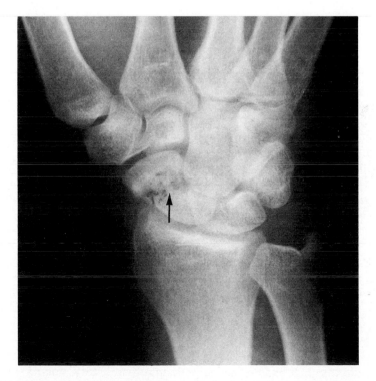

Fig. 112. Old fractures in the waist of the navicular bone show cystic changes, as in this patient, or show sclerosis at the margins of the fracture line in addition to cystic areas. The fracture line in this patient occurred several months prior to the date of this examination. No late sign of aseptic necrosis is present in the proximal fragment.

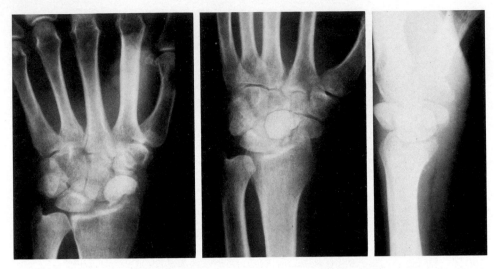

Fig. 113. Occasionally a fracture fragment is so displaced and rotated that it mimics the increased density of aseptic necrosis. In this patient the proximal portion of the fractured navicular bone has been displaced posteriorly. A carpal dislocation is also present.

Hand

Extensor tendon avulsion injuries are not uncommon in the so-called contact sports and sports in which a hard object or ball can strike the fingers directly.[10] The terms "mallet finger,"[22] "baseball finger," or "dropped phalanx"[8] have been applied to this injury. The distal phalanx is held in a flexed position (hence the term "dropped phalanx") and cannot be actively extended at the distal interphalangeal joint. Radiographs will show the abnormal attitude of the distal phalanx and may show a minute fragment of bone at the dorsal aspect of the distal interphalangeal joint (Figs. 114, 115).

The first metacarpal–carpal and first metacarpal–phalangeal joints are common dislocation points within the hand, as are the interphalangeal joints. One usually has no difficulty detecting the dislocation in the finger or thumb but may find the metacarpal subluxations a diagnostic challenge. Again, comparison views of the uninjured hand are most important in easing the examiner's dilemma.

Aneurysms of the palm occur in activities in which the hand is used as a hammer.[11,12,19] The two common sites for true aneurysms are at the hook of the hamate and at the thenar eminence, where branches of the ulnar and radial arteries are relatively exposed[17] (Fig. 116). Arteriography may be of value in showing that such an injury exists.[4,11,20]

Ulnar artery aneurysm and thrombosis have been reported in sports injury. A 16-year-old football player developed an ulnar artery aneurysm after the palm of his hand was jammed forcibly against an opponent's shoulder pads. Surgical removal of the aneurysm was successful. An ulnar artery injury led to

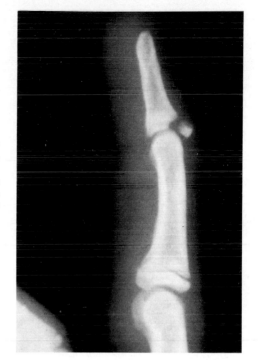

Fig. 114. A blow to the end of the finger can be of such force that the extensor tendon avulses from its insertion at the dorsum and base of the distal phalanx. This is the so-called mallet or baseball finger that features a dropped or partially flexed position of the distal phalanx.

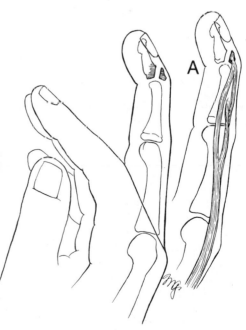

Fig. 115. The superimposed drawing (A) shows the site of insertion of the lateral bands of the extensor tendon on the avulsed fragment of the proximal phalanx.

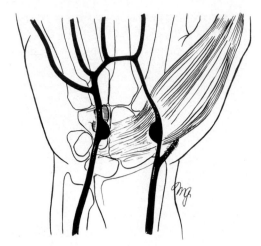

Fig. 116. The two most common sites of aneurysms in the palmar arch are shown. They occur at relatively unprotected sites over the hook of the hamate and at the base of the thenar eminence.

hypothenar tenderness, coolness, and paresthesia on exposure to cold in a 30-year-old bowler who had the habit of hitting the palm of his hand on his bowling ball while waiting for his turn to bowl.[19] Ulnar artery thrombosis was detected on physical examination. Rest alone led to relief of his symptoms. In addition to these cases karate and handball involve other potential causes of wrist and palmar arterial injury although actual examples have not been documented.

References

1. Adams JE: Injury to the throwing arm. A study of traumatic changes in the elbow joints of boy baseball players. Calif Med 102:127–137, 1965
2. Birch-Jensen A: Luxation of the distal radio-ulnar joint. Acta Chir Scand 101: 312–317, 1951
3. Brogdon BG, Crow NE: Little Leaguer's elbow. Am J Roentgenol 83:671–675, 1960
4. Calenoff L: Angiography of the hand: guidelines for interpretation. Radiology 102:331–335, 1972
5. Conwell HE, Reynolds FC: Key and Conwell's Management of Fractures, Dislocations and Sprains, 7th ed. St. Louis, Mosby, 1961, p 555
6. Curwen IHM: Golf. In Armstrong JR, Tucker WE (eds): Injury in Sport. London, Staples, 1964, pp 200–204
7. Cyriax JH: The pathology and treatment of tennis elbow. J Bone Joint Surg 18: 921–940, 1936
8. Editorial: Dropped finger. Lancet 2:958–959, 1968
9. Ellis JS: Smith's and Barton's fractures. J Bone Joint Surg 47B:724–727, 1965
10. Flatt AE: Athletic injuries of the hand. J La State Med Soc 119:425–431, 1967
11. Gaylis H, Kushlick AR: Ulnar artery aneurysms of the hand. Surgery 73:478–480, 1973
12. Green DP: True and false traumatic aneurysms in the hand. J Bone Joint Surg 55A:120–128, 1973
13. Head RW: Anterior dislocation of the distal ulna without accompanying fracture of the ulnar styloid. Br J Radiol 44:468–471, 1971

14. Heiple KA, Freehafer AA, Vant Hof A: Isolated traumatic dislocation of the distal end of the ulna or distal radio-ulnar joint. J Bone Joint Surg 44A:1387–1394, 1962

15. Hinkel CL: Fractures of the distal radius and ulna and dislocation of the proximal carpals. Radiology 69:809–814, 1957

16. Keats TR, Teesluik AD, Williams JH: Normal axial relationships of the major joints. Radiology 87:904–907, 1966

17. Kleinert HE, Burget GC, Morgan JA, Kutz JE, Atasoy E: Aneurysms of the hand. Arch Surg 105:554–557, 1973

18. Mazet R Jr, Hohl M: Carpal navicular fracture. J Bone Joint Surg 45A:82–112, 1963

19. Millender LH, Nalebuff EA, Kasdon E: Aneurysms and thromboses of the ulnar artery in the hand. Arch Surg 105:686–690, 1972

20. O'Connor RL: Digital nerve compression secondary to palmar aneurysm. Clin Orthop 83:149–150, 1972

21. Schultz RJ: The language of fractures. Baltimore, Williams, 1972

22. Stark HH, Boyes JH, Wilson JN: Mallet finger. J Bone Joint Surg 44A:1061–1068, 1962

23. Waris W: Elbow injuries of javelin throwers. Acta Chir Scand 93:563–575, 1946

24. Wiot JF, Dorst JP: Less common fractures and dislocations of the wrist. Radiol Clin North Am 4:261–278, 1966

25. Woodyard JE: A review of Smith's fractures. J Bone Joint Surg 51B:324–329, 1969

THORAX AND ABDOMEN

Thorax

Clavicle and rib fractures are common in sports injuries to the chest. Sternal fractures, sternoclavicular and shoulder dislocations, diaphragm rupture, pulmonary or cardiac contusion, pneumothorax, mediastinal emphysema, and bronchus or tracheal rupture can occur as well.

X-rays of the ribs and chest are the usual radiographic sample after thoracic trauma. As before, we must first ask ourselves are the radiographs adequate? Properly exposed and positioned views are a must (Fig. 117). The chest x-ray ideally consists of a posteroanterior view and a lateral view. On the posteroanterior and lateral views, the examiner should inspect the chest for rotation, adequate inspiration, and clarity of detail. Rotation is assessed on the posteroanterior view by noting the overlap of posterior and anterior midline structures such as the thoracic spinous processes and the clavicular sternal joints (Fig. 118). Inspiration is assessed by counting the number of posterior or anterior ribs above the hemidiaphragm. Clarity of detail can be obscured by respiratory motion during the exposure of the film and is assessed by inspecting the normal vascular markings in each lung.

Has the radiograph been exposed in an anteroposterior method rather than in the conventional posteroanterior one? The anterior intrathoracic structures such as the heart and ascending aorta may thereby be magnified. Do not confuse such a situation with cardiac or aortic enlargement.

When examining the ribs for a fracture remember to view the entire rib. Occasionally fractures occur at the posterior rib margins near the spine or at the anterior ribs near their cartilaginous articulations with the sternum (Fig. 119). Raney has emphasized that posterior rib injury may include subluxation in addition to the more common hematoma or fracture.[18] The costotransverse ligaments may be ruptured by forceful blows leading to superior subluxation of the third through tenth ribs. He has seen this injury in a skier who fell against a log and in a basketball player who was kneed in the back. Anterior or superior displacement of the eleventh and twelfth ribs are even more likely after blunt trauma. Raney has seen this following a diving-board injury. If nonoperative methods of treatment are unsuccessful he suggests that operative excision of the costotransverse joint and decompression of the intercostal nerve may relieve pain.

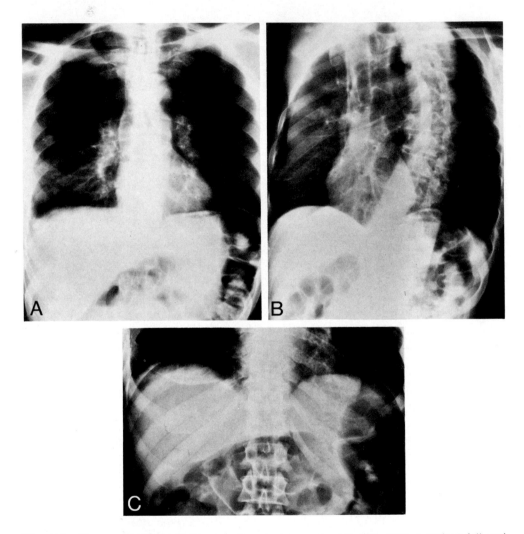

Fig. 117. The search for a rib fracture is not always an easy one. Here a patient fell and injured the right lower hemithorax. **A, B.** Rib films may not be helpful in showing fractures of the ribs if the views include the entire chest. The sudden change in radiographic density of the lung area and upper abdomen makes an even x-ray technique impossible. **C.** A focal view was made of the limited lower thoracic area in the same patient, showing fractures of the posterior parts of the right ninth, tenth, and eleventh ribs. These fractures were not shown on the views of the entire chest.

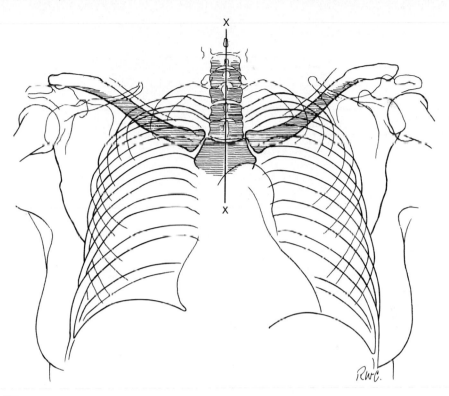

Fig. 118. A well-centered chest x-ray is a must. The midline of the posterior spinous processes of the lower cervical and upper thoracic spine (×—×) should project through the middle of the manubrium and between the two clavicles. This centering sets the stage for the evaluation of the chest and helps particularly in the study of the mediastinum, heart, and subdiaphragmatic areas.

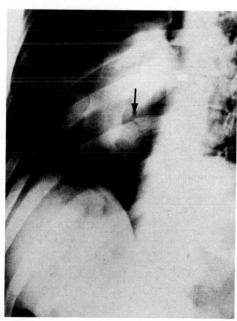

Fig. 119. A crushing tackle injured the chest of a quarterback. The arrow indicates the site of a posterior rib fracture in the left side of the chest. The figure has been reversed so that the patient's ribs are viewed from behind.

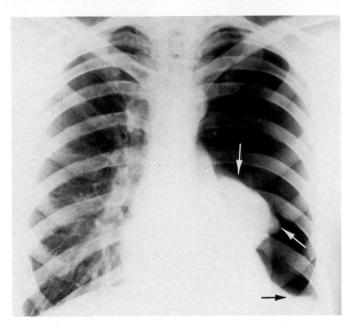

Fig. 120. The day after the injury shown in Figure 119 a chest x-ray was made because the quarterback had increasing shortness of breath. A total collapse of the left lung is present (white arrows) with pneumothorax and hemothorax. The straight line in the left costophrenic angle indicates the presence of air and fluid. The fluid in this hemithorax proved to be blood. (From Bowerman, McDonnell: Radiology 117:36, 1975)

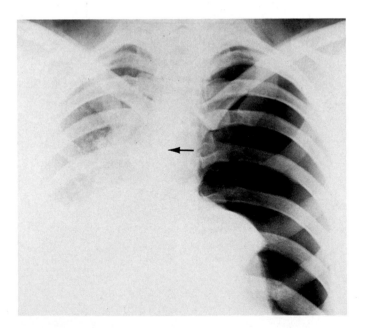

Fig. 121. Several hours after Figure 120 was made, the pneumothorax had increased, the mediastinum had shifted to the right, and the dyspnea had increased. A chest tube was subsequently placed in the left hemithorax, relieving the tension for all concerned. (From Bowerman, McDonnell: Radiology 117:33–36, 1975)

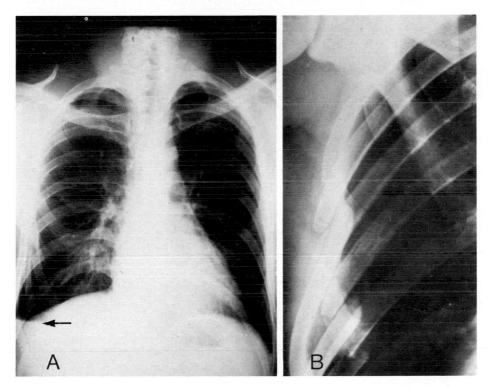

Fig. 122. An energetic guard in a game played in the National Basketball Association collided with an opposing center. The center's knee was thrust forward into the right side of the guard's chest. The guard had immediate severe chest and pleural pain. **A.** The posteroanterior chest view shows an air–fluid level (arrow) in the right costophrenic angle indicating a hemothorax and pneumothorax. **B.** The enlarged oblique view of the ribs shows four rib fractures with displacement of the fracture fragments. After a prolonged period of recovery the guard was able to resume play.

The associated pneumothorax should be anticipated (Figs. 120–122). Look for this as an arc of lucency at the margins of the lung. Air usually rises to the apex if the pleural space is free of adhesions. Occasionally the air will be confined by adhesions to the lateral inferior costophrenic region. Once a pneumothorax is detected we must further anticipate a possible shift of the mediastinum to the side opposite the leakage of air. A pneumothorax of major proportion with a mediastinal shift is a tension pneumothorax. Both lungs may then become compromised in a life-threatening situation. The judicious placement of a chest tube or catheter will prevent an uncomplicated pneumothorax from progressing to this state (Fig. 121).

Fractures of the lower ribs may be associated with rupture of the diaphragm, liver, or spleen. Clues to splenic injury on the chest x-ray include a medial displacement of the gastric air bubble by a splenic hematoma. An irregular contour of the hemidiaphragm usually occurs when the diaphragm is ruptured. Rupture of the diaphragm is usually visible on the chest x-ray but

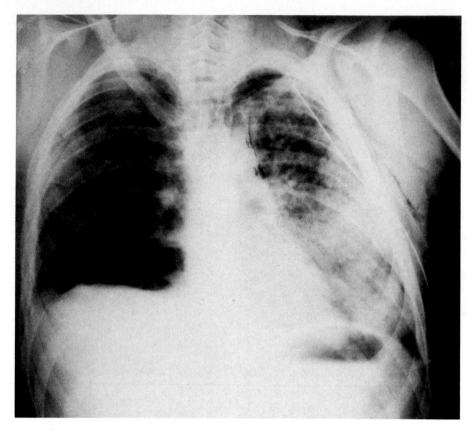

Fig. 123. A patient injured in a high-speed automobile crash sustained severe chest and abdominal injuries. The original chest x-ray showed pneumomediastinum, pulmonary contusions, bilateral pneumothorax, left clavicle fracture, and interstitial emphysema of the chest wall. A chest tube has been placed in the left pleural space.

often is not detected initially. In a study of diaphragm rupture by Wise et al the most common abnormalities shown on x-ray included hemothorax, herniation of a hollow viscus through the ruptured diaphragm, and an abnormal contour at the area of the hemidiaphragm.[22] In this report the left side of the diaphragm was injured in 22 to 25 cases of blunt injury. The liver is thought to act as a protective splint in sparing the right side of the diaphragm in most individuals with blunt abdominal and thoracic trauma. In a series of blunt injuries to the hemidiaphragm reported by Ebert et al 22 of 24 occurred at the left side.[5]

The tracheal shadow in the normal unrotated chest is in the midline or lies slightly to the right of midline. Hemorrhage in the mediastinum or in the lower neck can displace the trachea. Air leakage along the mediastinal tissue planes may be the only sign of tracheal or bronchial rupture. To anticipate this look for vertically oriented linear streaks of radiolucency along the mediastinal shadows (Figs. 123, 124).

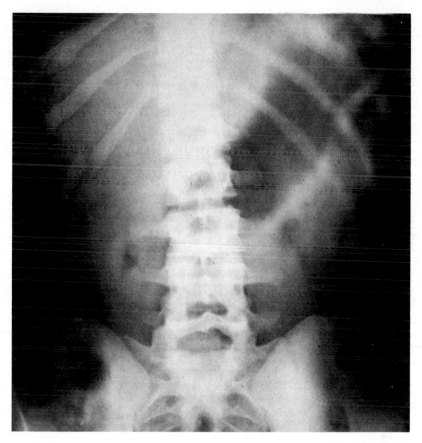

Fig. 124. The abdominal film on the same patient as shown in Figure 123 shows fractures of the posterior aspects of the lower right ribs involving the ninth through the twelfth ribs. The right psoas shadow is partially absent and a retroperitoneal hemorrhage is present.

Compression fractures of the thoracic spine usually present no diagnostic difficulty. In the adolescent, however, vertebral endplate irregularities occur normally and are often puzzling when evaluating the thoracic spine of an active young person. Alexander contends that vertebral disc margin irregularities often attributed to infection or to an unknown cause are due to trauma.[1] He points out that the sites of maximum stress to the thoracolumbar endplates in flexion correspond to the sites of so-called juvenile discitis. The effects of repeated compression forces in certain sports such as tumbling, diving, horseback riding, trampolining, and football warrant further study.

Occasionally sudden death occurs in an athlete. The cause of death may not be easy to determine despite autopsy findings. Extensive postmortem studies of the heart were done by James et al in two young soldiers, ages 19 and 25, who died suddenly and unexpectedly.[9] Both men proved to have fibrosis within the cardiac conduction system and a narrowed main coronary artery or branching artery. In addition, one of these young men had extensive myocarditis. He had been hospitalized for episodes of easy fatiguability, exertional dyspnea, and chest pain that he attributed to a series of injuries to the head, chest, and abdomen during football one year previously. Trauma is a possible explanation for his myocarditis but remains only one of several theoretical considerations.

Traumatic rupture of the aorta with aneurysm formation or fracture of the aorta from the shearing forces of blunt injury is another potential cause of fatality. This injury usually occurs in a setting involving motor vehicles.[17] This setting of high-velocity impact provides the necessary forces for the shearing injury. The aorta usually ruptures at the aortic isthmus, ie, at the descending arch of the thoracic aorta distal to the branching of the left subclavian artery. One theory holds that this isthmus is a relatively fixed point in the descending arch because the ligamentum arteriosum acts as a tether.

A less common point of rupture and a second site of relative fixation is the aortic root or supravalvular portion of the aorta. Rupture here can lead to aneurysm, cardiac tamponade, and rapid death. Lundevall's measurements of the tensile strength of the aorta indicate that the weakest portion of the aortic wall is the isthmus, followed by the supravalvular portion.[12] The diagnosis of post-traumatic aneurysm of the descending arch can be difficult. Those who keep their eyes on the mediastinal shadows, including the aortic outline on chest radiographs, after blunt trauma to the chest are the first to suspect the injury. Widening of the aortic shadow is a characteristic finding, particularly at the descending arch (Fig. 125). Harsh systolic murmurs may be present either in the interscapular space to the left of the spine or at the anterior left second intercostal space.[7] The murmurs are usually explained by turbulence. Aortography is of diagnostic use in showing the aneurysm and its extent[11] (Figs. 126, 127). Since 25 to 35 percent of patients with aortic rupture die during the first 24 hours post injury,[7,17] we must suspect the injury, arrange for aortography if our suspicions are high, and be willing to accept some negative arteriographic examinations all in a short period of time. Replacement grafts of woven dacron have been successfully employed at the time of surgical removal of the injured segment of aorta.

Abdomen

In Gonzales' report of sports deaths in New York City, several examples of blunt trauma to the abdomen were recorded.[8] Both hollow and solid viscera can be ruptured. McCort's[14] and Zatzkin's[25] texts deal extensively with radiographic findings in abdominal injury.

The most common serious intra-abdominal injury following blunt trauma to the abdomen is rupture of the spleen. Splenic injury often includes subcapsular hematoma, retroperitoneal hemorrhage, or intrasplenic hematoma. Plain film diagnosis can be difficult, and isotopic, ultrasonic, or angiographic diagnostic studies are usually required. Left upper quadrant tenderness may be the only physical finding in some cases. If the diagnosis is made early and surgery per-

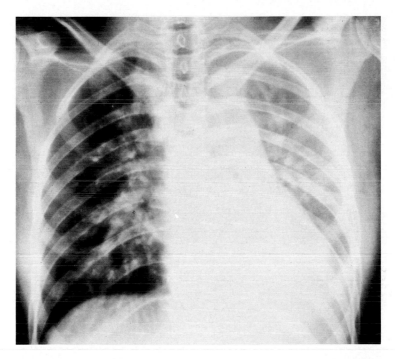

Fig. 125. The mediastinal widening and the haziness of the left lung field due to a left pleural effusion in this patient are clues to an underlying aortic or esophageal rupture. The patient fell from a motorcycle and suffered shearing forces of the chest. Her subsequent vascular studies are shown in Figures 126 and 127.

formed without delay, the mortality of treated patients is in the range of 1 to 2 percent.[16] Untreated cases have a mortality approaching 80 to 100 percent.[16] The former practice of prolonged observation of patients with blunt trauma has been replaced by an aggressive approach combining the techniques of observation, peritoneal lavage, isotope scanning, and arteriography.[16] All of these modalities are useful for the evaluation of injury to the liver as well as the spleen.

The psoas muscle margin may be obscured in retroperitoneal hemorrhage (Fig. 124). Bowel gas displacements and soft tissue masses may be seen on plain radiographs of the abdomen. Hepatic and renal ruptures have the same potential to produce abnormal x-ray findings and, like splenic injury, show variation in the extent and the presence of diagnostic signs.

If blunt injury occurs to a child's abdomen the cause is usually a fall in play or in sports activities rather than an automobile accident. Tank et al reported that sledding produced 13 injuries and bicycling 10 in a study of 74 patients up to 14 years old.[19] In these 74 patients, 82 organs were injured, with the spleen (30 cases) and the kidney (18 cases) leading the list. Trauma brought to light coexistent renal tumors in three children who had operation following injury.

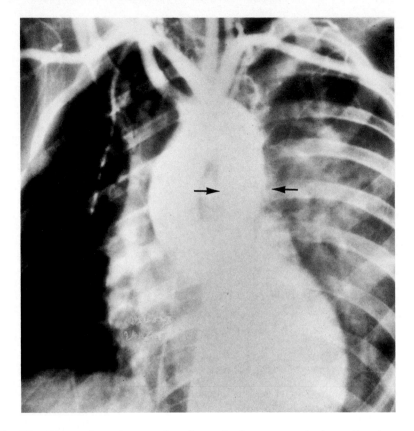

Fig. 126. The retrograde aortogram via a femoral artery approach shows the abnormal focal widening of the aorta in this patient. The widened area is only slightly widened in a fusiform fashion (arrows). (See also Figures 125 and 127.)

Blunt trauma to the liver usually damages the right hepatic lobe.[13] Disruption of the intrahepatic branches of the hepatic artery has been shown radiographically in experiments with blunt trauma to cadavers in which barium had been injected intravenously within the liver prior to the injury. Lobar arterial and venous ligations may be necessary to control hemorrhage. Sepsis is the second most common cause of death in hepatic trauma after hemorrhage. Drainage of perihepatic spaces is usually required. Mays suggests that an especially effective means of draining the perihepatic space on the right is removal of the twelfth rib.[13] This creates a posterior defect for dependent drainage through that costal bed.

Hemorrhage into biliary paths is called hemobilia. This condition generally causes hematemesis or melena, but occasionally produces occult bleeding. The source of bleeding may be in the liver, bile ducts, gallbladder, or pancreas. Blunt trauma is the most common cause of hemobilia.[3] Bismuth estimated that approximately 2 percent of liver injuries are complicated by hemobilia.[3] Ar-

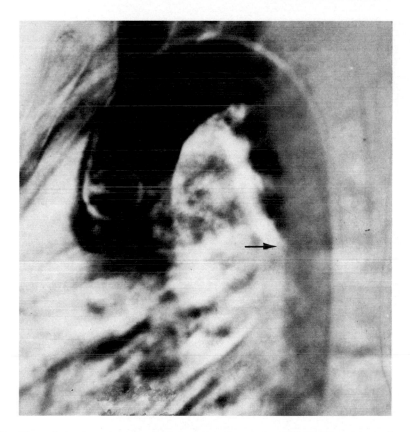

Fig. 127. The subtraction view shows the abrupt change in caliber of the descending portion of the aortic arch (arrow). This indicates an aneurysm at the distal arch centered at the site of maximal fixation of the arch by the ligamentum arteriosum. Shearing forces of impact at the time of the fall produced this traumatic aneurysm. (See also Figures 125 and 126.)

teriography is useful in showing arterial injury and false aneurysm and in indicating the site of the major vascular damage.[3]

How useful is the presence or absence of the psoas muscle shadow on abdominal x-rays after injury to the abdomen? One would expect normal patients to show both shadows and expect obliteration of the psoas margin in patients with massive retroperitoneal bleeding. In addition, intraperitoneal hemorrhage or ascites can obliterate the psoas shadow by creating an overlying haze. Elkin and Cohen studied scout films of the abdomen in 200 normal people.[6] The right psoas shadow was clearly visualized in 138 patients (69 percent) and the left was clearly seen in 159 (75 percent). In addition, the right and left shadows were present but visualized with difficulty in 44 (22 percent) and 30 (15 percent) patients, respectively. Absent psoas shadows occurred normally in 18 patients (9 percent) on the right side and in 11 patients (6 percent) on the left. In another group of patients with rupture of the spleen the psoas margins were

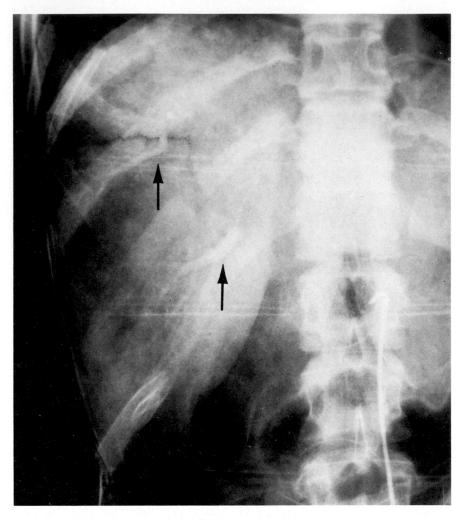

Fig. 128. Blunt trauma to the right upper quadrant produced a lacerated liver. This preoperative celiac arteriogram shows (in the capillary phase) the laceration extending horizontally across the lateral margin of the right lobe of the liver. Two post-traumatic arteriovenous fistulae are shown as well (arrow). (See also Figures 129 and 130.)

absent once. This occurred bilaterally because of 3500 cc of bloody fluid in the peritoneal cavity found at laparotomy. Wyman found loss of the left psoas shadow in 2 of 15 patients with rupture of the spleen.[24] However, the left kidney was also ruptured in one of these two patients. Wang and Robbins reported obliteration of the left psoas margin in 14 of 43 patients with a ruptured spleen.[21] Thus obliteration of the margin of the psoas muscle can occur in approximately 5 to 10 percent of normal patients, and the margin is normal in most patients with a ruptured spleen.

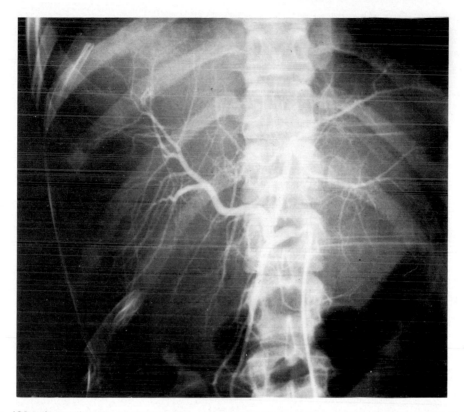

Fig. 129. An earlier phase of the celiac arteriogram showed normal major arteries in the liver (see Fig. 128). The major arteries are not displaced or lacerated. The tip of the catheter is at the level of L1.

Two examples of blunt abdominal trauma in athletes are described in a report on splenic trauma by Owens et al.[16] In one instance, a 22-year-old skier on the University of Utah team fell on a mogul while skiing and injured his left chest and upper abdomen. His chest x-ray and rib films were normal. Left upper quadrant tenderness persisted in the presence of a fall of the hematocrit from 52 to 42 percent over a period of several hours. A lavage catheter was introduced into the peritoneal cavity and returned blood. At laparotomy a 2-cm laceration was found in the upper pole of the spleen. In the second example a 38-year-old woman skier fell while skiing and had persistent left upper quadrant pain. She was admitted to a hospital and underwent splenic arteriography. No abnormality was noted and the patient was able to leave the hospital after an overnight stay. This particular hospital lacked the capability of isotope scanning but was equipped for arteriography leading to a short hospitalization time and no surgery for the patient.

Liver–spleen scans are usually performed prior to the arteriography when possible. Technetium 99m is the usual radionuclide used in a sulfur colloid ve-

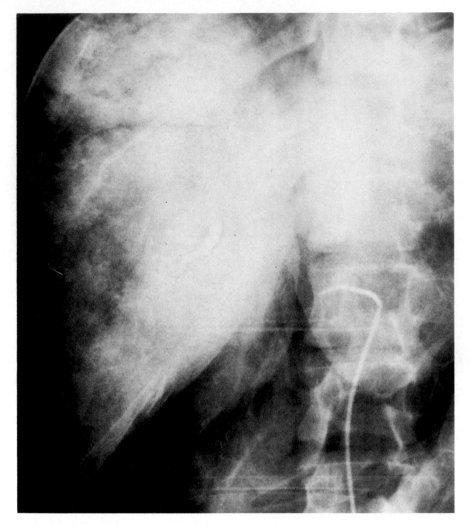

Fig. 130. A later hepatic capillary phase of the preoperative celiac arteriogram shows more clearly the 5 cm laceration in the right lobe of the liver (see Figs. 128, 129). The two post-traumatic arteriovenous fistulae are barely discernible.

hicle. The labeled colloid is injected intravenously and is phagocytized by reticuloendothelial cells in the liver and spleen. Multiple views of both organs are obtained by a gamma camera or a rectilinear scanner. Typical scans following trauma usually show an abnormal margin or a filling defect. The spleen may be displaced or, rarely, fail to visualize. The abnormal results at arteriography following trauma include leakage, transection, and displacement of vessels as well as arteriovenous shunting and organ enlargment (Figs. 128–130). The mucosal blush of vessels in the wall of a distended stomach may be mistaken for extravasation of splenic vessels in arteriography done to evaluate the possibility

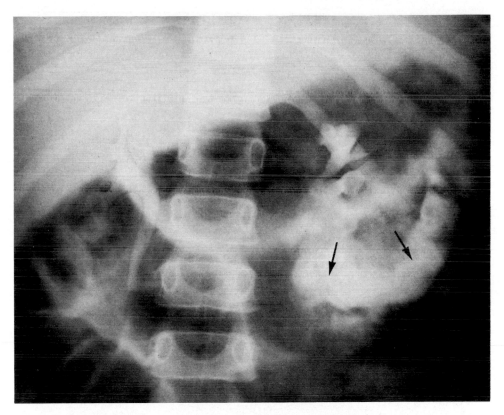

Fig. 131. Blunt trauma followed by hematuria led to an intravenous pyelogram in a child. Contrast material (arrows) extravasates from the lower pole of the ruptured kidney. The calyces of the left upper pole are dilated. The arteriographic findings are shown in Figure 132.

of splenic injury. Tuttle suggests that gastric suction be performed prior to arteriography to avoid this pitfall.[20]

Blunt trauma in sport may produce serious injury to the pancreas. Wohl wend and Hirata remind us that this organ enjoys a protected retroperitoneal position,[23] citing the fact that only 1 to 2 percent of all abdominal injuries involve the pancreas.[10] They describe an example of traumatic pancreatitis with rupture of the tail of the pancreas in a football player[23]:

> This 19-year-old reserve linebacker was running full speed away from the line of scrimmage in direct pursuit of a pass receiver, following completion of a short pass "under" the left corner back. With full attention devoted toward maintaining both angle and over-taking speed, he remained totally unaware of an opponent-blocker approaching obliquely at full speed from the blind side to his left. Said blocker, with perfect angle and execution, forcefully impacted a right shoulder deep into his left epigastrium, accomplishing total deceleration within the space of two yards.

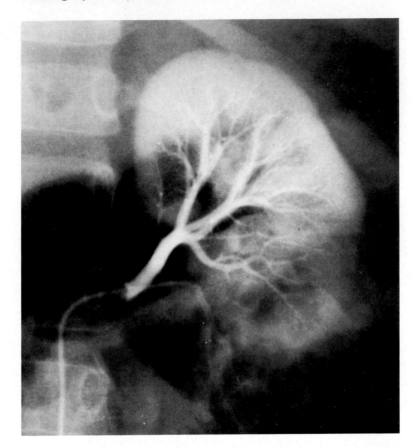

Fig. 132. A selective left renal arteriogram of the patient shown in Figure 131 shows lack of arterial filling in the lower pole. A prior aortogram showed a single artery to this left kidney so that the changes are not a function of a dual blood supply that is otherwise a common normal variant.

Pain and tenderness persisted following the injury and led to the patient's aforementioned operative findings. The young man had a complicated post-operative course and developed a pancreatic fistula expected to require further surgery. In another report a pseudocyst of the pancreas developed after blunt trauma to the upper abdomen of a 29-year-old woman injured in an accident at a go-kart track.[2] Postoperatively a gastric and pancreatic fistula occurred with subsequent hemorrhage and multiple emergency operations that finally led to the patient's recovery.

How common is renal injury after blunt trauma in a contact sport? Boone et al addressed this issue in a report on hematuria in the members of a college football team.[4] Urines were collected on the opening day of training, each Wednesday after practice, and following Saturday's game throughout the season. A total of 874 urine specimens were evaluated in 58 players. Attrition due to prolonged illness and other factors reduced the number of players to 37 regular subjects. Albuminuria, casts, and microscopic hematuria were noted after

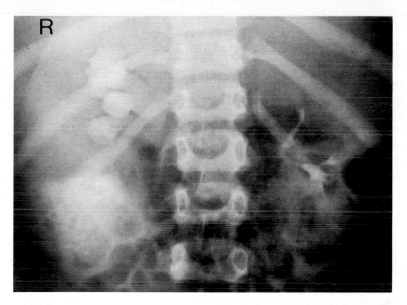

Fig. 133. In a patient with trauma to the right flank there is extravasation of contrast material at the right lower pole. The right calyces and renal pelvis are dilated and displaced partially by a hematoma. The arteriographic findings are shown in Figure 134.

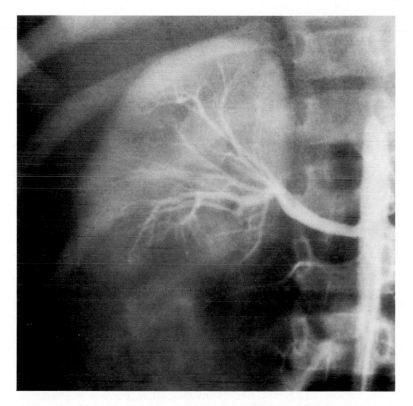

Fig. 134. The right renal arteriogram of the patient shown in Figure 133 shows transection of the right lower pole of the kidney. The vessels in the midportion of the kidney are draped over the hematoma.

early training conditioning exercises and increased after body contact work. Hematuria was found in every player studied and reached a peak after each Saturday's game. Microscopic hematuria occurred as often as 19 times in 24 specimens in one player. Gross hematuria was recorded in six men who continued to play regularly. Their urines returned to "football normal" within three to four days. No blood pressure recordings or further renal evaluations were mentioned in this enlightening report.

Mitchell suggests that the most common cause of renal injury in England is an accident in sport and that rugby football produces the majority of such injuries in boys.[15] Intravenous pyelography should be performed at the earliest opportunity followed by arteriography if an injured kidney is functionless on the pyelogram. Mitchell has found that 40 percent of pyelograms done for renal trauma show no abnormality at all.[15] Intravenous pyelography will show displacement of the kidney and ureter and gross intrarenal abnormalities when they are present (Figs. 131–134).

References

1. Alexander CJ: The aetiology of juvenile spondylarthritis (discitis). Clin Radiol 21: 178–187, 1970
2. Baker R: Pseudocyst of the pancreas due to trauma: spontaneous intraperitoneal rupture. Proc R Soc Med 67:115–116, 1974
3. Bismuth H: Hemobilia. N Engl J Med 288:617–619, 1973
4. Boone AW, Haltiwanger E, Chambers RL: Football hematuria. JAMA 158: 1516–1517, 1955
5. Ebert PA, Gaertner RA, Zuidema GA: Traumatic diaphragmatic hernia. Surg Gynecol Obstet 125:59–65, 1967
6. Elkin M, Cohen G: Diagnostic value of the psoas shadow. Clin Radiol 13:210–217, 1962
7. Freed TA, Neal MP Jr, Vinik M: Roentgenographic findings in extracardiac injury secondary to blunt chest automobile trauma. Am J Roentgenol 104:424–431, 1968
8. Gonzales TA: Fatal injuries in competitive sports. JAMA 146:1506–1511, 1951
9. James TN, Armstrong RS, Silverman J, Marshall TK: De subitaneis mortibus VI. Two young soldiers. Circulation 49:1239–1246, 1974
10. Jones RC, Shires GT: Pancreatic trauma. Arch Surg 102:424–430, 1971
11. Lipchik EO, Robinson KE: Acute traumatic rupture of the thoracic aorta. Am J Roentgenol 104:408–412, 1968
12. Lundevall J: The mechanism of traumatic rupture of the aorta. Acta Pathol Microbiol Scand 62:34–46, 1964
13. Mays ET: Hepatic trauma. N Engl J Med 288:402–405, 1973
14. McCort JJ: Radiographic Examination in Blunt Abdominal Trauma. Philadelphia, Saunders, 1966
15. Mitchell JP: Trauma to the urinary tract. N Engl J Med 288:90–92, 1973
16. Owens ML, Brantigan J, Chang F: Splenic trauma. Rocky Mt Med J 72:114–117, 1975
17. Parmley LF, Mattingly TW, Manion WC, Jahnke EJ: Nonpenetrating traumatic injury of the aorta. Circulation 57:1086–1101, 1958
18. Raney FL, cited in: Editorial: Care urged in treating injury to rib cage in young athlete. Hosp Trib, p 22, April 22, 1968
19. Tank ES, Eraklis AJ, Gross RE: Blunt abdominal trauma in infancy and childhood. J Trauma 8:439–448, 1968

20. Tuttle RJ: Splenic trauma—a pitfall in diagnosis. J Can Assoc Radiol 22:160–162, 1971
21. Wang CC, Robbins LL: Roentgenologic diagnosis of ruptured spleen. N Engl J Med 254:445–449, 1956
22. Wise L, Connors J, Hwang YLH, Anderson C: Traumatic injuries to the diaphragm. J Trauma 13:946–950, 1973
23. Wohlwend D, Hirata I Jr: Pancreatic injury in intercollegiate football. J Am Coll Health Assoc 23:223–224, 1975
24. Wyman AC: Traumatic rupture of the spleen. Am J Roentgenol 72:51–63, 1954
25. Zatzkin HR: The Roentgen Diagnosis of Trauma. Chicago, Year Book, 1965

LUMBAR SPINE, PELVIS, AND HIPS

Lumbar Spine

Radiographs of the spine, as elsewhere in the body, must be tailored to the injury situation and to the anatomy being examined. The anatomy in the lower lumbar spine changes drastically compared to the upper lumbar spine with respect to vertebral body, appendage, and disc space alignment at hand. Furthermore, the x-ray tube, if angled so that it looks directly at the disc space or vertebral appendage in question, will yield the best display of the anatomy. Views of the lumbar spine in the weight-bearing positions of neutral, flexion, and extension can be obtained with the patient standing or sitting and give a better idea of disc and bone relationships than do radiographs taken in the supine or prone positions. As mentioned in the discussion of the cervical spine, interpretation is most complete when each view is analyzed in its component parts: the vertebral bodies, vertebral appendages, intervertebral discs, paraspinal soft tissues, sacrum, pelvis, and sacroiliac joints (Fig. 135).

Spondylolysis is an acquired defect in the pars interarticularis of the lumbar spine (Fig. 136). Because of the high incidence of trauma and strenuous activity in patients with spondylolysis the defect very likely represents a post-traumatic one[1,13] (Figs. 137, 138). Freiberger[6] and Murray[10] have observed patients with documented acquired pars defects and examples of defects that were followed by healing. Newman classified spondylolysis and spondylolisthesis and allowed for etiologic congenital factors in addition to trauma.[12] Beeler has recently discussed the evidence for trauma as a cause in this condition.[1] Football and gymnastics played a prominent part in the activities of 12 patients with pars defects reported by Wiltse et al.[13] Nearly all the defects in this group healed with corset, brace, or body cast treatment.

Spondylolisthesis is an anterior or posterior slip of one vertebral body on another (Fig. 139). This malalignment can follow traumatic pars defects as well as facet joint degenerative disease.[5] The unstable spine is often associated with disc degeneration at the level of the spondylolisthesis (Fig. 140). The lower lumbar spine is the most common site of spondylolysis and spondylolisthesis. Most commonly, the fifth lumbar vertebral body is displaced anteriorly on the body of the first sacral segment.[5]

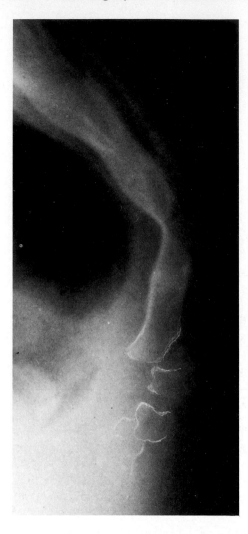

Fig. 135. A young woman fell on her bottom while ice skating. She had severe pain at the sacrum. This lateral view shows a transverse fracture in the sacrum. The fracture fragments are partially displaced.

In several professional football players in the United States, fractures of multiple lumbar transverse processes have been observed.[2] Transient hematuria occurred in one of these players. For further information, see the section on injuries in American football in Part II.

Pelvis and Hips

Avulsion sites of injury at the pelvic margins have been discussed in the chapter dealing with soft tissues. Instability of the symphysis pubis and the sacroiliac joint is a hazard of the scissoring kicking actions of professional soccer players.[8] Radiographs of the symphysis pubis in the athlete with pain at that site should be obtained in the weight-bearing position as the player first stands on one foot and then the other (see the section on soccer in Part II).

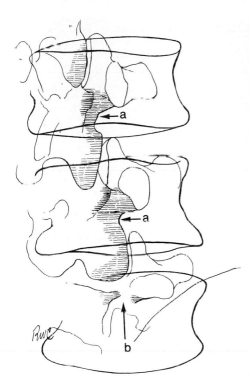

Fig. 136. The oblique view of the lumbar spine is useful for showing the pars interarticularis (a). This is the site of a fracture defect (b) in L5 in this drawing.

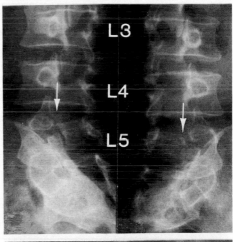

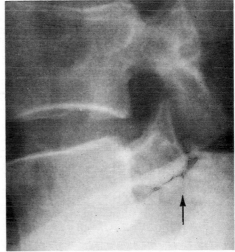

Fig. 137. The fracture defects (arrows) of the pars interarticularis areas of L5 in this patient are easy to see on these oblique views. In some patients it may be necessary to obtain cephalad-angled oblique views or tomograms to show spondylolysis. The pars defects may be prominent enough so that they appear on a lateral view of the lower lumbar spine (lower enlargment). Usually, however, an oblique view is needed to show the pars defects.

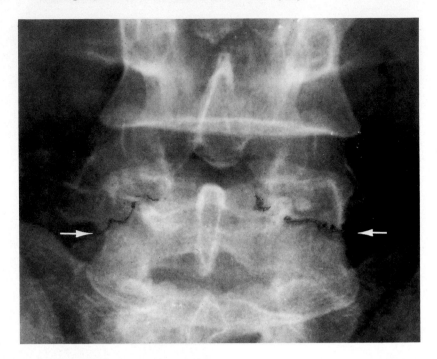

Fig. 138. Occasionally bilateral spondylolysis is visible, although faintly, on an anteroposterior view of the spine.

Murray has studied adults in England with degenerative disease of the hip and has found many outstanding former athletes with a configuration of the femoral head and neck that suggests a prior slipped capital femoral epiphysis[9] (Fig. 141). Extending these observations to school boys, Murray and Duncan found a higher incidence of slipped capital femoral epiphysis in boys who were active in sports than in a group of age-matched students who participated infrequently in sports.[11] These observations point the way to the recognition of a form of degenerative hip disease in certain individuals that is secondary to a rearranged femoral–acetabular articulation (Figs. 142–145).

In evaluating hip fracture and pelvic fracture the possibility of postischemic changes in the femoral head must be realized. When ischemic necrosis involves the femoral head the superior and anterolateral weight-bearing portion of the head is the site of the irregularity, subchondral collapse, and subsequent sclerosis (Fig. 146). The so-called abduction or frog leg view, the lateral hip view, and the anteroposterior view of the partially flexed hips are best for showing the profile of the necrotic head (Fig. 146). Hip dislocation without fracture can lead to aseptic necrosis.[7] Furthermore, avascular necrosis can occur as a delayed complication of hip injury several months after the initial injury.[3] Therefore, in viewing radiographs of the hip, the examiner should inspect the femoral head on early and follow-up radiographs after hip or pelvic injury. It is a mistake to assume that a radiodense femoral head is a necrotic

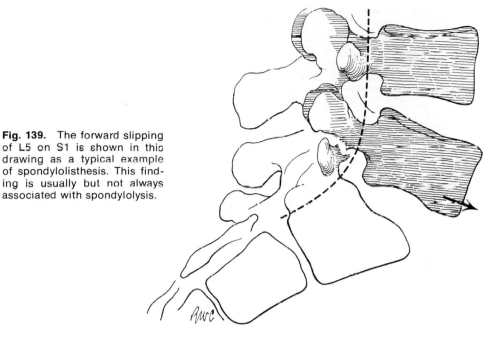

Fig. 139. The forward slipping of L5 on S1 is shown in this drawing as a typical example of spondylolisthesis. This finding is usually but not always associated with spondylolysis.

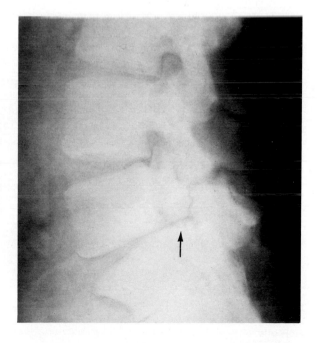

Fig. 140. Lower back pain prompted these x-rays in a 30-year-old athlete. There is bilateral spondylolysis of L5 (arrow), spondylolisthesis of L4–L5, disc space narrowing of L4–L5, and sclerosis at the lower lumbar facet joints. The patient has been an all-around athlete and was especially proficient at football.

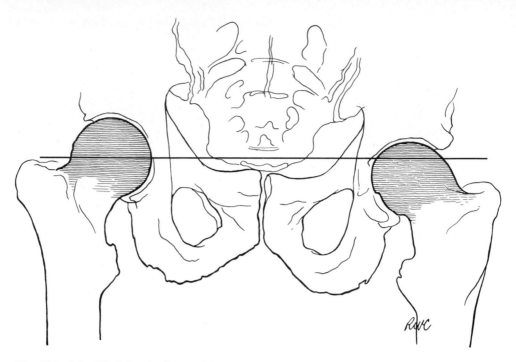

Fig. 141. The tilt deformity is a residual feature of a minimal slip of the capital femoral epiphysis. The right femoral head is seated in a normal position on the femoral neck. The left femoral head sits eccentrically on the neck in a tilted or drooping position. Note that the horizontal line runs through the center of the normal femoral head.

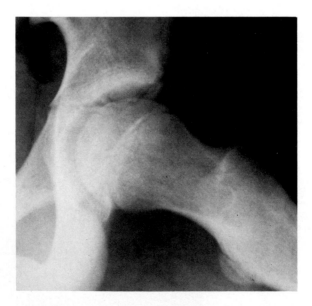

Fig. 142. The normal adolescent hip is shown in this view of a 14-year-old. The femoral capital epiphysis is seated evenly on the physis and neck of the femur. These normal relationships are important in evaluating the possibility of a slipped capital femoral epiphysis.

112

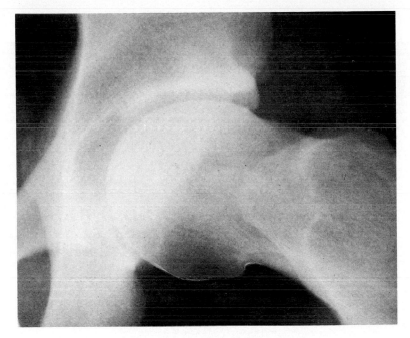

Fig. 143. An overweight 19-year-old football and basketball player complained of mild hip pain. His pelvic radiograph showed degenerative disease of the hips in the form of osteophytic flanges on the femoral heads. The slightly eccentric placement of the femoral head on the femoral neck indicates that a partial slip of the capital femoral epiphysis had occurred in the past.

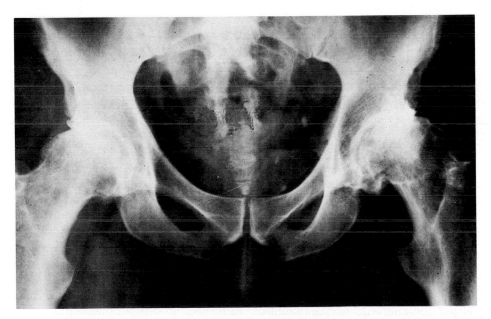

Fig. 144. This patient was an accomplished sprinter and distance runner as a young man. He now exhibits the minimal tilt deformity of the femoral heads described by Murray.[9] Murray recognized that certain patients with degenerative joint disease of the hip showed this tilt deformity and that nearly all of those with a tilt deformity were former athletes.

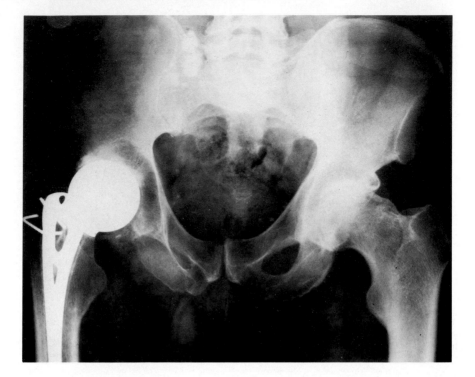

Fig. 145. This x-ray was obtained in an Englishman who had been a champion schoolboy runner. Degenerative joint disease led to a femoral replacement operation at the right hip. The left femoral head shows the tilt deformity described by Murray,[9] reflecting an old partial slip of the capital femoral epiphysis. Murray and Duncan have linked this deformity with the heavy athletic schedules of certain English school children.[11]

femoral head. Histologic evidence of bone necrosis precedes any alteration in the radiodensity of bone.[4] Hence bone ischemia exists in some patients—after injury or vessel compromise—in the presence of a normal radiograph. The reparative sclerosis of new bone laid down on necrotic trabeculae, the so-called creeping substitution, accounts for most of the density seen in radiographs following ischemia to a bony part. Other contributing factors include an osteoporosis to the nonischemic zone that can accentuate the radiodense zone as well as occasional microfractures or foci of trabecular collapse that attenuate the x-ray beam. A radiodense zone of bone can be thought of as an area involved in a battle and not necessarily yielding to a lethal or nearly lethal blow.

The common injuries shown as x-ray abnormalities at the hip include fractures and dislocations. Both can lead to the delayed onset of avascular necrosis of the femoral head. Fractures are usually recognized easily. Shenton's line may be disturbed after fracture and the awareness of this landmark can facilitate the detection of fracture in injuries with minimal displacement (Fig. 147).

Dislocation of the hip is sometimes overlooked after injury to the pelvis

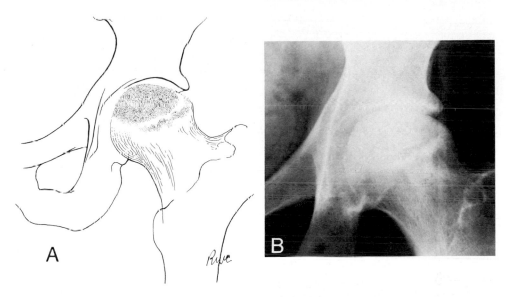

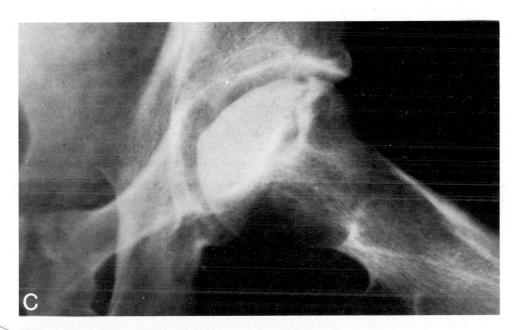

Fig. 146A, B. Aseptic necrosis nearly always affects the superolateral area of the head of the femur. Partial collapse of the cortical margin of the femoral head has helped define the articular limit of the zone of necrosis. This example is an advanced form of necrosis. Milder forms with patchy sclerosis in the same zone of the femur are more common, especially in patients with trauma or with systemic disease leading to infarction. C. An abduction view of the same hip is valuable in presenting another profile of the zone of necrosis.

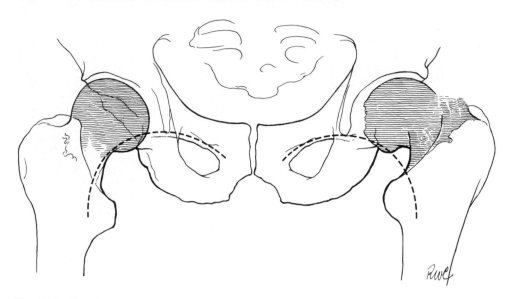

Fig. 147. The dotted line drawn at the right hip along the medial margin of the neck of the femur and arching gracefully to connect with the inferior margin of the superior pubic ramus is known as Shenton's line. On the left the same landmarks are altered because of a fracture in the femoral neck. The left femoral head and upper femoral neck fragment protrude down into the arch of what would be Shenton's line. A graceful arch does not exist on the left side to match that on the right. At times, because of the subtlety of fracture lines in the proximal femur, disturbances in Shenton's line may provide the main clues to the diagnosis of a fractured proximal femur.

and leg. The femoral head usually dislocates posteriorly so that the leg on the affected side is shortened, adducted at the hip, and internally rotated.[3] Anterior dislocation of the hip occurs rarely. The anterior capsule of the hip is reinforced by Bigelow's ligament, a major blockade for the femoral head. Remember that with the dislocation force, the femoral head may be driven through the posterior acetabulum or into the central acetabulum. Hence pelvic fractures and fragments of the acetabulum may be present. Particularly difficult to diagnose is the posterior fragment of the acetabulum. This is commonly associated with posterior dislocation of the hip. Occasionally a fragment of bone or cartilage prevents adequate or complete relocation of the hip. A fracture of the margin of the femoral head due to an impaction injury can be difficult to diagnose. One must examine the joint margins of the injured hip for unusual densities or focal alterations of contours. Arthrography is often of assistance in this situation in showing a cartilaginous and osseous defect. Similarly, tomography may show the injury site. Comparison views are essential in such a plain film and tomographic search. Oblique and stereoscopic views of the injured acetabulum or femoral head can be valuable in identifying the position and extent of the fracture fragments.

References

1. Beeler JW: Further evidence on the acquired nature of spondylolysis and spondylolisthesis. Am J Roentgenol 108:796–798, 1970
2. Bowerman JW, McDonnell EJ: Radiology of athletic injuries: football. Radiology 117:33–36, 1975
3. Brav EA. Traumatic dislocation of the hip. J Bone Joint Surg 44A:1115–1134, 1962
4. Catto M: Histological study of avascular necrosis of the femoral head after transcervical fracture. J Bone Joint Surg 47B:749–776, 1965
5. Epstein BS: The Spine. Philadelphia, Lea, 1969
6. Freiberger RH: Personal communication, 1971
7. Funk FJ Jr: Traumatic dislocation of the hip in children. J Bone Joint Surg 44A:1135–1145, 1962
8. Harris NH, Murray RO: Lesions of the symphysis in athletes. Br Med J 4: 211–214, 1974
9. Murray RO: The aetiology of primary osteoarthritis of the hip. Br J Radiol 38: 810–824, 1965
10. _____: Stress fractures of the pars interarticularis. Proc R Soc Med 61:555–557, 1968
11. _____, Duncan C: Athletic activity in adolescence as an etiologic factor in degenerative hip disease. J Bone Joint Surg 53B:406–419, 1971
12. Newman PH: The etiology of spondylolisthesis. J Bone Joint Surg 45B:39–59, 1963
13. Wiltse LL, Widell EH, Jackson DW: Fatigue fracture: the basic lesion in isthmic spondylolisthesis. J Bone Joint Surg 57A:17–22, 1975

KNEE, LOWER LEG, ANKLE, AND FOOT

Knee

The knee is the most publicized joint of the professional athlete. At this site ordinary radiographs are often of little assistance in the diagnosis of acute ligament or meniscus injury. For this reason, arthrography has had a resurgence of use in the detection of knee abnormalities in many hospitals.[3,7,10,16,28] Arthroscopy has its proponents as well and has advanced following recent developments in the manufacture of lenses and the design of improved arthroscopes.

Arthrography is the examination of the articular surfaces of a joint by radiographic means. The procedure requires the placement of a needle within the joint under study using aseptic technique. In using this technique, one has a choice of air, carbon dioxide, or iodinated contrast material (water-soluble compounds such as Renografin-60) to outline tears in menisci and knee ligaments. In usual practice, a combination of room air and iodinated contrast material is employed. Leakage of contrast material can occur in abnormal areas to show a rupture of a joint or the extension of synovial contents posteriorly into a popliteal (Baker's) cyst.

The usual site for needle placement, after careful aseptic preparation of the skin, is at the midportion of the patella and at its lateral or medial margins. A nonfluoroscopic technique can be employed with the use of a horizontal x-ray beam.[16] The patient usually lies on one side and the knee is also positioned on its side. This position displays the uppermost meniscus and compartment of the knee. Air or carbon dioxide will rise in the joint and contrast material will fall after coating the meniscal surface. Alternatively a vertical x-ray beam can be used at fluoroscopy.[3] With this method, which is highly recommended over the other, the examiner is able to study the menisci as he positions the knee during fluoroscopy. The volume of contrast material used varies in different reports from 4 to 10 cc. Some examiners use 10 to 20 cc air and 4 cc of contrast material. Others use this combination plus 30 to 40 cc carbon dioxide. Several examples of fluoroscopic views of the knee made at arthrography are shown in Figures 148 through 152.

In addition to meniscus tears and ligament ruptures, synovial cysts can be detected at arthrography (Figs. 153–155). A chronic post-traumatic effusion can

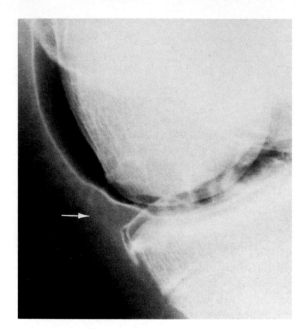

Fig. 148. The normal medial meniscus in the arthrogram is a wedge-shaped structure outlined by contrast material at its upper and lower margins.

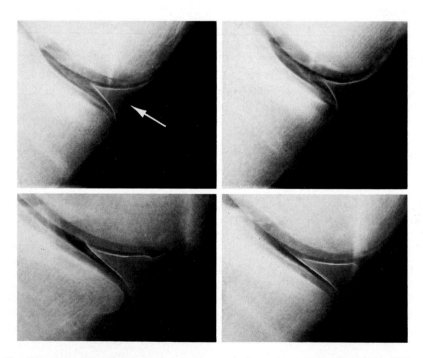

Fig. 149. The normal medial meniscus is shown in four views made at slightly different degrees of knee rotation.

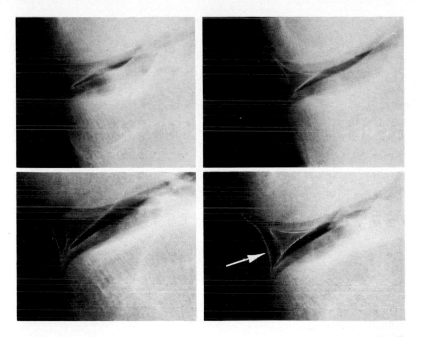

Fig. 150. The lateral meniscus is shown in four views made at slightly different degrees of knee rotation. The normal synovial attachment (arrow) of the popliteus tendon is shown at the lateral joint margin.

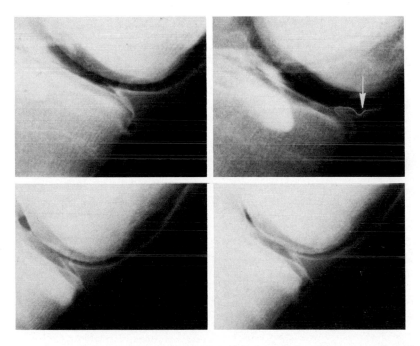

Fig. 151. In three of these views the margins of the medial meniscus are normal. In the remaining view the superior margin appears indented (arrow), suggesting a damaged meniscal surface.

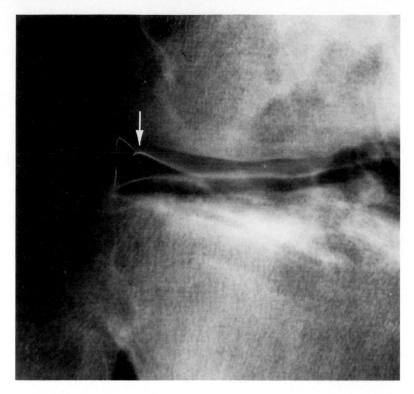

Fig. 152. In a different patient from the one shown in the preceding figures, a small peripheral tear is present at the superior margin of the lateral meniscus. The synovial attachments of the popliteus tendon are present at the extreme lateral margin of the lateral meniscus. These lateral-most synovial attachments are not to be misinterpreted as a torn meniscus.

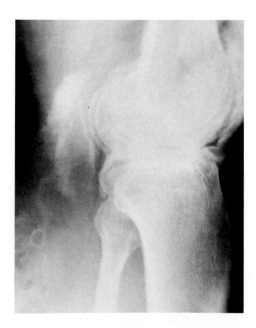

Fig. 153. The popliteal cyst is an extension of the synovial fluid and/or synovial disease via the popliteal bursae. The bursae usually involved are the semimembranosus and the gastrocnemius bursae. The popliteal cyst may extend further into the area of the calf and produce symptoms there mimicking thrombophlebitis.

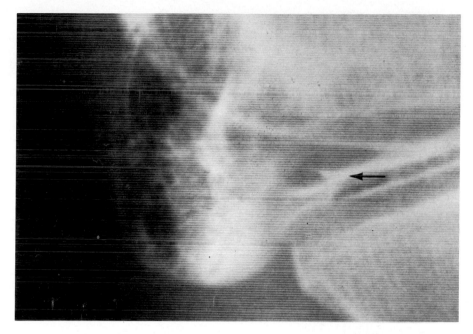

Fig. 154. A transverse tear is shown by a linear leak of contrast material (arrow) into the medial meniscus in this magnified view. A popliteal cyst overlaps the meniscus.

be of sufficient volume to distend the semimembranosis gastrocnemius bursal complex in the popliteal region. This bursal area acts as a decompression chamber and can be symptomatic and swollen, producing a typical Baker's cyst.[12] Such cysts are named for W. Morrant Baker of St. Bartholomew's Hospital in London, who described synovial cysts in multiple forms of arthritis.[1,5] The orthopedic surgeon encounters synovial cysts as frequent companions of injury and meniscus tear. The rheumatologist encounters synovial cysts as companions of rheumatoid arthritis and other arthritides. Dixon and Grant[11] and Good[17] have described examples of calf pain due to downward extension of synovial cysts that have produced symptoms of thrombophlebitis. Such patients have often been misdiagnosed as having thrombophlebitis without consideration of joint injury or disease as a cause.[7]

The plain radiographs of the knee normally include anteroposterior and lateral views. A complete array of plain radiographs should include a tangential view of the patella, weight-bearing views (Fig. 156), and a tunnel view of the intercondylar notch (Fig. 157). The latter view presents the picture that would obtain if you stooped down viewing the knee from the front and looked through the knee joint at its intercondylar notch. It is a helpful adjunct to the two basic views. It is invaluable in showing articular margin defects as compression fractures of the femoral condyles. An alteration of the articular margin of the femur is most commonly seen at the lateral aspect of the medial femoral condyle. In a young person a bony defect at this site is usually referred to as os-

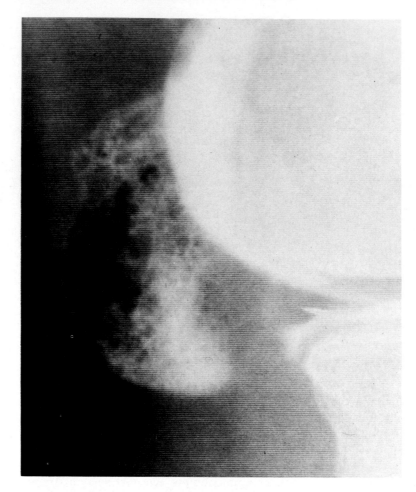

Fig. 155. This view of the same abnormal knee as shown in Figure 154 is nearly a true lateral view of the posterior portion of the knee. The transverse tear extends into the medial meniscus. A 3 × 4-cm popliteal cyst extends posteriorly due to chronic effusion. The knee was injured in jogging by a 50-year-old athlete in good condition who is devoted to tennis and jogging.

teochondritis dissecans. The condition is named inappropriately, as if it were a dissecting form of inflammatory lesion involving bone and cartilage. Osteochondritis dissecans is often associated with a history of trauma or sports activity and probably represents a form of compression fracture.[1,2]

Soft tissue signs of injury may be the only abnormal radiographic finding at the knee after an injury to that joint. The reader is referred to the chapter on soft tissue injuries in Part I, specifically to the sign of suprapatellar effusion.

Stress views of the knee are of value in documenting ligamentous ruptures and fractures (Figs. 158–161). If the medial collateral ligament of the knee has torn completely, then the knee can hinge open medially in an abnormal way

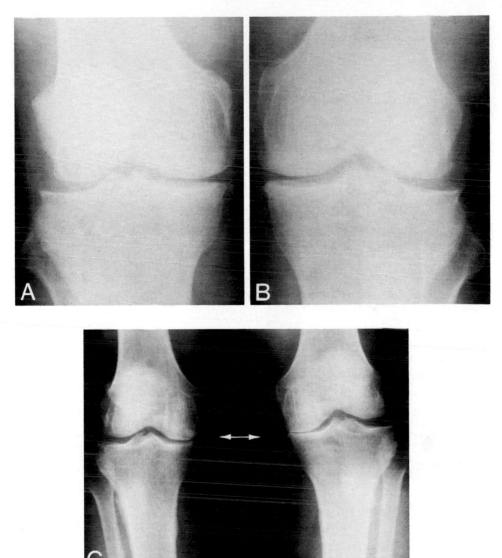

Fig. 156A. The left knee in a non-weight-bearing view shows minimal narrowing of the medial compartment and spur formation of its articular edges. **B.** The right knee in a non-weight-bearing view also shows minimal narrowing of the medial compartment with articular spur formation indicating degenerative joint disease. **C.** Weight-bearing views of both knees in the same patient show the marked narrowing and full extent of degeneration and narrowing of both medial compartments (arrow).

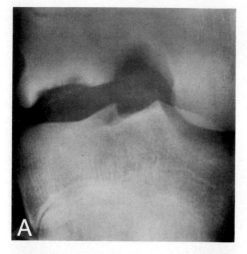

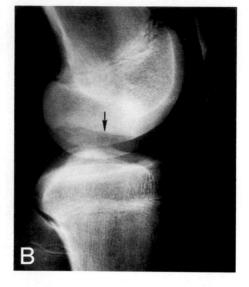

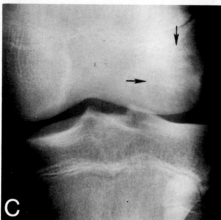

Fig. 157A. This view of the intercondylar notch shows a large zone of osteochondritis dissecans in the lateral femoral condyle of a 15-year-old cross-country runner. He complained of pain in this knee after prlonged running. **B.** The lateral view. **C.** The anteroposterior view. Both these views show the same condylar defect (arrows) but less prominently. The anteroposterior view is reversed so that the condylar defect appears on the reader's right.

when a valgus force is placed on the knee. On rare occasions we have recognized ligament rupture by recording abnormal knee motion under stress in cineradiography. The higher levels of radiation exposure in cine recordings make this a tool for only certain diagnostic problems. It should not be used in place of plain radiographic examinations or ordinary stress views obtained in a static-knee position.

The patella and the patellofemoral joint must not be neglected on physical and radiographic examinations. In evaluating the patella remember its normal variants of ossification (Fig. 162). Hughston considers subluxation of the patella to be the second most common cause of knee derangement in athletes.[18] Only meniscus lesions and collateral ligament injury are more common.[18] The radiographic examination may be normal after subluxation of the patella, but generally some abnormality is detected to support the clinical diagnosis. Abnormal findings include either a malpositioned patella, a tilt of the patella, or an

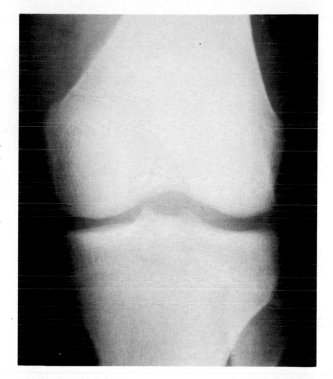

Fig. 158. This anteroposterior view of the knee is apparently normal following a clipping injury in football in an 18-year-old boy. A major fracture is present but nearly obscure on this view. (See also Figures 159 161).

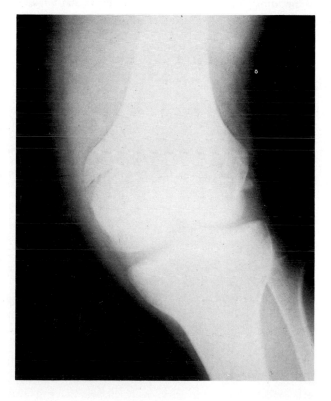

Fig. 159. A stress view made with the patient under anesthesia shows a hingelike femoral fracture opening at the medial condyle. One examiner initially misinterpreted the findings at physical examination and believed that instead of fracture the knee contained a severe ligament injury with separation of the medial aspect of the joint. (See also Figures 158, 160, and 161.)

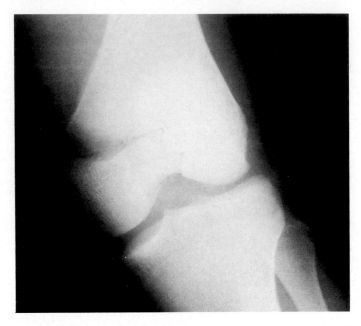

Fig. 160. A valgus stress view shows the fracture site more clearly crossing the medial condyle and extending to the joint at the intercondylar notch. The cleavage plane represents part of the former line of the epiphyseal cartilage and hence is a form of a delayed Salter III type injury. (See also Figures 158, 159, 161.)

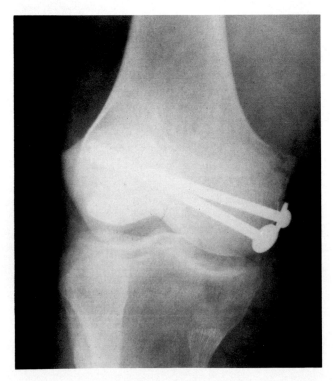

Fig. 161. The crossed screws used to repair the fracture are shown in a frontal view. (See also Figures 158–160.)

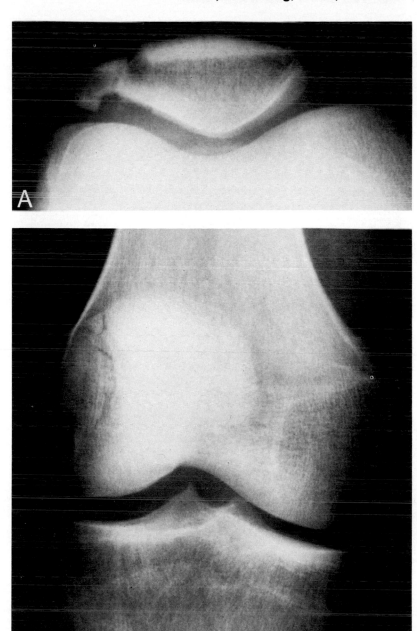

Fig. 162A. Occasionally a bipartite or tripartite (as in this case) patella will show irregular margins exactly mimicking a fracture. **B.** The upper outer quadrant location of the separate ossification centers on the frontal view helps in deciding for a patellar anomaly rather than an injury. The tripartite patella contains two separate ossification centers at the upper lateral quadrant of the patella. The bipartite patella contains one separate ossification center at the upper lateral quadrant.

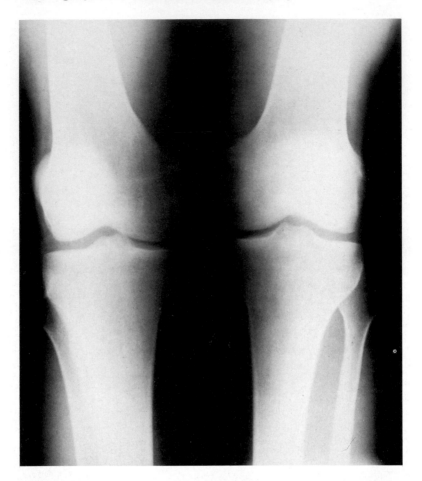

Fig. 163. A waterskier injured his left knee suddenly when the tip of his left ski dipped beneath the water. He suffered an acute twisting flexion injury of the knee but made little of this injury. Subsequently knee pain led to a medical appointment where a tumor or occult lesion of the knee was suspected. The pain was localized at the upper end of the left fibula. He was admitted to a hospital for evaluation of this problem, including an anticipated radioisotopic bone scan and arteriography. These tests were never performed because the plain film showed an abnormality. (See Figures 164–166.)

osteochondral fracture. The patella is usually displaced laterally and may be shifted proximally so that a patella alta is present on the lateral view. Tangential views of the patella are invaluable in showing the lateral or medial malposition and the patella surfaces. Ficat,[13] Ficat and Hungerford,[14] and Hughston[18] have emphasized that this tangential view must be recorded in a position of normal patellofemoral contact. The knee should be flexed only up to 50° or 60°. Flexion beyond this point shifts the patella away from the femur and away from the femoropatellar joint that is the focus of the investigation.

Fractures of the medial patellar margin occurred frequently in association with traumatic dislocation of the patella in 72 patients reported in a five-year study by Scheller and Martenson.[26] Osteochondral fracture of the femoral condyles were also noted. The compression forces that create such osteochondral fractures in the femur are discussed by Kennedy et al.[20] They showed that axial compression loads of from 300 to 400 pounds per square inch were needed to produce cartilage defects in the femoral condyles of cadaver knees. They also emphasized that loose fragments of bone may not be shown on x ray in the knee with an osteochondral fracture. Remember that the ossicles of the tibial tubercle may be projected over the patella or femoral margins on a tangential or axial view of the patella and mimic a loose body or osteochondral fracture.[19]

Occasionally cortical irregularities with focal indentation, cortical thickening, or periosteal reaction may be found on knee radiographs in young patients, especially in the 10- to 15-year-old group. The changes are usually found at the medial posterior metaphyseal margin at the supracondylar ridge of the femur. These findings are normal and should not be confused with disease. Kimmelstiel and Rapp originally described these changes and showed desmoplastic tissue on histologic examination.[21] They referred to the findings as "periosteal desmoids" because the fibrous tissue and abundant intercellular material resembles the tissue found in desmoid tumors of the abdominal wall. Other authors have used other terms, including "avulsive cortical irregularity," "benign cortical irregularity," and "distal irregularities of the femur."[8,9,27,32] Barnes and Gwinn have shown that the aponeurosis of the adductor magnus inserts along the linea aspera of the femur and that this normal ridge produces the radiographic appearance that may cause confusion following injury.[6]

Pain localized to the proximal end of the fibula or near that fibular head after a violent or twisting injury of the knee should not only suggest the possibility of fracture, but dislocation of the upper fibula as well. This author has seen two fresh examples of this often overlooked injury—one in a waterskier and the other in a basketball player (Figs. 163–166). A high index of suspicion of the injury plus careful comparison of symmetric views of both knees should lead to the diagnosis. Ogden discusses this subject extensively, classifies 43 patients in various subgroups, and suggests that proximal fibular resection is useful for the patients who develop the complications of chronic subluxation or chronic posttraumatic arthritis of the proximal tibiofibular joint.[24]

Lower Leg

Shin splints are painful overstretchings or tears of the muscle and fascial attachments of the anterior lower leg. (See the section on track and field in Part II.) The radiographic counterpart of the chronic form of this frequent condition is tibial cortical thickening or periosteal reaction of minimal extent. The entire process appears to be a phenomenon of the mid and lower tibial anterior surface. Do not assume that all leg pain in this region is a soft tissue or surface effect. Stress fractures can occur as a result of the wobble of the tibia or fibula by the repeated contractions of the muscles of the leg (Fig. 167).

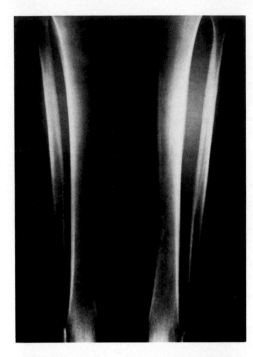

Fig. 164. Comparison views were made of both knees with the legs positioned in exactly the same manner. This view shows an asymmetry of tibiofibular interosseous spaces due to displacement of the left fibula in a lateral direction. This shift has occurred with dislocation of the proximal left fibula. (See also Figures 163, 165, and 166.)

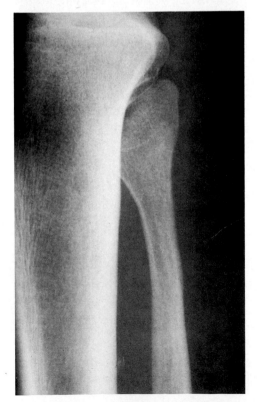

Fig. 165. The lateral view of the waterskier's uninjured knee is useful in showing the normal position of the fibula. (See also Figures 163, 164, and 166.)

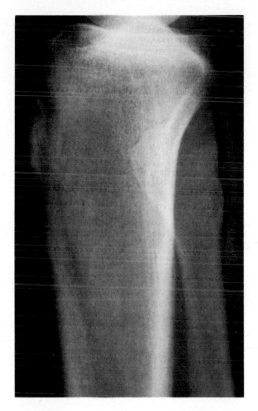

Fig. 166. This lateral view of the water skier's injured knee shows the anterior position of the dislocated fibula. (See also Figures 163–165.)

(See the section on track and field in Part II.) Stress fractures can occur in the professional athlete's tibia whenever training exceeds the structural strength of the bone. Periosteal reaction in a focal area, rarely exceeding 1 cm in length, is a prominent early x-ray sign of stress fracture. Subsequently, resorption of the fracture margin occurs and a radiolucent defect appears in a linear fashion. The fracture line can be ill defined or may involve only one cortex.

Ordinary radiography is not the only diagnostic tool for the detection of stress fractures. Soft tissue radiography, xeroradiography, and bone scanning are also useful for this purpose. Each of these techniques is likely to be better than conventional radiography in locating and defining a fracture site.

Ankle and Foot

The base to the athlete's movement is the soft tissue and bone of the foot and ankle. Ankle injuries plague the athlete as much as knee injuries (Figs. 168–170). Here, fractures of the malleoli require careful scrutiny of anteroposterior, lateral, and oblique radiographs for detection of injury. Occasionally only the oblique view will show the fracture gap. Stress views should be obtained whenever significant ankle ligament injury is suspected. In such

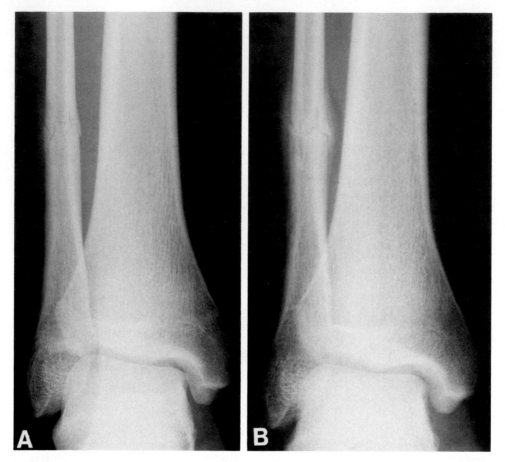

Fig. 167A. A painful lower leg was x-rayed in a young man who is a long-distance runner. What is your diagnosis? **B.** Periosteal new bone reaction of the distal fibula indicates the correct diagnosis of a stress fracture. The periosteal response developed in a three-week period after the injury. (From Murray, Jacobson: The Radiology of Skeletal Disorders, 1971. Courtesy of Churchill Livingstone.)

views the ankle is everted and inverted in an effort to show abnormal motion of the talus within the ankle mortise on the frontal view. A small percentage of normal ankles will show laxity of ligaments and permit approximately 5 degrees of deflection of the superior surface of the talus on the stress views.[15,24]

In a study from the Dartmouth Affiliated Hospitals in Hanover, N.H., sports injury produced ankle injury of significant degree in 27 athletes with an average age of 19.7 years.[29] Approximately half of the injuries occurred in basketball. Ankle arthrography was used as part of the evaluation of 26 of the patients. All but one showed a massive lateral extravasation of contrast material beyond the normal joint margins. The exception was a faulty injection involving leak of contrast about the injection needle. Operative repair of the ruptured

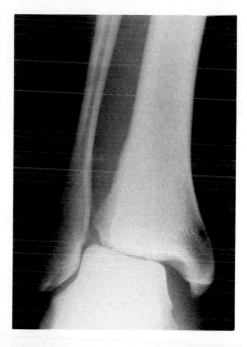

Fig. 168. The talus is displaced in the ankle mortise of this athlete who injured his ankle. The talus and fibula have been shifted laterally. The fibular shift is discernible as a slight widening of the distal interosseous space between the fibula and tibia. This fibular shift indicates a rupture of the interosseous membrane. Occasionally the blood supply to the talus can be compromised in this type of injury and subsequent follow-up ankle views will show patchy sclerosis or possible collapse of the superior margin of the talus. Fortunately no gross evidence of avascular necrosis of the talus was discovered in this patient.

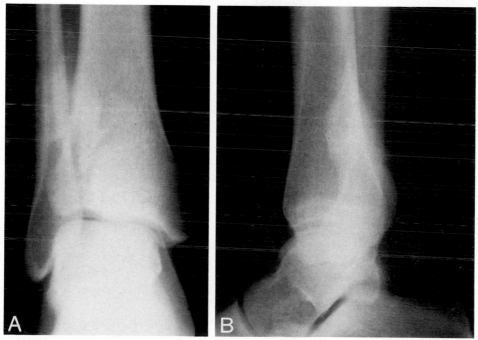

Fig. 169AB. An ankle injury in football season in a high school player troubled him again in the spring when he ran track. These views were taken during track season and show interosseous membrane ossification at the distal tibia and fibula following prior ankle injury.

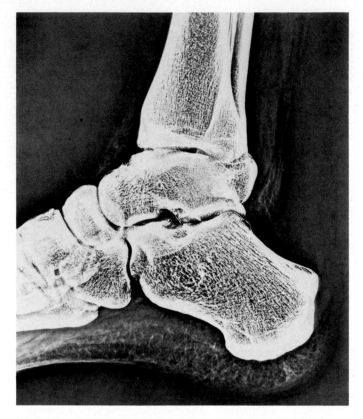

Fig. 170. This xeroradiographic view was made in evaluation of ankle pain in a marathon runner. He also complained of limited dorsiflexion. The dorsum of the talus and its overlying soft tissue were inspected carefully but no traction spur or loose body was detected. An ankle arthrogram was normal and is not shown here.

ankle ligaments was performed in each case. Within an average of 11.4 post-operative months all but three patients recovered fully. These three were able to return to sports despite occasional ankle stiffness and swelling. The results in these patients with surgical repair were significantly better in the author's opinion than a comparison group of 68 patients treated by cast immobilization for three to eight weeks. Only 40 (58.8 percent) of the group treated by cast only were without any symptoms or limitations. The author concludes that immediate surgical repair is best for the young athlete with a fresh rupture of anterior and lateral ankle ligaments, especially if the patient expects to resume strenuous athletic activity. Following the rupture of collateral ligaments, the talus can be grossly unstable and show unusual displacement in the mortise (Fig. 171).

The talus can also be the site of fracture and avascular necrosis. Fractures usually occur in the midportion or in the posterior part of the bone (Fig. 172). The os trigonum is an accessory ossicle with rounded margins at the posterior margin of the talus. After ankle injury be certain to examine the margin of a

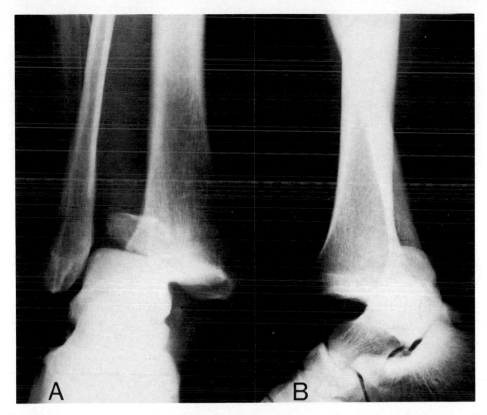

Fig. 171AB. A soccer player was injured in rough play and suffered this disabling injury. His fibular fracture and dislocated ankle indicate an eversion injury of the foot and ankle.

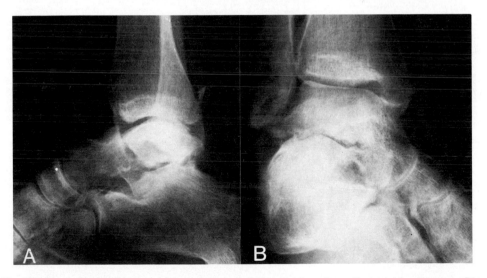

Fig. 172A. A young woman rider was thrown against a tree by a thoroughbred horse. She injured her ankle severely as it was entrapped in the stirrup. **B.** A fracture is present across the midportion of the talus. This resulted in nonunion and required operative treatment for the relief of persistent pain. An ankle fusion was subsequently performed in which a sliding graft was placed at the anterior tibiotalar joint.

137

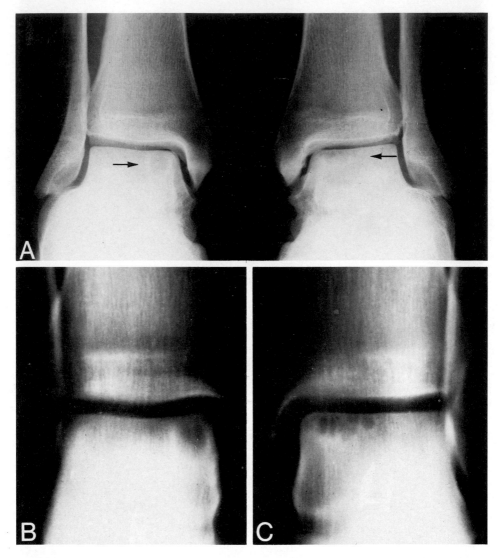

Fig. 173A. A keen squash player and fencer complained of bilateral ankle pain. The ankle x-rays show abnormalities in each talus. The cystic areas (arrows) in each talus are post-traumatic subchondral cysts that affect weight-bearing joints. They often form in association with joint swelling and degenerative disease and can be found in some athletes after repeated knee and ankle stress. **B.** A tomographic view showing a single cyst in the right talus. **C.** A tomographic view showing multiple subchondral cysts in the left talus.

separate ossicle in this area. It may represent a fractured fragment of the posterior portion of the talus in some instances. The fracture fragment is recognized by its ragged or sharp edge as it breaks away from the part of the talus. Avascular necrosis, as elsewhere in the skeleton, first rears its ugly head as a radiolucent crescent beneath the articular margin of bone. The sclerotic ap-

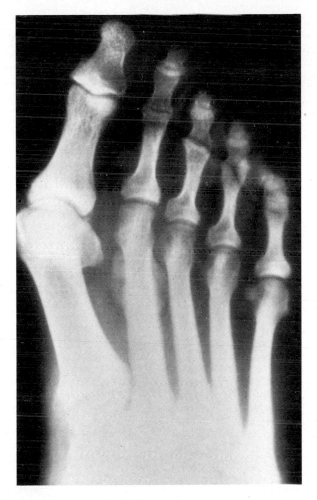

Fig. 174. Repeated play at basketball led to severe foot pain in a 19-year-old boy. The second metatarsal contains a stress fracture. The abundant periosteal reaction is characteristic of the injury. A hallux valgus deformity is present.

pearance of reparative efforts occurs subsequently.[22(p203)] In extensive necrosis, collapse of the articular bony margins occurs at the superior part of the talus. The anteroposterior view of the ankle best shows the abnormal area in the talus. The lateral view can be confusing because of the overlapping malleoli. In addition, tomographic views can be of value in demonstrating avascular necrosis of the talus.

Cysts within the margin of the talus occur following repeated stress and weight bearing. Other weight-bearing joints, such as the knee and hip, occasionally show similar cysts. Various names have been applied to these radiolucent defects that occur at the margin of the talus, tibia, or femur and include "post-traumatic subarticular cyst," "intraosseous ganglion," and "degenerative cysts."[22(p187)] The joint space adjacent to the cyst is usually narrowed, but not invariably. Tomographic views usually best define the margins of the cyst and display its extent for the interested physician or surgeon (Fig. 173).

Narrowing of the subtalar joint and talonavicular spurs are also post-traumatic abnormalities seen after extensive ankle injury. Recurrent talonavicular ligament stresses also occur in sports that require rapid change of direction, speed afoot, and jumping, such as basketball and soccer.

Variations of normal foot structure, including the syndrome of the short first metatarsal described by Morton, have important ramifications to athletes. Sheehan[26] and Subotnick[30,31] have emphasized the frequent association of these variations in symptomatic runners. (See the section on track and field in Part II.) The most common site of stress fracture in the foot is the second metatarsal. The stress fracture may be associated with an abnormality in foot structure as shown in Figure 174.

References

1. Aichroth P: Osteochondritis dissecans of the knee. J Bone Joint Surg 53B:440–447, 1971
2. _____: Osteochondral fractures and their relationship to osteochondritis dissecans of the knee. J Bone Joint Surg 53B:448–454, 1971
3. Angell FL: Fluoroscopic technique of double contrast arthrography of the knee. Radiol Clin North Am 9:85–98, 1971
4. Baker WM: On the formation of synovial cysts in the leg in connection with disease of the knee joint. St Barth Hosp Rep 13:245–261, 1877
5. _____: The formation of abnormal synovial cysts in connection with the joints. St Barth Hosp Rep 21:177–190, 1885
6. Barnes GR Jr, Gwinn JL: Distal irregularities of the femur simulating malignancy. Am J Roentgenol 122:180–185, 1974
7. Bowerman JW, Muhletaler C: Arthrography of rheumatoid cysts of the knee and wrist. J Can Assoc Radiol 24:24–32, 1973
8. Brower AC, Culver JC, Keats TE: Histological nature of medical posterior distal femoral metaphysis in children. Radiology 99:389–392, 1971
9. Bufkin WJ: The avulsive cortical irregularity. Am J Roentgenol 112:487–492, 1971
10. Butt WP, McIntyre JL: Double contrast arthrography of the knee. Radiology 92:487–499, 1969
11. Dixon A St J, Grant C: Acute synovial rupture of the knee joint in rheumatoid arthritis. An arthrographic study. Lancet 1:742–745, 1964
12. Doppman JL: Baker's cyst and the normal gastrocnemio-semimembranosus bursa. Am J Roentgenol 94:646–652, 1965
13. Ficat P: Pathologie Femoro-Patellaire. Paris, Masson, 1970
14. _____, Hungerford DS: Disorders of the Femoro-Patellar Joint. Baltimore, Williams, (in press)
15. Fordyce AW, Horn CV: Arthrography in recent injuries of the ligaments of the ankle. J Bone Joint Surg 54B:116–121, 1972
16. Freiberger RH, Killoran PJ, Cardona G: Arthrography of the knee by double contrast method. Am J Roentgenol 97:736–747, 1966
17. Good AE: Rheumatoid arthritis, Baker's cyst and "thrombophlebitis." Arthritis Rheum 7:5664, 1964
18. Hughston JC: Subluxation of the patella in athletes. In: Symposium on Sports

Medicine, American Academy of Orthopaedic Surgeons, Oklahoma City, Okla, Aug 1967, St. Louis, Mosby, 1969, pp 162–177

19. Jacobs P: Osgood-Schlatter's disease: cause of a misleading radiographic sign. Clin Radiol 22:487–489, 1971
20. Kennedy JC, Grainger RW, McGraw RW: Osteochondral fractures of the femoral condyles. J Bone Joint Surg 48B:436–440, 1966
21. Kimmelstiel P, Rapp IH: Cortical defect due to periosteal desmoids. Bull Hosp Joint Dis 12:286–297, 1951
22. Murray RO, Jacobson HG: The Radiology of Skeletal Disorders. London, Churchill, 1971
23. Ogden JA: Subluxation and dislocation of the proximal tibiofibular joint. J Bone Joint Surg 56A:145–154, 1974
24. Olson RW: Arthrography of the ankle: its use in the evaluation of ankle sprains. Radiology 92:1439–1446, 1969
25. Scheller S, Martenson L: Traumatic dislocation of the patella. Acta Radiol [Suppl] 336, 1974
26. Sheehan GA: Personal communication, 1975
27. Simon H: Medical distal metaphyseal femoral irregularity in children. Radiology 90:258–260, 1968
28. Staple TW: Extrameniscal lesions demonstrated by double contrast arthrography of the knee. Radiology 102:311–319, 1972
29. Staples OS: Ruptures of the fibular collateral ligaments of the ankle. J Bone Joint Surg 57A:101–107, 1975
30. Subotnick SI: Orthotic foot control and the overuse syndrome. Physician Sports Med 3:75–79, 1975
31. _____: The abuses of orthotics in sports medicine. Physician Sports Med 3:73–75, July, 1975
32. Young DW, Nogrady MB, Dunbar JS, Wigglesworth FW: Benign cortical irregularities in distal femur of children. J Can Assoc Radiol 23:107–115, 1972

PART II
INJURY IN SPORT

The material that follows in this section is listed alphabetically by sport. The information available on some activities is meager despite an extensive search of the literature. In some instances only one or two reports can be quoted on a specific sport. Certain sports such as baseball and football have commanded so much attention from a medical viewpoint that the problem here has been to exclude some material yet include valuable and representative studies in these sports. What is sport to some is not sport to others; some activities might fit more easily into a category of recreation. Finally, this is not an exhaustive list of sports or activities, so that some athletes may not find their particular sport listed.

AIRCRAFTING

A study of the patterns of injury and death in light aircraft accidents identified by the Armed Forces Institute of Pathology between 1944 and 1962 showed several interesting factors.[1] Of 210 accidents listed with autopsy data only 178 had complete information suitable for review. Light aircraft were defined as those under 12,500 pounds in weight and numbered approximately 105,000 in the United States in 1970. Toxicologic information on alcohol and carbon monoxide levels in pilots and passengers was difficult to obtain because often fresh samples of tissues and blood were not taken or were contaminated or not preserved. In eight accidents elevated postmortem blood and/or tissue alcohol were found. Two additional crashes were suspected of being related to alcohol use, but this suspicion could not be confirmed because of mishandled blood samples.

Of 51 burn victims, 10 died from the effects of fire that occurred after the crash. Only 148 cases had sufficient autopsy material for further study of skeletal and visceral injury. Lethal visceral injury occurred without skull fracture in 12 people, pointing up the need for a complete postmortem examination after severe trauma. An external examination alone would have failed to explain death in these individuals. Included among this group were ruptures of the heart, aorta, liver, and spleen. The skeletal injury in the entire study group included 104 skull fractures, 52 spinal fractures and dislocations, and 110 lower extremity injuries.

Reference

1. Reals WJ, Davidson H, Karnitschig HH: Pathology of light aircraft accidents. Aerosp Med 35:133–135, 1964

BADMINTON

Badminton has its ocular hazards. These are amply illustrated in a report by Chandran from Kuala Lumpur, Malaysia.[3] The sport is very popular there and throughout Southeast Asia. In a five-year period 63 eye injuries from badminton were seen at the Eye Clinic of the University Hospital. Other sports contributed an additional 33 eye injuries in the same time period. Of the 63 patients, 9 had injuries from a direct blow from a partner's racquet. The remaining 54 individuals were struck in the eye by the shuttlecock after a "smash" hit. The shuttlecock is almost cone shaped and measures ¾ inches at its striking end. The eye injuries included hyphema (49 patients), traumatic mydriasis (34), commotio retinae (12), lid hematoma (9), corneal abrasion (8), vitreous hemorrhage (8), subconjunctival hemorrhage (4), and lid laceration (2). There were 35 complications of trauma in this group, including 5 patients with cataract and 4 with glaucoma. Most of the injuries occurred in inexperienced or nearsighted players; however, a peak of 17 cases was noted in a three-month period in 1970 during the Thomas Cup finals held in Kuala Lumpur. Chandran concludes that myopes and novices should wear safety glasses in this usually safe sport.

Benjamin reported a case of black heel (pigmented areas on the posterior heel secondary to petechial hemorrhage) in a 23-year-old woman who played badminton and tennis regularly.[2] She experienced pain in the right heel following such activity. The condition has also been noted in basketball and soccer and is usually painless.[1,4,5]

References

1. Ayers S Jr, Mihan R: Calcaneal petechiae, letter to the editor. Arch Dermatol 106:262, 1972
2. Benjamin ES: Black heel. S Afr Med J 47:919–920, 1973
3. Chandran S: Ocular hazards of playing badminton. Br J Ophthalmol 58:757–760, 1974
4. Crissey JT, Peachey JC: Calcaneal petechiae. Arch Dermatol 83:501, 1961
5. Verbov J: Calcaneal petechiae, letter to the editor. Arch Dermatol 107:918, 1973

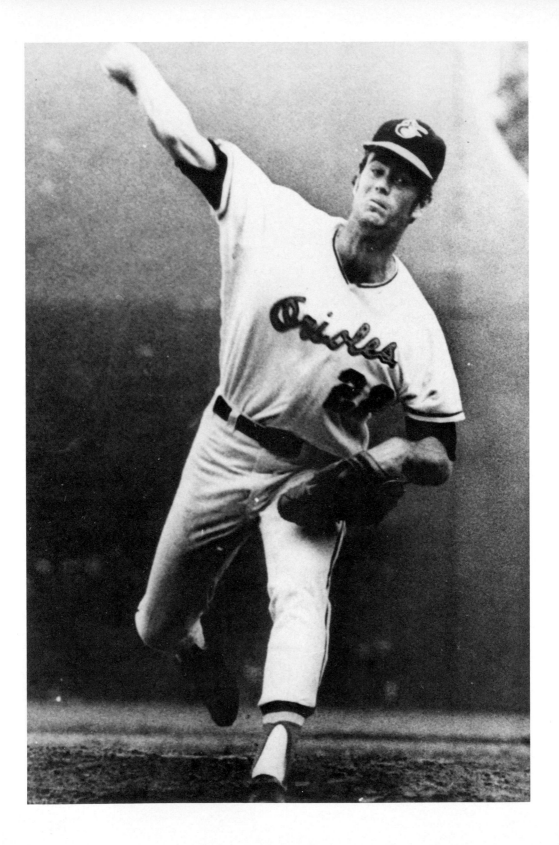

BASEBALL

In the American game of baseball there is a mixture of athletic activity: swinging a wooden bat, sudden sprints of running, sliding on various parts of the body, and, occasionally, colliding with barriers or opponents in pursuit of the game (Figs. 175, 176)

Arm and Shoulder Injuries

A dominant activity in baseball is throwing the ball, and the pitcher is most prone to the effects of stress from throwing. The pitching motion has been analyzed by several authors.[6,7,10,13,20,27] The initial phases of throwing include a smooth sequence of elevation, abduction, and external rotation of the upper arm. This movement leads quickly to a sudden, forceful, forward flexion, abduction anteriorly, and internal rotation of the shoulder associated with extension of the elbow and flexion of the wrist and fingers. At the center of the initial sequences lies the shoulder, or glenohumeral joint, which is surrounded throughout its circumference by the muscles of the rotator cuff (Fig. 177). These muscles extend from the trunk in short, thick pathways to insert on the humerus. They act to rotate the humerus—hence the rotator cuff. Brewer refers to these muscles as the most important muscles involved in throwing.[10] The chief internal rotator is the subscapularis muscle, which inserts on the lesser tuberosity of the humerus. External rotators include the supraspinatus, infraspinatus, and teres minor attached to the greater tuberosity.

Bennett classified throwing injuries into those of the anterior and posterior shoulder muscle groups.[7] He recognized some anterior abnormalities confined to the supraspinatus or to the long head of the biceps tendon in the intertuberous groove or tunnel. He was the first to recognize a lesion peculiar to the throwing motion that involved the origin of the long head of the triceps brachii muscle (Fig. 178). The long head originates from the scapula at the infraglenoid tubercle and merges with the rest of the triceps muscle to continue into the elbow at the olecranon process. Brewer noted that the triceps muscle is intrinsically related to the effort of throwing in two ways.[10] First, the triceps is the strong extensor muscle of the elbow, and, second, the long head of the triceps acts as a rein when the shoulder stretches as the pitcher throws his arm toward home plate. Bennett observed several pitchers—some late in their careers and

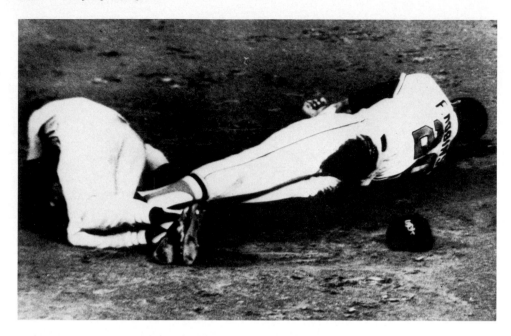

Fig. 175. Baseball can be a sport of collisions. This is the aftermath of a collision at second base that produced a serious injury in each player. (Photograph taken by Morton Tadder)

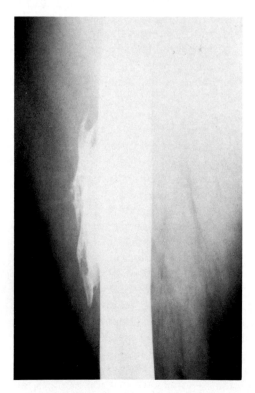

Fig. 176. This spike-laden zone of myositis ossificans is attached to the femur. The injury that produced the ossification occurred several months prior to the time of this radiograph as an outfielder collided with the wall of Yankee Stadium in New York City. This added bone interfered with the motion of the quadriceps muscle and was subsequently removed at surgery. (From Bowerman, McDonnell: Radiology 116:614, 1975)

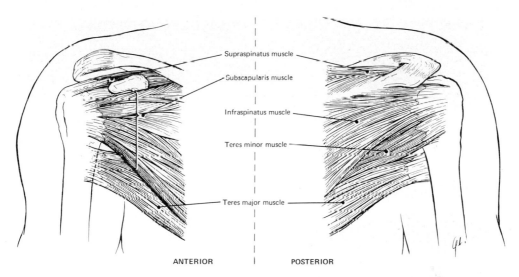

Supraspinatus muscle

Subscapularis muscle

Infraspinatus muscle

Teres minor muscle

Teres major muscle

ANTERIOR   POSTERIOR

Fig. 177. The rotator cuff muscles that are heavily involved in throwing are well beneath the overlying pectoralis and trapezius muscles. Here the overlying muscles have been removed and are not included in the anterior or posterior views.

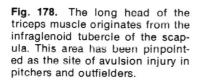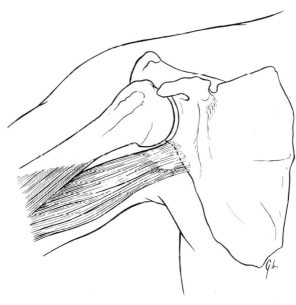

Fig. 178. The long head of the triceps muscle originates from the infraglenoid tubercle of the scapula. This area has been pinpointed as the site of avulsion injury in pitchers and outfielders.

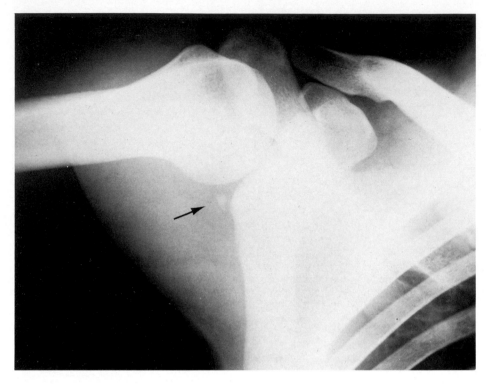

Fig. 179. This abduction view of a pitcher's shoulder shows a fragment of bone adjacent to the infraglenoid tubercle. The fragment has been produced by a throwing injury of an avulsion type. The abduction view is needed to demonstrate the injury, which often is missed on standard anteroposterior views of the shoulder. The view is made with the arm at a right angle to the body or nearly so. The opposite shoulder should be elevated to give a partial profile of the axillary margin of the scapula to be studied. The central beam of the x-ray tube is centered at the axilla and directed 5° cephalad. (From Bowerman, McDonnell: Radiology 116:611–615, 1975)

some early—who had avulsion injuries at the infraglenoid tubercle, detected on x-ray examination[7] (Figs. 179, 180).

THE ADOLESCENT PLAYER.   The effects of stress in pitching on the developing shoulder and elbow are varied.[3,26] In the adolescent skeleton cartilage growth proceeds to bone at the zones of epiphyseal cartilage and at centers of ossification that form the articular ends of bones in the adult. Fracture of the proximal humeral epiphyseal cartilage was described by Dotter in Little League players in 1953.[14] Brogdon and Crow described radiographic abnormalities of the medial epicondyle, including fragmentation as a result of avulsion injuries, in two Little League pitchers.[11] Adams compared the x-ray findings of the elbow in pitchers and other players to those of a control group of boys who did not participate in organized baseball.[2] The boys ranged in age from 9 to 14 years and included 80 pitchers, 47 nonpitchers, and 35 boys in the control group. Accelerated closure of the epiphyseal cartilage occurred in 76, 7, and 3 members of these groups, respectively. Fragmentation of the medial

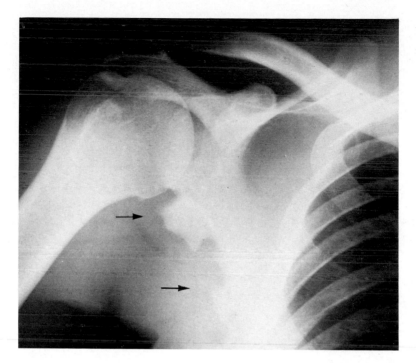

Fig. 180. Myositis ossificans is present at the axillary margin of the scapula in this professional outfielder. This has developed after an avulsion injury involving the origin of the long head of the triceps at the Infraglenoid tubercle of the scapula and after lower scapular avulsion injury as well, probably involving the teres musculature. This type of injury was originally described by Bennett in professional pitchers and often tolled the death knell of a player's career. Both outfielders and pitchers may face this injury due to forceful throwing. (From Bowerman, McDonnell: Radiology 116:612, 1975)

epicondylar epiphysis occurred in 39, 6, and 2 members, respectively (Fig. 181). Irregular ossification of the capitellum and head of the radius occurred in six of the pitchers and in none of the other groups. In further work, Adams commented that without adult supervision such young athletes usually do not overexert themselves and healing following injuries usually progresses normally.[4] With adult supervision, overexertion does occur and treatment methods are then in the hands of the responsible adults. He cited Hale,[18] who presented data on 15,444 injuries among 771,310 Little League baseball players.[4] In this group, 52 percent of the injuries were contusions and abrasions, 19 percent were fractures, and 13 percent were sprains.

As a result of his observations, in 1970 Adams recommended the restriction of pitching times to two innings a week in Little League and to three innings a week in Pony League.[5] He also proposed that the league be divided into a younger and an older age group, that throwing of curve balls be abolished, and that practice throwing at home be avoided. In addition, he suggested that the season be shortened in the hope that all these steps would reduce the incidence of so-called Little League elbow—Brogdon and Crow's term[11]—that

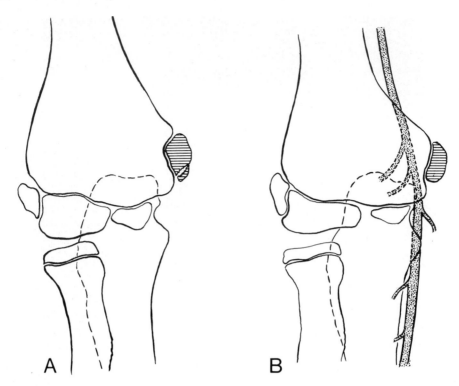

Fig. 181A. The immature elbow has multiple ossification centers that may be confusing when radiographed. This outline drawing shows the fragmentation of the medial epicondylar ossification (shaded) in a symptomatic elbow. **B.** The normal adolescent elbow is shown for comparison and the path of the ulnar nerve is indicated. Occasionally ulnar nerve compression occurs after chronic injury to the medial epicondyle.

had reached epidemic proportions in southern California. These suggestions have had varying degrees of acceptance and enforcement. The author has recently witnessed Little League play among boys 10 to 12 years old in which the pitcher was allowed to pitch seven innings in each league game.

The path of the ulnar nerve is near the medial epicondyle (Fig. 181). Because spur formation is common at this epicondyle, it is not surprising that repeated pitching can lead to traumatic ulnar neuropathy. In 1971, Godshall and Hansen reported two examples of teenage pitchers with paresthesias of the ulnar nerve after league play in Pennsylvania.[15] Both patients had fragmentation and partial avulsion of the medial epicondyle on x-ray examination. Both players underwent operations that showed ruptures of ligaments that normally stabilize the ulnar groove, giving rise to paresthesias. The ulnar nerve was transposed anteriorly in both individuals. One returned to baseball but never regained full effectiveness as a pitcher.

THE PROFESSIONAL PLAYER.   As the successful adolescent player gains attention with his skill, he has an ever increasing chance of becoming a profes-

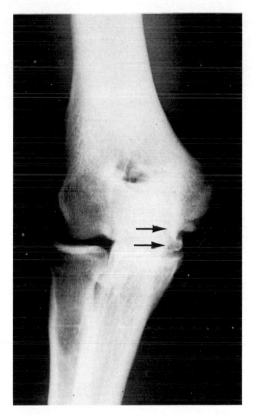

Fig. 182. Two traction spurs have developed at the medial margin of the elbow following chronic overuse injury in pitching in a professional baseballer. Stress to the common flexors at their origin from the medial epicondyle produces the injury. (From Bowerman, McDonnell: Radiology 116:612, 1975)

sional pitcher. He also increases his chance of having elbow abnormality. King et al estimated that two of every three professional pitchers have an abnormal elbow.[20] They examined 50 minor and major league professional pitchers and studied radiographs of both elbows in each player. In some instances motion pictures were taken of those with abnormal elbows or those with classic deliveries of certain pitches. Hypertrophy of the arm and forearm was the rule, and flexion contractures of the elbow were present in over 50 percent of the pitchers examined. On all radiographs hypertrophy of the humerus was present and in some there were traction spurs and loose bodies of bone within the joint (Fig. 182). Bennett observed similar elbow lesions of varying stages of players' careers.[7] He reported loose bodies of bone in the olecranon fossa, near the tip of the coronoid process of the ulna, and near the medial epicondyle, where they caused irritation of the ulnar nerve.

In reviewing radiographs of professional players, Bowerman and McDonnell found loose bodies within the elbows of two outfielders[9] (Figs. 183–185). In one of these players a fracture of the olecranon tip occurred as he swung forcefully in batting and missed the ball (Fig. 185). In another, an intra-articular loose body was detected at tomography of the elbow (Fig. 184). Similarly, abnormalities of the shoulder are not confined to pitchers. One outfielder in

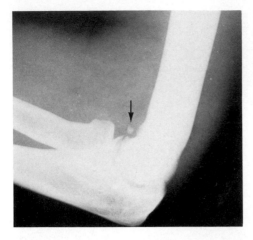

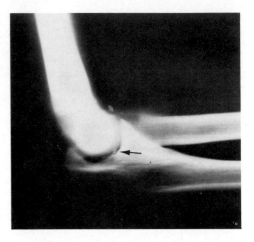

Fig. 183. An outfielder in professional baseball complained of elbow pain and showed signs of joint "locking." This plain radiograph shows a bone fragment in the antecubital fossa and a traction spur at the coronoid process of the ulna (cf Fig. 184). (From Bowerman, McDonnell: Radiology 116:612, 1975)

Fig. 184. This lateral tomographic view of the elbow shown in Figure 183 demonstrates a second intra-articular bony fragment (arrow) that was not shown on previous plain radiographs. The fragments were removed at surgery. Following surgery, the player continued to perform brilliantly at bat and in the field. (From Bowerman, McDonnell: Radiology 116:613, 1975)

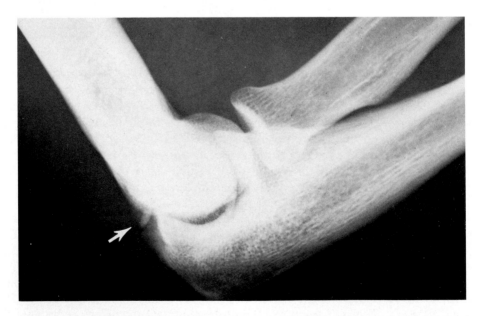

Fig. 185. A baseball batter had sudden pain in the elbow after missing a ball and overswinging. The pain occurred as his elbow reached full extension during the follow-through. The arrow indicates a small fracture fragment at the proximal tip of the olecranon process. (From Bowerman, McDonnell: Radiology 116:613, 1975)

this group had extensive calcification at the infraglenoid margin of the scapula following a throwing injury (Fig. 180; Table 1).

**TABLE 1. Common Sites for
Radiographic Examinations
in Professional Baseball
Players***

Site	Number of Players with Injury
Shoulder	307
Elbow	186
Knee	92
Lumbar Spine	71
Ankle	57
Hand and Fingers	50
Cervical Spine	44
Ribs	34

*These athletes were examined in one orthopedic practice between 1930 and 1968. (Courtesy of Dr. E. J. McDonnell)

Unusual lesions of the pitching arm were discussed extensively by Tullos et al.[27] These lesions include thrombosis at the axillary artery, avascular necrosis of the radial head, stress fracture of the olecranon process and the first rib, fracture of the humerus, and stress fracture of the anterior tips of the lowest three ribs. The arterial injury occurred in a 36-year-old left-handed professional pitcher who had a two-year history of easy fatigability of the left arm. He had absent left brachial, radial, and ulnar pulses and had thrombosis with total occlusion of the left axillary artery. He was treated by a transthoracic cervicodorsal sympathectomy. He still experienced symptoms in cold weather and during night games and had recurrence of easy fatigability two years after surgery. A repeat arteriogram showed the same occlusive findings. A venous bypass operation was performed to relieve the thrombosed artery. He played one more season following surgery.

The stress fracture of the olecranon process occurred in a 20-year-old professional pitcher.[27] Because of non-union he later received bone grafting with subsequent healing of the fracture. The mechanism of injury suggested that of extensor overload of the triceps brachii muscle, as in the injury classification suggested by Slocum.[24] One of the patients reported by Tullos et al was an 18-year-old left-handed professional pitcher with the insidious onset of localized discomfort at the base of the neck on the right side, with pain radiating to the right interscapular region.[27] This problem occurred shortly after the onset of spring training. Radiographs showed a nondisplaced fracture of the middle third of the right first rib. Tomography showed callus formation at the margins of the rib fracture. A similar example was observed by Meaney[22] (Fig. 186). The

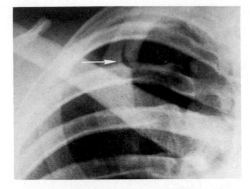

Fig. 186. The violent force of throwing rarely produces a stress fracture of the first rib. This injury hampered the career of a professional player known as a fast ball pitcher. He threw right handed and developed this fracture in his right first rib. The muscle pulls of the scalenus anticus and the scalenus medius are probably involved in producing the fracture. Both muscles insert on the first rib.

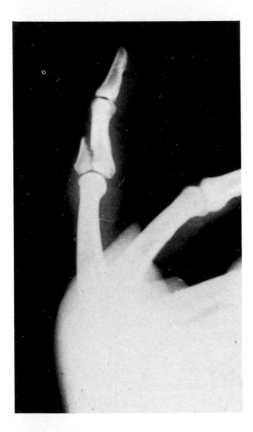

Fig. 187. The catcher, like the wicketkeeper in cricket, is prone to injury of the fingers and hand. This fracture of the middle phalanx of the index finger extends into the articular margin of the proximal interphalangeal joint. The injury occurred as a professional catcher attempted to catch a fluttering pitch thrown as a "knuckle ball."

mechanism of injury is not clear. The injury occurs on the side opposite the throwing arm, according to Tullos et al, and at the thinnest area of the rib in the subclavian groove between the attachments of the scalenus anticus and scalenus medius muscles. The serratus anterior muscle also attaches at this level and may be involved in the process.

The examples of fracture of the humerus are unusual in that both occurred

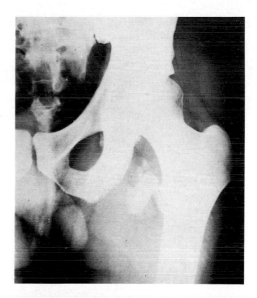

Fig. 188. Ossification is present in the thigh following an avulsion injury of the insertion of the iliopsoas muscle that occurred while this infielder was running. The bone fragments were removed surgically.

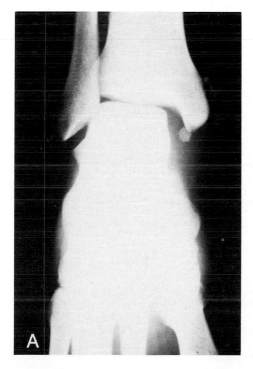

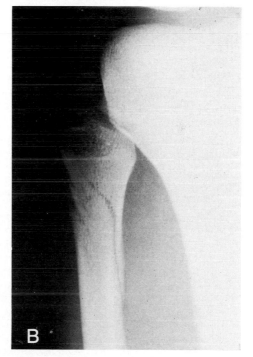

Fig. 189A. This ankle is that of a baseballer who was injured in a slide into home plate. The talus is shifted laterally and superiorly in the ankle mortise, indicating medial collateral ligament rupture. **B.** This player also had pain at the proximal fibula. The eversion injury of the ankle produced the fibular fracture by transmitting force to the proximal fibula. (From Bowerman, McDonnell: Radiology 116:614, 1975)

in semiprofessional pitchers.[27] The mechanism is sudden contraction of muscles. Callender suggested that the action of the deltoid muscle, in suddenly stopping the motion of the humerus, was responsible for the injury.[12] The injury has occurred in untrained athletes as a rule, and it has been reported in men and women throwing softballs, javelins, European handballs, and hand grenades.[8,17,23] The fracture is a spiral fracture of the mid or lower third humeral shaft and is sometimes comminuted.

Other Injuries

The terms "baseball finger," "cricket finger," "mallet finger," and "dropped finger" all refer to loss of extension of the distal interphalangeal joint following injury.[21] Both extensor tendon abnormalities and phalangeal fractures can produce this lesion. If a fracture is present a fragment of bone is usually noted at the dorsum of the articular margin of the distal phalanx (Fig. 187). In a series of 163 such injuries studied by Stark et al only 19 were caused by a ball.[25] The majority of injuries were produced by bumping or striking the finger on an object or on the ground. Of the ball-associated injuries only a few were due to baseballs—volleyballs, footballs, soccerballs, and basketballs were included. Some authors recommend surgery[25] and others recommend splintage.[1]

The pelvis and lower extremities of the baseball player are subject to injury as well as the arm and hand (Figs. 188, 189). The author has observed at least one injury from sliding in which the medial malleolus was fractured, the ankle dislocated, and the proximal fibula fractured[9] (Fig. 189). Godshall and Hansen reported the incomplete avulsion of a portion of the iliac apophysis in a 14-year-old male.[16] He rounded third base and suddenly reversed direction to return to third base. As he did so, he felt a sudden pain over the anterior part of the left iliac crest. Radiographs showed a separation of the anterior 2 cm of the left iliac apophysis. This healed with rest and the use of crutches.

References

1. Abouna JM, Brown H: The treatment of mallet finger. Br J Surg 55:653–667, 1968
2. Adams JE: Injury to the throwing arm. A study of traumatic changes in the elbow joints of boy baseball players. Calif Med 102:127–132, 1965
3. _____: Little League shoulder. Osteochondrosis of the proximal humeral epiphysis in boy baseball pitchers. Calif Med 105:22–25, 1966
4. _____: Bone injuries in very young athletes. Clin Orthop 58:128–140, 1968
5. _____, cited in: Little–Pony Leaguers urged to restrict use of pitchers. Hosp Trib, June 1, 1970
6. Bateman JE: Athletic injuries about the shoulder in throwing and body contact sports. Clin Orthop 23:75–83, 1962
7. Bennett GE: Shoulder and elbow lesions of the professional baseball pitcher. JAMA 117:510–514, 1941
8. Bingham EL: Fractures of the humerus from muscular violence. US Armed Forces Med J 10:22–25, 1959
9. Bowerman JW, McDonnell EJ: Radiology of athletic injuries: baseball. Radiology 116:611–615, 1975

10. Brewer BJ: Injury to the shoulder in throwing sports. Proceedings of the Sixth National Conference on the Medical Aspects of Sports, AMA Committee on Medical Aspects of Sports, Division of Socio-Economic Activities, Miami Beach, Fla, Nov, 29, 1964

11. Brogdon BG, Crow NE: Little Leaguer's elbow. Am J Roentgenol 83:671 675, 1960

12. Callender CL, cited by Weseley MS, Barenfeld PA. Ball thrower's fracture of the humerus. Clin Orthop 64:153–156, 1969

13. Dively RL, Meyer PW: Baseball shoulder. JAMA 171:1659–1661, 1959

14. Dotter WE: Little League shoulder fracture of the proximal humeral epiphyseal cartilage due to baseball pitching. Guthrie Clin Bull 23:68–72, 1953

15. Godshall RW, Hansen CA: Traumatic ulnar neuropathy in adolescent baseball pitchers. J Bone Joint Surg 53A:359–361, 1971

16. _____, Hansen CA: Incomplete avulsion of a portion of the iliac epiphysis, an injury to young athletes. J Bone Joint Surg 55A:1301–1302, 1973

17. Gregersen HN: Fracture of the humerus from muscular violence. Acta Orthop Scand 42:506–512, 1971

18. Hale CJ: Injuries among 771,810 Little League baseball players. J Sports Med Phys Fitness 1:80–83, 1963

19. King JW, cited in: Tribune sports report: two-thirds of pro pitchers seen with pathologic elbow. Hosp Trib, p 23, June 2, 1969

20. King JW, Brelsford HJ, Tullos HS: Analysis of the pitching arm of the professional baseball pitcher. Clin Orthop 67:116–123, 1969

21. Leading article: Dropped finger. Lancet 2:958–959, 1968

22. Meancy T: Personal communication

23. Peltokallio P, Peltokallio V, Vaalasti T: Fractures of the humerus from muscular violence in sport. J Sports Med Phys Fitness 8:21–25, 1968

24. Slocum DB: Classification of elbow injuries from baseball pitching. Tex Med 64:48, 1968

25. Stark HH, Boyers JH, Wilson JN: Mallet finger. J Bone Joint Surg 44A:1061–1068, 1962

26. Tullos HS, King JW: Lesions of the pitching arm in adolescents. JAMA 220:264–271, 1972

27. _____, Erwin WD, Woods GW, et al: Unusual lesions of the pitching arm. Clin Orthop 88:169–182, 1972

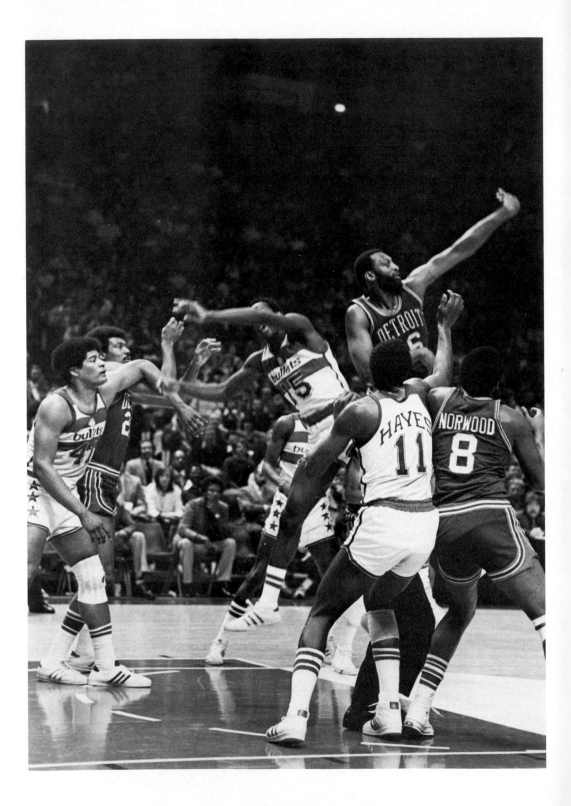

BASKETBALL

Several studies suggest that the ankle sprain is the most common injury to the basketball player.[1,3,4] Lunceford pointed out that the injury usually occurs under the backboard during the process of rebounding the ball.[4] Finger injuries, including sprains, fractures, and dislocations, are also common in his experience.

Blazina and Westover reported ankle abnormality in a high proportion of freshman college basketball candidates at the University of California at Los Angeles.[1] Nearly one-third showed bony spurs of the anterior talus at the ankle joint on x-ray. Almost half of 44 athletes examined as first-year candidates for the football and basketball teams had abnormal ankle joints.

The findings in 13 professional basketball players who were injured were reviewed by Spence and the author.[3] Knee and ankle injuries had an equal incidence (five each) and were the main sites of complaint (Figs. 190–193). Four players had recent or prior surgery for knee meniscus tears. Two had surgical repair for a ruptured Achilles tendon. Six players had either recent or prior ankle injury or both. The majority of these players showed spurs at the margins of the talus, especially at its dorsal margin on ankle radiographs (Fig. 193). One player collided with an opponent's knee and sustained multiple rib fractures and a pneumothorax (Fig. 122).

Many are not aware of the frequency of x-ray findings of chronic ankle joint abnormality in basketball players. Morris[6] and, later, McMurray[5] reported similar findings in soccer players. They considered the spurs and degenerative changes to be a direct result of kicking the ball with the dorsum of the foot and the term "footballers ankle" was used by McMurray.[5] It is likely that the common features of basketball and soccer, such as running with sudden stops, changes of pace and direction, and jumping, account for the stress to the ankle and foot. The dorsal surface of the talus is the anchor site for part of the capsule of the ankle joint. Capsular tears and tears of the ligamentous covering of the dorsal surface of the talonavicular joint are the likely mechanisms involved. Two of McMurray's patients returned to world class soccer after removal of bone spurs that were intracapsular.

There are several other areas of injury in the basketball player that are worth consideration. Patellar or quadriceps tendonitis (the so-called jumper's knee), Achilles tendonitis, and stress fractures of the tibia are mentioned by

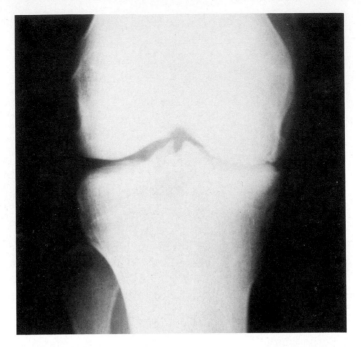

Fig. 190. This abnormal knee radiograph would not be very remarkable in an elderly person. The knee, however, belongs to a 23-year-old university athlete who was able to achieve All-American status in basketball. The findings of premature degenerative changes with joint space narrowing and spur formation have also been observed in squash and football players.

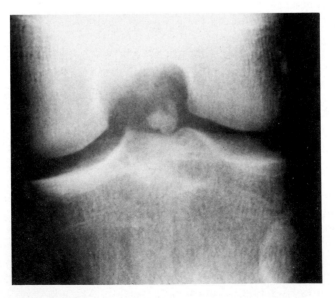

Fig. 191. This zone of ossification appeared after repeated knee injury in a professional basketball player. The ossification was subsequently removed at surgery and was found in the tissue of the patellar tendon. Tendon injury in the anterior portion of the knee was followed by hemorrhage and ossification. This represents one of the types of tendon and bone injury in the quadriceps mechanism that are collectively referred to as "jumper's knee."

162

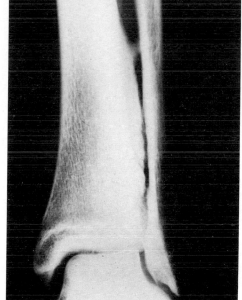

Fig. 192. The irregular projections of bone along the lateral margin of the tibia have formed following hemorrhage along the interosseous membrane. The injury occurred as this center in basketball severely sprained his ankle, producing a tibiofibular diastasis several months prior to the time of this radiograph.

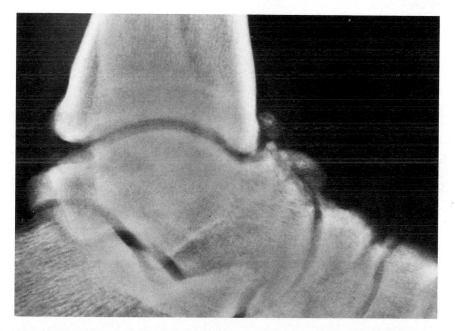

Fig. 193. Marked spur formation at the dorsal margin of the talus is shown in this professional center in basketball. This post-traumatic spur formation has been reported previously in college basketball and football players and in professional soccer players. The sudden stopping, starting, and changing of direction required at advanced levels of these sports are likely causes of the spur formation. The capsule of the ankle joint attaches at this talar margin.

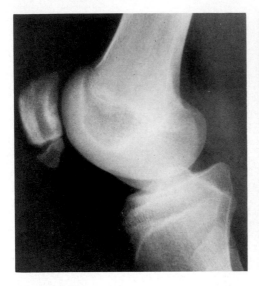 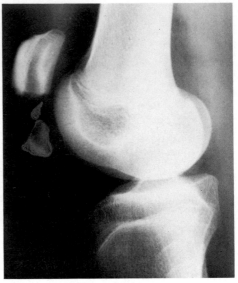

Fig. 194. A fall while jumping in basketball produced an avulsion injury to the patella of this young man. The lower pole is separated as a fracture fragment. The injury did not occur as a direct blow to the patella.

Fig. 195. The same player as shown in Figure 194 subsequently injured the opposite knee. A patellar fragment is shown following another fracture that occurred in an off-balance landing while jumping in basketball. There was no direct blow to the patella, although such a blow is the usual cause of patellar fracture.

Blazina et al.[2] In a 17-year period they estimated that they encountered 300 players with partial or complete rupture of the patellar or quadriceps tendon. The majority (186) had pain only after activity; however, 18 had pain during and after play at basketball and 4 had pain all the time. Achilles tendon problems plagued another 33 players. Eight of these players had a prolonged period of pain and discomfort in the Achilles tendon prior to rupture. The number of players with tibial stress fracture is not stated. Most of these athletes had been misdiagnosed as having soft tissue injury or shin splints. Serial x-rays eventually showed periosteal new bone formation in the form of periosteal thickening along the medial border of the tibia. The authors recommended modification of activity, arch supports, and physical therapy as treatment. Cast treatment was not employed. Jumping motions can be so forceful that avulsion fractures of the patella occur from the contraction of the quadriceps muscle (Figs. 194, 195).

Eye injury can be disastrous in basketball. It seems from a few incidents that the most vulnerable players are the forwards and the centers; they are most apt to be in the middle of furious scrambles for the ball that is rebounding or in flight at eye level. The author knows of at least two players at forward and center who have suffered this type of injury—in one there was a permanent loss of vision in one eye. Park et al reported a rare example of complete loss of vision in the left eye of a basketball player.[7] He complained of immediate complete loss of vision after being jabbed with an opponent's finger. Interestingly, his eye showed no external signs of injury. A rotational and dislocating force had been transmitted to the globe and optic nerve. This led to immediate vitreous hemorrhage, retinal edema, and laceration of the optic nerve.

The question of eye protection is again raised. The development of suitable safety glasses or goggles should help this predicament. Players, parents, coaches, and trainers must be warned of this hazard.

References

1. Blazina ME, Westover JL: Ankle joints of freshman college athletes. Clin Orthop 42:73–80, 1965
2. ————, Fox JM, Carlson GJ: Basketball injuries. In Craig TT (ed): The Medical Aspects of Sports, Vol 15. Chicago, AMA, 1975, pp 50–52
3. Bowerman JW, Spence K: Unpublished data
4. Lunceford EM Jr: Basketball. In Armstrong JR, Tucker WE (eds): Injury in Sport. London, Staples, 1964, pp 155–158
5. McMurray TP: Footballer's ankle. J Bone Joint Surg 32B:68–69, 1950
6. Morris LH: Athletes ankle. J Bone Joint Surg 25B:220, 1943
7. Park JH, Frenkel M, Dobbie JG, Choromokos E: Evulsion of the optic nerve. Am J Ophthalmol 72:969–971, 1971

BICYCLING

In 1967 the number of Americans using bicycles was estimated at 60 million.[2] The number of bicycles sold in the United States doubled between 1955 and 1966 from 3 to 6 million. Annually, 7000 lives were lost in pedal cycling accidents and 120,000 to 150,000 disabling injuries occurred. In 1971 the estimated total of injuries was placed at 1 million annually, including 120,000 fractures and 60,000 concussions.[10] Nearly three-fourths of the deaths are in the 5- to 14-year-old age group, and 90 percent of these youngsters are boys.[2] The great majority of the deaths are due to collisions with motor vehicles and involve errors on the part of the cyclist such as failure to yield the right of way, improper turning, etc. These tragic deaths and frequent injuries deserve more comment in terms of public safety announcements. Bicycle safety classes could become a requisite for bicycle owners.

McDermott surveyed the records of the emergency department at the University of Washington Hospital in Seattle for evidence of bicycle injury. Although the sample was small, he found that 4 percent of patients presenting in the emergency department after bicycle injury died of the effects of injury.[8] McDermott and Wood then studied bicycle injuries reported over a one-year period by the Seattle–King County area chapter of the Emergency Department Nurses Association.[8] A total of 613 cases were collected in this manner from various departments of the area hospitals. The age groupings of the injured featured 380 patients ages 4 to 14, 92 ages 15 to 20, 64 ages 21 to 30, and 52 over the age of 31. The injuries occurred as the bicyclist fell off the bicycle (480 patients), collided with an automobile (81), hit a motorcycle (2), hit another bicycle (3), caught the lower extremity in the spokes (3), or was caught in the chain (5). Nearly half the injuries involved soft tissues only, but 134 of the 613 injuries were fractures. The forearm (44 fractures) and the shoulder (39 fractures, including 29 fractures of the clavicle) were particularly vulnerable. The three deaths in the series had unusual aspects. One was a fatal cranial and thoracic injury as a result of a collision between a motorcyclist and a bicyclist. Another involved a fatal head injury in an elderly cyclist. The third victim was a 6-year-old child who was fatally injured at night.

In addition to the more severe injuries to bicyclists, there are other hazards of cycling. An uncommon overuse injury experienced by bicyclists is "handlebar palsy."[1,3,9] This is a neuropathy secondary to trauma of the deep palmar branch of the ulnar nerve. There is usually weakness and wasting in the intrinsic muscles of the hand without sensory involvement.[3] Cyclists and factory workers may experience this injury from pressure on handlebars or on industrial tools.

The case of a 22-year-old student who developed bilateral vulnar neuropathy on the tenth day of an ambitious bicycle trip was reported by Eckman et al.[1] In 30 days he crossed the United States and covered approximately 3000 miles. He noticed weakness in both hands without any sensory disturbance. On physical examination there was atrophy of the dorsal interossei, the abductor digiti minimi, and the abductor pollicis muscles. He was advised to abstain from cycling and improved as he did so. He showed less weakness and atrophy on a follow-up examination several months later. Hodges cites paresthesia of the pudendal nerve as a similar compression neuropathy in bicyclists.[4] This is produced by pressure on the perineum by the narrow saddles of bicycles and is manifested by scrotal and penile hypesthesia in the male.

Several riders complained of complex features of the bicycles such as the brakes and gears. Difficulty in controlling these features was directly related to many injuries. McDermott and Wood emphasize that simplicity in bicycle operation is needed as well as improvement of bicycle codes and the education of the public in these matters.[8]

While spoke injuries were not common in the emergency-room-oriented study by McDermott and Wood,[8] they have been severe enough to warrant special consideration. Izant et al reported experience with 60 patients under 14 years of age over a four-year period.[7] In nearly all cases the injury occurred while two children were on a bicycle built for one. The entrapped foot of the passenger suffers lacerations from the knifelike action of the spoke, crushing from the wheel and frame of the bicycle, and shearing from both forces combined. The widespread extent of soft tissue damage may not be immediately apparent. Debridement, elevation of the extremity, non–weight-bearing, and frequent dressing changes are suggested as the mainstays of treatment. Occasionally skin grafting is required.

Howell has recently reported an increasing incidence of craniofacial trauma related to bicycles with small front wheels, low-set front axles, long narrow seats, and high wide handlebars.[6] Two types of facial injury were described: fractures of the mandible, usually bilateral, from falls on the chin, and maxillofacial and nasal injuries, usually unilateral, due to falls on the side of the face. Eight cases (seven children and one adult) were described in which the rider was thrown over the handlebars when the progress of the front wheel was abruptly halted.

Unfortunately, some bicyclists are injured in stunt riding. Horwitz et al suggest that this practice is on the upsurge and is related to the publicity generated by the daredevil feats of Evil Knievel.[5] They noted an increase in bicycle accidents treated at the Long Island Jewish–Hillside Medical Center in the two-week period following the nationally telecast motorcycle-rocket jump at the Snake River Canyon in Idaho. A case history mentioned in this report is that of an 11-year-old boy who had always been a leader in his group of friends. He suffered a concussion, multiple abrasions of the face and arms, and a hematoma of the left eye lid when he fell while attempting to jump five automobile tires after bicycling up a wooden ramp.

References

1. Eckman PB, Perlstein G, Altrocchi PH: Ulnar neuropathy in bicycle riders. Arch Neurol 32:130–131, 1975
2. Editorial: Cycling fatalities on the rise. Stat Bull Metropol Life Ins Co 48:4–6, 1967
3. Finelli PF: Letter to the editor regarding handlebar palsy. N Engl J Med 292:702, 1975
4. Hodges SC: Letter to the editor regarding handlebar palsy. N Engl J Med 292:702, 1975
5. Horwitz J, Furman G, Nussbaum M, Shenker IR: Dangers of stunt riding. N Engl J Med 291:1194–1195, 1974
6. Howell TR: Accidents and those bizarre bicycles. Pediatrics 42:214, 1968
7. Izant RJ Jr, Rothman FB, Frankel VH: Bicycle spoke injuries of the foot and ankle in children: an underestimated "minor" injury. J Pediatr Surg 4:645–656, 1969
8. McDermott JE, Wood PA: Personal communication
9. Smail DF: Letter to the editor regarding handlebar palsy. N Engl J Med 292:322, 1975
10. Waller JA: The dangers of the bicycle. N Engl J Med 285:747–748, 1971

BOBSLEDDING

Allaria gathered information on prior reports of injuries in this sport.[1] He cited Fischer's report of 1909 that referred to a fractured pelvis and genital injury as typical bobsled injuries. In addition, Allaria reported 46 fractures, 5 dislocations, 16 bruises and sprains, and 7 lacerations in bobsledders. Eight patients had multiple fractures and four fractures were compound injuries. One 34-year-old man was injured fatally when he sustained a compound fracture of the frontal bone and nasal and mandibular fractures. Another example illustrated in his report is a severely comminuted, compound fracture of the proximal tibia and fibula. This injury, and another in which eight ribs were fractured, was produced by the skates of the bobsled hitting the individual in a fall from the sled. A fracture and dislocation of the cervical spine occurred in another sledder, 32 years of age, after he was crushed by the tumbling sled. Allaria mentions that sled speeds of 150 km per hour have been recorded at Alpe d'Huez, France.

Fry documented injury to 198 patients who were injured in sledding or tobogganing in Tahoe Valley, Calif., between 1967 and 1969.[2] Only 17 injuries occurred in controlled and relatively safe sledding areas. Of a total of 129 fractures there were 61 fractures of the spine, including 16 at the first lumbar vertebral body and 15 at the T-12 level.

Ryan recorded a fatality in Olympic bobsledding the 1964 Winter Games at Innsbruck.[3] A member of the British team went off the run on his sled and ruptured his aorta when he struck a tree.

References

1. Allaria A: Bobsleigh trauma. In Johanson O (ed): Sport and Health, Proceedings of the International Conference on Sport and Health, Oslo, 1952. Oslo, Royal Norwegian Ministry of Education State Office for Sport and Youth Work, 1952, pp 165–172
2. Fry PJ, cited in: Snow sledding sport on rise, hazards worse than skiing. Hosp Trib p 21, Jan 26, 1970
3. Ryan AJ: History of sports medicine. In Ryan AJ, Allman FL Jr (eds): Sports Medicine. New York, Academic, 1974, pp 13–29

BOWLING

There were 23 cases of "bowler's thumb," or ulnovolar neuroma, reported in five articles between 1965 and 1972.[1,2,4-6] The mechanism of injury is apparently related to trauma to the digital nerve from the edge of the hole in the ball.

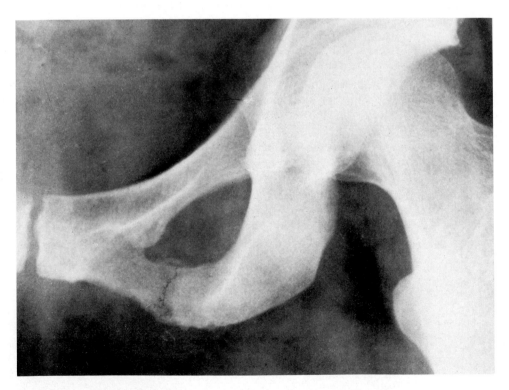

Fig. 196. A woman complained of chronic groin pain after bowling. She experienced maximum pain as she released the ball and ended her delivery motion at the foul line. The cortical interruption of the inferior pubic ramus represents a stress fracture. This occurred without systemic disease and is a most unusual finding secondary to bowling. (From Murray, Jacobson: The Radiology of Skeletal Disorders, 1971. Courtesy of Churchill Livingstone)

A proliferation of fibrous tissue occurs, and in some instances surgery is beneficial. Dobyns et al reported in 1972 that at least 20 million people regularly participate in bowling in the United States.[1] A variety of minor thumb and finger abnormalities occur after repeated bowling, including enlargement of the long and ring fingers and callous formation.

Although bowling is certainly a sport of little hazard, Hoon has reported three examples of acute avulsion injuries of the adductor muscles in bowlers.[3] The adductor muscle attachment zone at the inferior pubic ramus is rarely the site of stress fracture (Fig. 196). Each injury discussed in Hoon's paper occurred in a middle-aged man who either slipped or stopped suddenly while delivering the ball at the foul line. Each man overstressed the origin of an adductor muscle that was called upon suddenly in a moment of imbalance. One of these bowlers required surgery for his injury, which included rupture of the origin of the adductor longus, avulsion of part of the inferior pubic ramus, and laceration of the vessels to the right testis. The extent of injury to the spermatic cord and testis was such that removal of these structures was mandatory.

References

1. Dobyns JH, O'Brien ET, Linscheid RL, Farrow GM: Bowler's thumb, diagnosis and treatment. A review of 17 cases. J Bone Joint Surg 54A:751–755, 1972
2. Dunham W, Haines G, Spring JM: Bowler's thumb (ulnovolar neuroma of the thumb). Clin Orthop 83:99–101, 1972
3. Hoon JR: Adductor muscle injuries in bowlers. JAMA 171:145–147, 1959
4. Howell AE, Leach RE: Bowler's thumb, perineural fibrosis of the digital nerve. J Bone Joint Surg 52A:377–378, 1970
5. Minkow FV, Bassett FH: Bowler's thumb. Clin Orthop 83:115–117, 1972
6. Siegel IM: Bowling thumb neuroma. JAMA 192:263, 1965

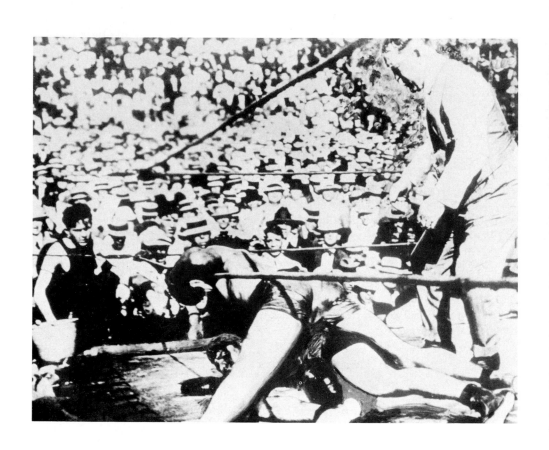

BOXING

The array of reports of injuries in boxing is centered about head injury. The hazards are greatest to the professional boxer or to the athlete with a prolonged amateur career. Amateur boxing has a relatively injury-free record. Novich has recently shown that no serious injuries occurred in 771 United States Amateur National Championship matches.[14] He cited a 1973 report from the Canadian Amateur Boxing Association that included 1030 bouts with an injury list of 24 eye contusions, 10 nosebleeds, 4 lacerations, and 1 fractured arm. During the 1963 Olympics there were 301 bouts and 305 boxers. There were three knock-outs, with no recognized aftereffects. Six boxers were conscious but late for the count. Five bouts were stopped because of lacerations, and there was one fractured fibula and one fractured nose.

Despite the recognition of cumulative trauma to the head, it is interesting to note that protective headgear is not yet required in Olympic and professional bouts. Information on chronic head injury in professional boxers has come from several sources. Martland is generally credited with the first important description of the "punch drunk" syndrome.[12] He observed the condition most often in fighters of the slugging type, who are usually poor boxers and take considerable head punishment in seeking to land a knockout blow. He also found it common in second-rate fighters used for training purposes. Boxing enthusiasts refer to such boxers as "cuckoo," "goofy," "cutting paper dolls," or "slug nutty."

The early symptoms are mental confusion and slight unsteadiness of gait. Progressively the patient may develop leg dragging, hesitant speech, hand tremors, head nodding, expressionless facial characterisitcs of Parkinsonism, vertigo, deafness, and finally marked mental deterioration. Nearly 50 percent of veteran fighters developed some form of this condition in Martland's view. In 1936 Carroll estimated that 5 percent of men who remained in professional boxing for a period of five years or more become punch drunk.[3] He noted that approximately 60 percent of fighters working five years or more will develop mental and emotional changes that are obvious to those who know them personally. Critchley referred to the condition as chronic, progressive, post-traumatic encephalopathy.[4]

On the subject of brain damage to boxers, Potter reminds us that following a knockout blow the head may be more seriously damaged by a second injury as it strikes the floor of the ring.[15] Van Den Bergh describes pitiful exboxers

173

that he has observed at boxing gymnasia and halls.[18] He reports that they were totally unemployable and could be seen shuffling through the corridors looking for handouts or offering to run errands for a few pennies.

Between 1954 and 1969, the postmortem pathologic and antemortem pathologic and neuroradiologic changes of this condition were described. Betti and Ottino cited the 1954 study of Brandeburg and Hallevorden in which an ex-middleweight boxer who had developed post-traumatic Parkinsonism and cerebral atrophy came to autopsy.[1] The hippocampus showed senile plaques and again changes were noted in the main and its vessels. Neurons showed typical Alzheimer's degeneration. They also site similar changes in a postmortem study by Grahmann and Ule of a veteran boxer who died of a thrombosis of the superior longitudinal sinus and its parietal afferents.

In 1959 Neuberger et al showed decreased cortical neurons and increased gliosis in two postmortem studies of boxers.[13] In one of these patients there was severe atrophy of the frontal lobes. Betti and Ottino reported results of a cerebral biopsy in an exboxer who had arm tremor, gait disturbance, dysarthria, and aggressive behavior.[1] Histologically there were numerous pyknotic, frontal cortical cells and intense perivascular gliosis of the white matter. The cortex showed severe atrophy of the pyramidal cells, especially at deep layers. A thalamotomy was performed with stereotactic apparatus yielding a good result. Spillane showed that defects in the septum pellucidum, demonstrated on pneumoencephalography, were present in four of five former professional boxers.[17] Four were studied because of chronic cerebral disorders and the fifth because of violent behavior. Isherwood showed that 23 of 28 former boxers had septum pellucidum defects on pneumoencephalography.[8] In addition, four boxers were found to have cerebral atrophy on postmortem examinations. Johnson showed that 13 of the 16 boxers had cortical atrophy on pneumoencephalographic examination.[9] He found that 11 had diffuse electroencephalographic changes of the type seen in presenile, nontraumatic dementia.

Whenever a death occurs after a head injury in boxing, the call to ban the sport is raised. Fortunately, such deaths are rare. In 14 years of boxing in the Royal Air Force, United Kingdom, there were 240 injuries and 2 deaths.[2] A leading article appeared in *Lancet* in 1969 after the death of Trinidad's heavyweight champion.[11] Between 1945 and 1969, six professional boxers died after contests in Britain. In Gonzales' study of deaths related to sports in New York City over a 32-year period, there were 21 boxing deaths.[6] (Of additional interest in that study were the 43 deaths due to baseball, some of which were in the prebatting helmet and preantibiotic era, and the 22 deaths in football.)

Helpern and Strassman reported a New York City medical examiner's study of four fighters, aged 19 to 25, who died 55 hours to 9 days after knockout.[7] All were unconscious from the time of knockout until death. Each boxer died despite surgical efforts to remove hematomas. The most prominent feature of the brain at autopsy in each instance was edema. Brain tissue had herniated through drill holes in three of the cases and in the fourth case there was herniation of one side of the base of the brain through the foramen magnum. Other features noted after gross and histologic examination included small residuals of subdural hemorrhage, areas of diffuse small hemorrhage within the brain, and thrombosis of superficial and deep vessels.

The so-called boxer's fracture is actually a "fistfighter's fracture" of the fourth or fifth metacarpals.[10] Perhaps the most common fracture in a true boxer is at the proximal third of the first metacarpal.[5] Farrow once x-rayed a boxer's hand in a boxing glove.[5] The resultant radiograph showed that the fist is not markedly clenched and that the first metacarpal lies in a position in which it may be injured.

An extremely unusual boxing injury was reported by Schwartz and Rankow.[16] A 24-year-old man developed a pulsating mass below the right side of the mandible. He had been struck at this site eight years previously by a gloved fist while boxing. That day, he noticed a small mass that subsequently enlarged. A palpable thrill and continous bruit were present. A selective arteriographic examination of the right external carotid artery showed an arteriovenous fistula. The major point of supply came from the facial artery. The fistula was removed successfully at surgery.

Obviously, in boxing, as in so many other sports, close medical supervision is necessary.

References

1. Betti OO, Ottino CA: Pugilistic encephalopathy. Acta Neurol Lat Am 15:47–51, 1969
2. Brennan TNN, O'Connor PJ: Incidence of boxing injuries in the RAF in the United Kingdom, 1955–1966. Br J Ind Med 25:326–329, 1960
3. Carroll EJ Jr: Punch drunk. Am J Med Sci 191:706–711, 1936
4. Critchley M: Medical aspects of boxing. Br Med J 1:357–362, 1957
5. Farrow R: Hand injuries. In Bass AL, Blonstien JL, James RD, Williams JGP (eds): Medical Aspects of Boxing. Proceedings of Conference, British Association of Sport and Medicine, London, Nov 1963. London, Pergamon, 1965, pp 43–50
6. Gonzales TA: Fatal injuries in competitive sports. JAMA 146:1506–1511, 1951
7. Helpern M, Strassman G, cited in: The puzzling punch drunk syndrome. Roche Med Image 11:14–17, 1969
8. Isherwood I: Pneumoencephalographic changes in boxers. Acta Radiol Diagn 5:654–674, 1966
9. Johnson J: Organic psychosyndromes due to boxing. Br J Psychiatry 115:45–53, 1969
10. LaRose JH, Sik KD: Knuckle fracture, a mechanism of injury. JAMA 206:893–894, 1968
11. Leading article: Hazards of boxing. Lancet 1:764, 1969
12. Martland HS: Punch drunk. JAMA 91:1103–1107, 1928
13. Neuberger KT, Sinton DN, Denst J: Cerebral atrophy associated with boxing. Arch Neurol Psychiatr 81:403–408, 1959
14. Novich MM: What really happens in boxing? Physician Sports Med 2:28–32, April 1974
15. Potter JM: Letter to the editor regarding boxers' brain damage. Lancet 2:1270, 1974
16. Schwartz GE, Randow RM: Traumatic arteriovenous fistula of the facial artery. Plast Reconstr Surg 40:453–456, 1967
17. Spillane JD: Cerebral disorders in former boxers. Br Med J 2:1205–1210, 1962
18. Van Den Bergh T: Letter to the editor regarding boxers' brain damage. Lancet 2:1270, 1974

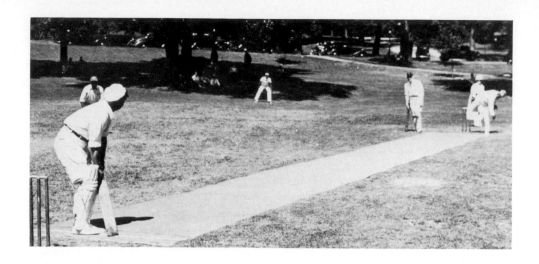

CRICKET

The hazards of cricket are not unlike those of baseball. The bowler is prone to shoulder injury and the wicketkeeper is vulnerable to finger injuries.[3,4] The ball weighs 5.5 ounces, is leather covered, and contains a hard cork composition material. Fielding in cricket is done barehanded and finger injuries are not uncommon. Batting in cricket is done without a protective helmet and usually with a light cap or bareheaded. Pye mentions that during the 1963 tour of the West Indian National Team one of their fast bowlers hit three batsmen on the head.[4] Two other batsmen had fractured wrists from bowled cricket balls.

A friend told the author that while umpiring he was hit by a batted ball and suffered a fractured skull.[1] Murray displayed an example of pelvic stress related to the forceful leg swinging and body torque in the motions of bowling performed by an All-England bowler.[2] The symphysis pubis became unstable and the instability was evident on stress–weight-bearing views of the symphysis. Vere-Hodge grouped injuries in cricket into three categories: (1) the usual muscle strains related to fast movement; (2) contusions and fractures from the ball; and (3) certain injuries related to special activity in cricket.[5] In the third group he included tendonitis of the supraspinatus tendon in bowlers and fatigue or stress fractures of the second metatarsal bone of the left foot of right-handed bowlers. The metatarsal fracture occurs as a result of the great force with which the foot is thrust down in bowling. Those not familiar with cricket should be reminded that the bowler runs toward the batsman before releasing the ball.

References

1. Hazra T: Personal communication, 1973
2. Murray RO: Personal communication, 1972
3. Petal MA: Game for the gritty. Physician Sports Med 2:79–80, 1974
4. Pye DW: Physiotherapy in cricket. Physiotherapy 51:121–124, 1965
5. Vere-Hodge N: Inuries in cricket. In Armstrong JR, Tucker WE (eds): Injury in Sport. London, Staples, 1964, pp 168–172

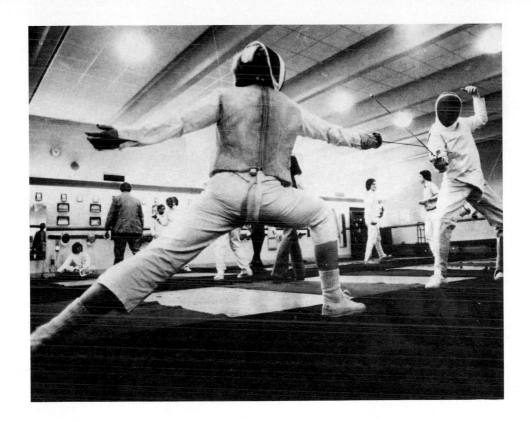

FENCING

Parfitt described three fatal accidents in fencing.[1] In one a blade broke and the sharp edge of the remaining portion penetrated the chest of a contestant in the 1937 World University Championship in Paris. In a second fatal case a blade plunged through the axilla of a fencer and penetrated the right lung, mediastinum, and left lung. This too occurred in a World Championship in Sweden in 1951. A third example is mentioned in which a broken blade pierced a mask. Minor musculotendenous arm, elbow, and back injuries are common, according to Parfitt, and include tears of the supraspinatus tendon at the shoulder in sabreurs, whose shoulder movements are wider than fencers using the foil or epee.

Reference

1. Parfitt R: The fencer at risk. In Armstrong JR, Tucker WE (eds): Injury in Sport. London, Staples, 1964, pp 173–190

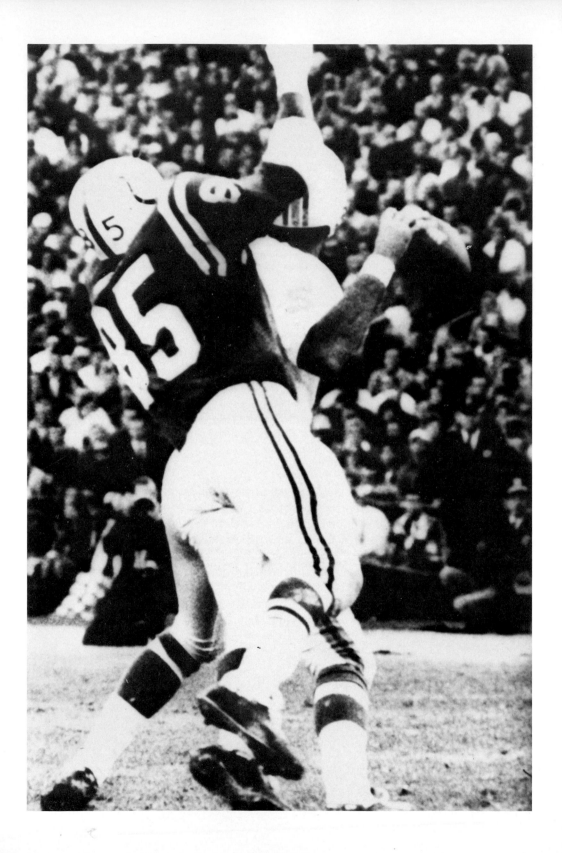

FOOTBALL

Amateur

The North American game of football is played by various age groups beginning with pre–high school children. According to Keefe, in 1965 more than 800,000 American children participated.[24] Castellanos and Green report that few injuries are observed at this level of competition.[11] Knee, ankle, shoulder, rib, and head injuries have been observed without a recorded fatality. Their study, based on participation as physicians to the Optimist Football League of Dade County, Miami, Fla., emphasizes concern for psychologic trauma that might be inflicted by overbearing coaches or parents, in disregard of the child's interest in playing for the sake of play alone.

Consider next what can happen to the pre–high school student if he continues to play football in high school. Data provided by two studies show that approximately one in five players will be injured each year.[18] A serious injury will occur in 1 in 13. Garrahan studied players in Rhode Island over a six-year period and compared his findings with those of McClellan in Ohio.[18] In 1965, Garrahan noted 575 total injuries in 2000 participants. Serious injuries (undefined) totaled 201. In 1964 McClellan recorded 550 total injuries in 2826 participants, including 210 potentially serious injuries. In the Rhode Island players, knee injuries ranged from 12 to 18 percent of all injuries, hand injuries were second in incidence at 12 percent, and ankle injuries were third at 8 percent.

In college football, two subgroups of play should be considered: intramural touch football and intercollegiate football. Touch football is perhaps a misnomer because the word *touch* implies a delicate use of the hands. This sport is in no way delicate. Play is usually without helmets, padding, or special footwear except for the use of cleated shoes in some leagues. Touch refers to the action of touching the ball carrier instead of tackling as in American football or rugby.

During the 1966 touch football season at the University of Minnesota, 283 injured players were observed in a group of 2650 students.[25] An injury rate of 1 in every 12 players occurred; 14 players had two separate injuries. Of the 297 total injuries, 160 (nearly 54 percent) were considered serious, including severe sprains, contusions, fractures, and head injuries. More than 7 percent of the injured players required hospitalization. Students with a history of a disabling injury in high school sports had a much higher injury rate than did players without such a history. The risk of foot and leg injuries was twice as great for players who wore touch football shoes (usually rubber cleated) than for those who wore ordinary tennis shoes. The authors note that "while the shoe gives the player a greater ability to stop quickly or turn sharply, these maneuvers may place unaccustomed stress on the foot, ankle, leg, or knee, thereby causing injury."

Injuries in intercollegiate football have not been studied extensively. A few reports do contain information regarding injuries to the spine and head in college players.[8,12,37] Schneider studied in detail the serious and fatal injuries of the spine and head collected by the Committee on Injuries and Fatalities of the American Football Coaches Association from 1959 to 1963.[37] Of a total of 225 such injuries (45 per year) occurring in all phases of organized football, there were 34 in college players. The total number of college players was estimated at 70,000 for that five-year period. The two major subcategories of injury in the total of 225 were subdural hematoma (69 cases with 28 deaths) and spine–spinal cord injury (78 cases with 16 deaths). Of additional concern in the latter category was a group of 56 cases with cervical spine fracture–dislocations in which 30 young men survived, but with complete paralysis. Greater than 88 percent of the entire study group—ie, collegiate and noncollegiate players—wore current equipment and could be presumed to be well equipped. The state of equipment design was not sufficient to prevent the injuries sustained.

Chrisman et al studied injuries to the neck over a five-year period (1959 to 1963) at Amherst College and at the University of Massachusetts.[12] The predominant group of neck injuries was described as being of the "nerve pinch" type, that is, a lateral flexion injury of the neck with nerve contusion or partial injury due to stretching. The symptoms are produced on the side on which the force is applied. There were 22 examples recorded, with 17 in football, 2 in basketball, and 1 each in wrestling, track (pit fall), and squash (collision against the sidewall). Each injury was similar, with neck and shoulder ache and neurologic changes in the arm. Some players showed decreased biceps or triceps reflexes and had numbness in the forearm for several months. Muscle weakness in the arm was common and persisted for more than six months in the majority of the injured. In three players, extensor–supination weakness and limitation of motion of the neck (toward the side of the injury) were present three years after the injury. These three also showed spur formation on cervical spine radiographs. Bateman has described similar injuries as those affecting the acromion–mastoid dimension, ie, between the top of the shoulder and the lower tip of the ear.[5] One would expect no positive x-ray finding on plain radiographs in such injuries. However, myelography of the cervical spine in severe injuries might show positive findings. The author has seen avulsion injury of nerve roots shown by myelography after a motorcycling accident. Contrast material leaked out into the area of the torn nerve root. (See the chapter on the cervical spine in Part I.)

Ferguson et al reported low back pain and abnormalities on lumbar spine radiographs in college football players.[17] Each of the players was an interior lineman accustomed to playing in a crouched stance with marked lumbar spine flexion and marked stress on sudden tension of the spine in blockage. Of the 25 interior linemen of the University of Pittsburgh team, 12 sought medical help for lower back pain in one year. Six of these players showed either spondylolisis or spondylolysthesis or both on x-ray examinations. Neurologic examinations were normal in each player.

Reid et al did a study of brain tolerance to impact in college football.[33] A single subject, a middle linebacker for the Northwestern University team in the 1970 season, was equipped with a special helmet. The helmet contained impact tranducers mounted on the suspension system at the midoccipital and at both temporal areas. Electrodes were sealed to the scalp with collodion and additional circuitry was mounted on the back of the player's shoulder pads. The transducer system was designed to serve as a measure of linear acceleration after brain impact. Electronic signals were detected in a receiver module in the stadium during play. The instrumented player participated in 418 plays of the seven conference games in 1970. He received 169 measured impacts on the head and peak accelerations ranged between 40 and 230 g forces with a time duration range between 20 and 420 msec. Almost all impacts had an appreciable frontal component. One of the five high-intensity impacts between 188 and 230 g forces produced a concussion. This force measured 188 g and lasted 310 msec. It is significant that such a study is feasible and can provide a quantitative indication of the extensive impact forces. The linkage of this method to the testing of new helmet designs would be an obvious step toward better head protection.

Rall et al submitted a questionnaire designed to gather information on the effects of knee injury to 350 former and present members of the University of Missouri football team.[31] Most of the players attended the university between 1954 and 1964 but a few dated back as much as 30 years. Radiographs of the knees were obtained in 44 of these players and 205 individuals contributed information in the questionnaire. This response group had a mean age of 28 years and an age range of 19 to 60 years. Repeated injury to the knee occurred during the playing careers of 105 players (51 percent). Persistent symptoms and radiographic changes of degenerative joint disease were reported in 83 of the injured (79 percent). The abnormal radiographic findings in the 44-player sample included degenerative joint disease (37 players, 84 percent) and ligamentous instability (14 players, 32 percent). The instability was judged by abnormal widening of the medial aspect of the joint space in comparison with x-ray films of the opposite side. The authors registered a plea for measures to reduce this "inordinate incidence of disability."

Allen reported the football injuries during two seasons (1965 and 1966) in players of the United States Air Force stationed at Clarke Air Base in the Phillippines.[2] The ages of the players are not stated but can be considered to be similar to the players of college age. The number of players competing was 465 and there was a total of 290 injuries. There were 16 abrasions–lacerations, 86 contusions, 42 strains (injuries adjacent to joints), 88 sprains (joint injuries), 10 dislocations, 18 fractures, and 38 miscellaneous injuries. The knee was the most frequently injured site and sprains were the most common type of disabling injury. There were no serious head injuries and no fatalities. Part of the fracture group included one at the spine, five of the ankle, one at the knee, and six at the forearm, wrist, and hand. Two of the ten dislocations were dislocations of the ankle.

If this report is a representative sample of football trauma in the armed services, then it seems that injuries are not uncommon and involved the majority of players. Of the total of 290 injuries in 465 men, 111 were considered major injuries: 38 players were hospitalized, 22 were operated upon, and 65 received injuries such that they were not able to finish the season.

Professional

What is the risk of injury to the professional player? Here a special set of circumstances is present. The players are a carefully selected group and they are outstanding in categories of desire, size, weight, speed, and skill. In addition, their livelihoods depend on avoidance of injury—in practice, in games, and away from their work. Craig calculated the exposure time to injury in game play in professional football by timing the length of each play in 11 games.[14] Active playing time constituted 22.6 percent (±0.7) of official time. Kicking plays—kickoffs and punts—had longer mean durations than running or passing plays. Field goals had the shortest mean duration, followed by running plays. Craig stated that the individual exposure time to possible injury averages 6.8 minutes per game if we assume that a player participates in an entire game working on either offense or defense.

From reports of injury, we know that significant injury can occur in those brief periods of time (Table 2). Virgin reported that in one year he had performed 11 knee operations on footballers.[26] Pisani, former team surgeon for the New York Giants, said that on one occasion in 1964, with a roster of 40 play-

TABLE 2. Common Sites for Radiographic Examinations in Professional Football Players*

Site	Number of Players with Injury
Knee	116
Hand and Fingers	56
Lumbar Spine	36
Shoulder	31
Cervical Spine	29
Ribs	28
Ankle	25

*These athletes were examined in one orthopedic practice between 1930 and 1968. (Courtesy of Dr. E. J. McDonnell)

ers, 28 were out because of injury and convalescence for six weeks or longer.[26] (The Giant's record for that year: won 1 game, lost 12, tied 1.) In 1970, overall league records indicated that of the 1222 players available to 26 professional teams more than 8 percent would undergo surgery in that year, predominantly for knee repair.[16]

Fortunately, fatalities are rare in professional and semiprofessional football. In Blyth and Arnold's annual survey of fatalities directly related to football there have been 15 deaths in the past 20 years in the pro and semipro ranks.[8] In 1973, there were no fatalities in this group, although there were two in sandlot football and seven in high school football. Their data are divided into direct fatalities and indirect fatalities. The former are those deaths directly related to participation in football, ie, collision or contact injury. The indirect fatalities are related to a body system failure as a result of exertion, eg, heat stroke. In 1973, there were eight indirect fatalities due to football. Since 1931, when such records were first kept, the majority of indirect fatalities have been related to heart failure, infections, and heat stroke. In the direct category, nearly 60 percent of all football deaths are due to head injury, nearly 19 percent are due to spinal injury, and nearly 18 percent are due to abdominal injury. For the time period 1931 to 1973, the average incidence of direct fatalities per 100,000 players is 1.6 for high school footballers and 2.51 for college footballers.

The work of Blyth and Arnold,[8] Schneider,[37] and others[36] has led in some areas to increased effort in strengthening neck muscles in an effort to reduce head and neck injuries, to enforcement of rules prohibiting "spearing" (the use of the head as a battering ram), and to emphasis on the need for improvement in helmet design.

The author had the opportunity to review the x-rays of a group of professional football players evaluated for injury by McDonnell.[10] There were 33 injuries in 25 players on one team evaluated over a period of several years. In looking for a pattern of injury it was found that there was no pattern per se and that injuries occurred from head to foot (Figs. 197–201). A number of knee injuries had no x-ray abnormality on plain radiographs. Within the group of injuries with abnormal radiographs there were two important minor themes: forearm injury and lumbar spine injury. Two linebackers and one center had direct trauma to the forearm of sufficient force to fracture the radius (Fig. 199). In one of these three the distal radioulnar joint was separated as well. All three had sustained direct blows to the unpadded forearm. In four flanker backs or pass receivers there were fractures of multiple transverse processes of the lumbar spine (Figs. 200, 201). Each player gave a history of a sudden injury to the lower back, usually as a result of a forceful tackle. One of the four players had transient hematuria.

Jackson reported a similar injury in an 18-year-old football player who injured his right flank while throwing a cross-body block in a high school football game.[23] He was unable to finish the game and had warmth and swelling of the back for four weeks following injury. Lumbar spine x-rays made several weeks later showed fractures of the right third and fourth transverse processes and

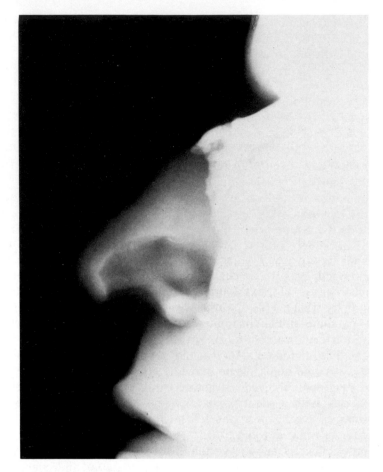

Fig. 197. The comminuted remains of a nasal bone fractured several times in football remind us of the value of the faceguard attachment to the present-day helmet. This man played in the National Football League prior to the use of the faceguard. Note how little of the nose is composed of bone. Most of the nose is made of cartilage, and this too has been fractured in this player judging from the depression in the outer profile of the nose.

bone bridging the right second, third, and fourth transverse processes. An intravenous pyelogram and urinalysis were normal. Back pain persisted for three years and led to a surgical excision of the dense body adjacent to the spine. The author considers this an example of myositis ossificans or excess callus at the transverse process fracture sites. The patient was able to resume basketball, football, and boxing without disability.

Conwell and Reynolds mention such isolated fractures of the transverse processes of the lumbar spine.[13] They state that this injury is not infrequent and is usually the result of direct trauma to the back, a fall from a height, or a sudden violent muscular exertion. A violent movement of the quadratus lumborum muscle is indicted and the second, third, and fourth transverse processes are most frequently involved.

Himmelwright[22] and, later, Garrick[19] emphasized the value of on-the-field examination of the injured athlete. Exact localization of pain and tenderness at the injury site can be accomplished with immediate examination before swelling or joint effusion complicates the picture. At some stadiums in North America, x-ray equipment is available so that rapid radiographic examination supplements the early evaluation of those injured on the playing field.

Several additional reports of injury in football have been grouped according to body site, beginning with injuries of the head and neck and continuing through the body to the foot and ankle. We must remember that the majority of such reports do not reflect the total picture of injuries but rather are a series of injury events.

Head and Neck Injury

The most detailed work on head and neck trauma in football is that of Schneider,[37] which covered high school and college players mainly. In a 1964 report that covered a five-year period he listed 225 craniospinal injuries that included skull fracture (11), extradural hematoma (5), subdural hematoma (69), intracerebral hemorrhage (14), pontine lesions (17), cerebral contusions and lacerations (17), spine–spinal cord injury (78), basilar artery thrombosis (1), and internal carotid artery thrombosis (1). Seventy-seven of these young men died.

Marks and Freed studied a 16-year-old boy who was injured while tackling a runner.[27] He became quadriplegic immediately but remained conscious. Cervical spine radiographs showed a fracture through the anterior portion of the C5 vertebral body with a slight posterior displacement of C5 on C6. After 36 hours he developed weakness of the left facial nerve distribution, bilateral palsies of the abducens nerve, tongue paralysis, aphonia, and dysphagia. Arteriography showed occlusions in both vertebral arteries. The cranial nerve sign resolved during the next two months except for residual diplopia on extreme right lateral gaze and mild dysarthria. The paraplegia was unchanged. A repeat arteriogram again showed occlusion of both vertebral arteries. The authors postulated that disruption of the spine affected the vertebral artery walls so that a clot formed within each vessel.

Borowiecki et al reported an unusual injury to the cervical esophagus and larynx associated with a dislocation of the left sternoclavicular joint.[9] The patient, a 14-year-old boy, injured the left side of his chest and left shoulder while playing sandlot football. He was running a pass pattern and was hit from the right side. The force of the blow knocked him to the ground and he tried to extend his left arm to break his fall. As he hit the ground he experienced severe sharp pain over the mid-upper chest. He was taken to a hospital on the following day, where he complained of severe pain of the left sternoclavicular joint and of pain on swallowing (odynophagia). Chest x-rays showed a widened mediastinal shadow and dislocation of the left sternoclavicular joint. On the second day after hospitalization he was unable to swallow and noted a change in the quality of his voice. He developed massive subcutaneous emphysema around the cervical esophagus, larynx, and pharynx and the cervical trachea

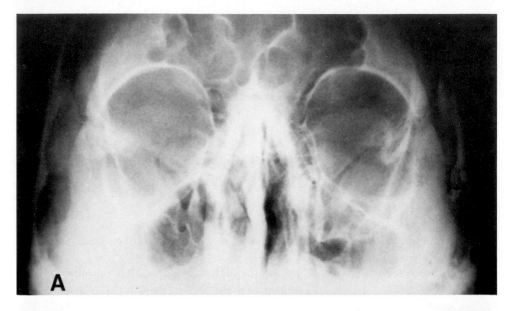

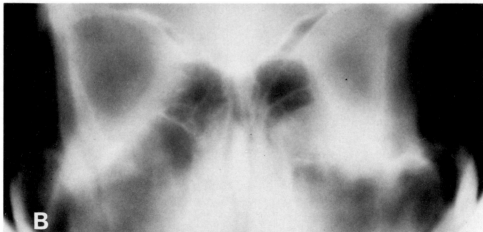

Fig. 198. A young professional football player was struck as he crossed the goal line for a touchdown. The elbow of his tackler hit his left eye as the elbow penetrated between the edge of the helmet and the upper margin of the nose guard. The patient has double vision. **A.** Waters view of the orbits. **B.** Tomographic view. The curvilinear calcification in the left eye is probably hemorrhage from an old injury. This calcification was present prior to the current injury.

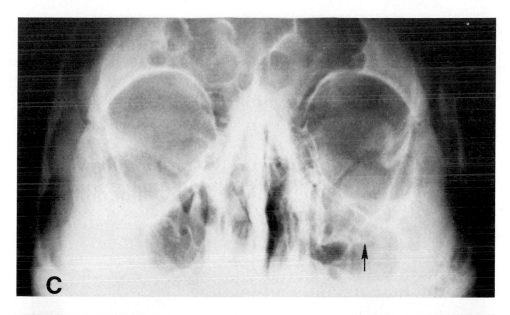

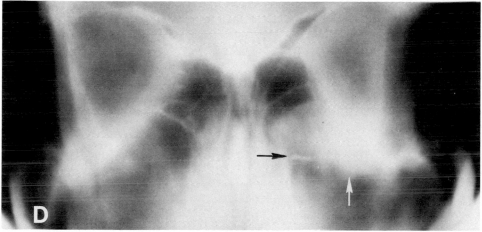

Fig. 198 *(cont.)* **C, D.** An orbital floor fracture or blow-out fracture is present at the left eye. The normal orbital floor landmarks are obliterated and a soft-tissue bulge protrudes inferiorly from the lower margin of the orbit. A fragment of bone is displaced at the medial margin of the orbital floor (horizontal arrow).

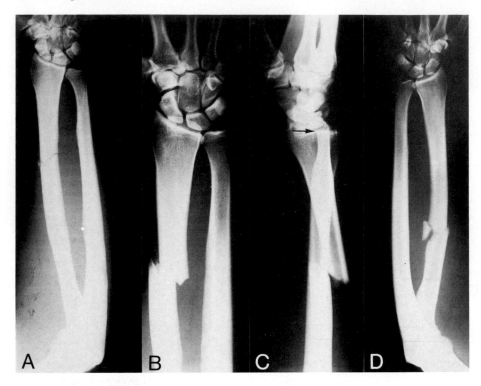

Fig. 199. A direct blow to the radius with fracture of the radius is an unusual fracture in sport. Three such fractures occurred in a group of professional football players and are shown here. In one injury (**B**) the distal radioulnar joint was disrupted and the distal ulna was displaced posteriorly at the wrist. All three injuries occurred in a time prior to the widespread use of extensive forearm padding. (From Bowerman, McDonnell: Radiology 117:34, 1975

was displaced to the right side. Three days following the injury, he developed a fever of 104 degrees and both anterior and posterior chest pain. The left arytenoid fold was found to be dislocated anteriorly on direct laryngoscopy. Esophagoscopy showed a small laceration on the left anterolateral esophageal wall at the lower portion of the cricopharyngeus muscle. Pus poured into the esophageal lumen at the tear. Surgical exploration of the left side of the neck was performed and large abscess cavities in the neck and superior mediastinum were opened. Apart from an additional episode of fever one month later that was followed by debridement of the clavicle, he made an uneventful recovery.

Arm and Hand

Aufranc et al reported a single example of a 15-year-old football player who fractured the proximal humerus at the cartilage growth plate.[3] This occurred as he blocked an opponent and fell on the left shoulder. Their report reminds us to carefully examine the growth plates on radiographs of the adolescent athlete.

Wenger reported four cases of rupture of the flexor digitorum profundus tendon of the ring finger in football and added these to Gunter's eight cases reported in rugby players from Australia.[40] The mechanism of injury is explained as an avulsion injury produced by the ring finger being caught in the jersey of an opponent. The long flexor of the ring finger allows the least independent extension of the fingers. The x-ray often shows on lateral view a tiny fracture fragment produced by a small fleck of bone avulsed just volar to the interphalangeal joint.

Blunt trauma to the chest can produce sternal fracture, rib fracture, pneumothorax, and cardiac abnormalities in football. Rose et al reported the case of a young man who was struck in the chest by the helmeted head of an opposing lineman.[36] He sustained a linear fracture of the sternum and developed pulse irregularity. An electrocardiogram showed a periodic atrioventricular block of the Wenckebach type as well as precordial V1–V4, T wave inversions, and ST segment shifts. The electrocardiographic changes disappeared predominatly. (See the chapter on the thorax and abdomen in Part I.)

Pelvis and Hip

Major muscle groups about the hip and thigh can produce large avulsion fracture fragments. (See the chapter on soft tissue injuries in Part I.) When

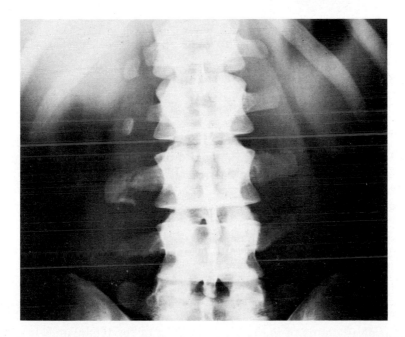

Fig. 200. Fractures of the three upper transverse processes occurred on the right side of the lumbar spine in an offensive end. They occurred as a result of blunt trauma inflicted in a tackle as he was hit by two opposing players. (From Bowerman, McDonnell: Radiology 117: 33, 1975)

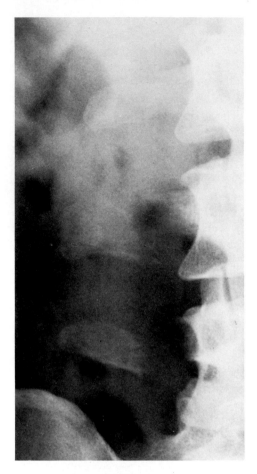

Fig. 201. This enlargement shows three fractured lumbar transverse processes damaged when a halfback was tackled. He had transient hematuria without further difficulty. (From Bowerman, McDonnell: Radiology 117: 33, 1975)

such bone margin lesions are encountered months to years after the injury they may be mistaken for neoplasm. Barnes and Hinds reported an example of a 23-year-old man who developed a 9 × 5-cm bony mass at the ischial apophysis following an injury in football six years earlier.[4] The mass was excised and showed "grossly deformed bone" on histology. Prior radiographs from the time of injury were sought and showed apophyseal injury. The authors found 39 examples in the English literature. The majority of the fragments did not unite with the pelvis. Ten were excised because of pain.

Dimon collected 30 examples of patients who had sudden sharp pain while running and developed a limp, stiffness and limited flexion of the hip, palpable tenderness of the thigh, and inability to raise a straight leg.[15] All 30 had isolated avulsion fractures of the lesser trochanter of the femur on x-ray examination. This number included 25 teenagers, and most of the patients (22) were engaged in some sports activity when the injury occurred. Seven of the injuries occurred in football players and five were in track athletes. The patients usu-

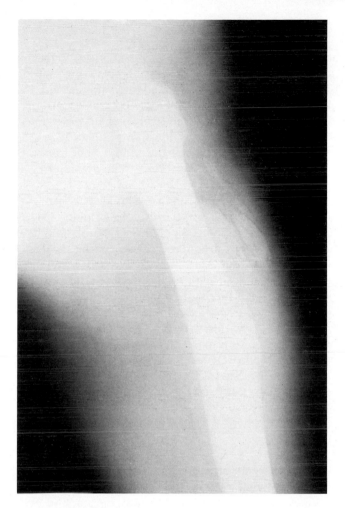

Fig. 202. An offensive end suffered a series of blunt injuries to the thigh in football. Two islands of myositis ossificans are indicated by the small arrows. An older zone of myositis ossificans projects from the surface of the midshaft of the femur (large arrow). (From Bowerman, McDonnell: Radiology 117:35, 1975)

ally returned to full activity in 12 weeks without surgery. This fracture site is the insertion point of the iliopsoas muscle.

Traumatic dislocation of the hip is an unusual injury that occurs in football, but is more common after automobile, motorbike, or motorcycle accidents. Pearson and Mann reported 24 examples, including 6 in patients who were 6 to 10 years old.[30] Of these 6 injuries, 4 occurred in football and one in a fall on a diving board. There were 14 patients ages 11 to 16, with only 2 injuries occurring in football; 6 were caused by automobile accidents and 5 by motorcycle or motorbike mishaps. Avascular necrosis is a recognized complication of this injury and is more common in patients with a delay in reduction of the hip.

Thigh

In addition to bony lesions of muscle and connective tissue, fibrotic masses can develop within the quadriceps muscle following muscle rupture. The rupture occurs during some uncoordinated forceful activity without a direct blow to the muscle from an external object. Rask and Lattig reported five examples, three of which had surgical removal of the fibrotic mass with good return of quadriceps function.[32] One of the five patients was a 15-year-old high school football player who experienced the injury while running. A 20 × 3-cm fibrotic tissue mass was excised seven weeks following injury. Three of the five patients were injured in track.

Myositis ossificans is apt to occur in the thigh because of its vulnerability to collision and because of its massive muscular volume (Fig. 202). The pitfall with this lesion is that, as in avulsion injuries, the history of trauma may be considered incidental or even forgotten. In this setting the lesion may be mistaken for neoplasm. Histologic interpretation of biopsy material of this fibrous vascular tissue can be confused with osteosarcoma at certain stages (Fig. 203). This is especially true if the biopsy is done early, when the post-traumatic lesion has not organized into a well-circumscribed bony mass. The x-ray appearance of myositis ossificans varies with the duration of the lesion from an early cloud of mineralized tissue to a mass of bone with a definite cortical rim which contains trabeculae of bone. Occasionally post-traumatic masses of bone develop on the surface of the shaft of a long bone (Figs. 204, 205). In this situation, bone has formed in a periosteal locus following a direct blow to the bone. (See the chapter on soft tissue injuries in Part I.)

Knee

The reports on knee abnormalities include advice on x-ray studies of the adolescent knee. Following injury, the epiphyseal cartilage or growth plate again may be separated and the separation may be a subtle finding. If such an injury is suspected, Rogers et al suggest additional views including oblique and intercondylar notch views for thorough evaluation.[35]

Reynolds and trainer Bruce Melin examined all the knees of the players on the Washington University football team, St. Louis, Mo., prior to each training session.[34] The knees were classified into stable and unstable groups. Between 1961 and 1963, there were 30 injuries in 137 players. The majority of injuries occurred in those with instability or relaxation.

The relationship between the incidence and severity of knee injuries in high school football players and the type of football shoe and cleat length is clearly shown in a paper by Torg and Quedenfeld.[38] They give credit to others who have studied this relationship, notably D. Moyer,[38] R. A. Nedwidek,[28] and D. F. Hanley.[21] Conventional football shoes have seven cleats that are ¾ inch in length with a ⅜-inch cleat tip diameter. The soccer-type shoes have cleat lengths of ⅜ inch with a cleat tip diameter of ½ inch. Thus the conventional shoe has longer, spikelike cleats which penetrate turf more deeply than the

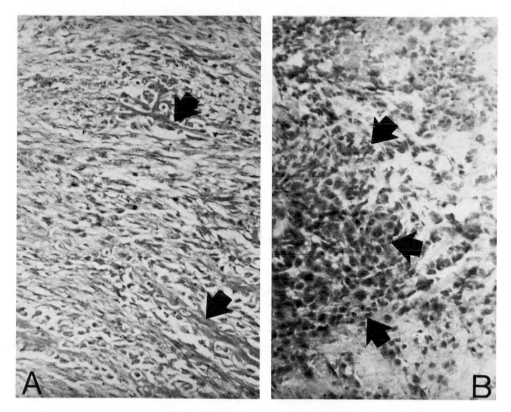

Fig. 203. Areas of bone formation are present in both microscopic fields of tissue. **A.** The bone forming in the fibrous strands of linearly oriented cells is developing following an injury to the thigh as myositis ossificans. **B.** The bone formation associated with plumper cells is part of an osteosarcoma of the femur. Although the cell patterns in these two fields are dissimilar, occasionally confusing patterns arise making it difficult to decide for or against malignancy.

soccer shoe due to a greater force through each cleat. (The force is estimated at 3.5 times the force exerted through a soccer cleat.)

In 1968, players from 18 Philadelphia public high school teams wearing the conventional football shoe had 51 knee injuries in 155 games, or 0.33 injury per team per game.[38] In the following year, the players wore the soccer-type shoe. There were 24 knee injuries at a rate of 0.14 injury per team per game. The severe knee injuries, ie, those with complete ligament tears, patella dislocation, meniscus tear, or osteochondral fracture, or those requiring more than 21 days to resolve, decreased from 29 in 1968 to 7 in 1969. The authors thus condemn the use of the conventional shoe.[38] They recommend that shoes have a synthetic molded sole, at least 14 cleats per sole, a minimum cleat tip diameter of ½ inch, and maximum cleat length of ⅜ inch.

Injury just distal to the knee is reported in the form of avulsion of the tibial tubercle in boys ages 14 to 16. In a report of seven patients with this injury,

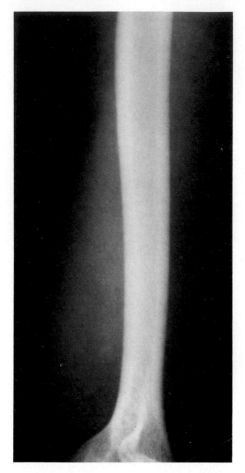 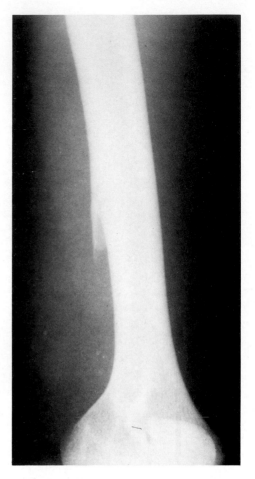

Fig. 204. A high school football player injured his arm by striking at an opponent instead of blocking with his shoulder and body. He had immediate pain and swelling of the distal part of the arm. This radiograph was made several days later and showed a faintly mineralized soft tissue swelling compared to the original radiograph (cf Fig. 205).

Fig. 205. Nine months after the radiograph shown in Figure 204, the soft-tissue swelling had regressed, leaving a zone of ossification partly attached to the humeral margin.

Hand et al discussed four that occurred in football and three that occurred in jumping.[20] Immediately after injury each patient was unable to extend the knee. The site of injury is the insertion of the quadriceps muscle. Each of the injuries in football showed a displaced bone fragment that involved the articular surface of the tibia on x-ray. The mechanism of injury is that of violent flexion of the knee against a tightly contracted quadriceps muscle. This is recounted in one instance in which a player was hit on the lower leg by a tackler while he carried two other tacklers on his back. Six of these patients had surgical repair.

Leg

Care of the bones and muscles of the leg after injury demands care of the nerves and vessels of the leg. Two examples will illustrate this point. Novich described a 16-year-old defensive back who received a body blow that twisted his knee.[29] A foot drop deformity ensued in one day. At operation an avulsed peroneal nerve was found in addition to a torn lateral capsule and torn insertion of the biceps femoris at the fibular head. At a subsequent operation a neuroplasty was performed. In another incident, an 18-year-old defensive halfback sustained a fractured tibia and fibula.[6] In the process of injury, fracture reduction, or casting, the patient developed pain and tissue loss. Subsequently a below-knee amputation was done. This case became a landmark of legal medicine and is known as the Darling case.

Ankle and Foot

The foot and ankle of the college and professional footballer have been evaluated in two reports. Blazina and Westover radiographed and examined the ankle joints of freshman college football and basketball players at the University of California at Los Angeles.[7] Nearly half the players had abnormal x-rays and a considerable number had a history of prior ankle injury. The x-ray abnormalities included spur formation at the margins of the ankle joint. Vincellette et al studied ankle and foot abnormalities in a group of professional footballers in Canada.[39] They were able to detect a higher incidence of foot and ankle abnormality in linemen than in backs, ends, or flankers. The constant crouching position and protracted blocking position of the lineman were considered possible determinants.

Does the condition of the playing surface or the type of playing surface influence the rate of injury in football? These questions were answered by Adkison et al in a study of injury to high school players.[1] Data were collected from 660 high school varsity football games, including 424 played on grass and 236 played on synthetic surfaces. Astroturf and Tartan Turf were used in 183 and 53 games, respectively.

Injuries were defined as "traumatic medical conditions resulting from participation in a football game that resulted in the player not finishing the game and/or missing two or more subsequent practices and/or any subsequent game or games." Severe injuries were defined as those in which a player missed "two or more subsequent games." Playing fields were considered "wet" if an open palm of the hand pressed on the 50-yard line at the center of the field was wet when removed from the playing surface. The playing surfaces were located in Seattle and Spokane, Wash., and in Portland, Ore. There were 357 games played on wet fields and 303 played under dry conditions.

The injury rates were generally lowest in games played on wet surfaces. The only exceptions occurred in the 53 games played on Tartan Turf. There were ten injuries in 24 games played on Tartan Turf under wet conditions, compared to five injuries in 29 games played on a dry Tartan Turf surface.

The injury rates following play on three Astroturf fields were usually higher than those played on grass. This difference was accentuated under dry conditions. In 44 games played under dry conditions on Astroturf there were 40 injuries—an injury rate of 0.91 injuries per game. In 230 games played on grass under similar conditions there were 128 injuries—an injury rate of 0.57 injuries per game. Severe injuries were tabulated by considering the injury rates in all games played under all weather conditions. The injury rate in 424 games played on grass was 0.19. The injury rate in 183 games played on Astroturf was 0.25 compared to a rate of 0.17 for 53 games on Tartan Turf.

The authors emphasized that not all synthetic surfaces are alike and that injury rates will vary with wet and dry field conditions. Two differences in the design of the synthetic surfaces are mentioned, namely, the fiber form in the synthetic surface and the system of underlying padding beneath the upper portion of the playing surface. The authors indicate that the fiber form in Astroturf is round and a flat fiber is used in Tartan Turf. In addition, different padding system designs are used, although they are not described in this report.

References

1. Adkison JW, Requa RK, Garrick JG: Injury rates in high school football. Clin Orthop 99:131–136, 1974
2. Allen ML: Air Force football injuries in clinical and statistical studies. JAMA 206:1053–1058, 1968
3. Aufranc OE, Jones WN, Bierbaum BE: Epiphyseal fracture of the proximal humerus. JAMA 207:727–729, 1969
4. Barnes ST, Hinds RB: Pseudotumor of the ischium. A late manifestation of avulsion of the ischial epiphysis. J Bone Joint Surg 54A:645–647, 1972
5. Bateman JE: Nerve injuries about the shoulder in sports. J Bone Joint Surg 49A:767–773, 1967
6. Bergen RP: The Darling case. JAMA 206:1665–1666, 1968
7. Blazina ME, Westover JL: Ankle joints of freshman college athletes. Clin Orthop 42:73–80, 1965
8. Blyth CS, Arnold DC: The Forty-Second Annual Survey of Football Fatalities 1931–1973. American Football Coaches Association, National Collegiate Athletic Association, and National Federation of State High School Athletic Associations, 1970
9. Borowiecki B, Charow A, Cook W, Rozycki D, Thaler S: An unusual football injury. Arch Otolaryngol 95:185–187, 1972
10. Bowerman JW, McDonnell EJ: Radiology of athletic injuries: football. Radiology 117:33–36, 1975
11. Castellanos A, Green P: Tackle football in pre high school children. J Sports Med Phys Fitness 6:187–190, 1966
12. Chrisman OD, Snook GA, Stanitis JM, Keedy VA: Lateral-flexion neck injuries in athletic competition. JAMA 192:117–119, 1965
13. Conwell HE, Reynolds FC: Key and Conwell's Management of Fractures, Dislocations and Sprains, 7th ed. St. Louis, Mosby, 1961, p 295
14. Craig AB Jr: Exposure time to injury in professional football. Res Am Assoc Health Phys Educ 39:789–791, 1968
15. Dimon JH: Isolated fractures of the lesser trochanter of the femur. Clin Orthop 82:144–148, 1972
16. Editorial: Pro football, the doctor's trauma lab. Med World News 11:24–30, 1970

17. Ferguson RT, McMaster JH, Stanitski CL, cited in: Low back pain held common in football interior linemen. Med Trib, p 22, May 1, 1974
18. Garrahan WF: The incidence of high school football injuries. RI Med J 50: 833–835, 1967
19. Garrick JG: Clues to knee injuries in athletes. Am Fam Physician 8:128–133, Oct 1973
20. Hand WL, Hand CR, Dunn AW: Avulsion fractures of the tibial tubercle. J Bone Joint Surg 53A:1579–1583, 1971
21. Hanley DF: Controlled external factors in lower extremity injuries. Paper presented at the Medical Society of the State of New York Symposium on Medical Aspects of Sports, 1969
22. Himmelwright GO: Field decisions—diagnosis in football. Md State Med J 16: 50–58, 1967
23. Jackson DW: Unilateral osseous bridging of the lumbar transverse processes following trauma. J Bone Joint Surg 57A:125–126, 1975
24. Keefe WF: Helping hands for peewee sports. Physicians Management, p 54, Sept 1965
25. Krauss JF, Gullen WH: An epidemiologic investigation of predictor variables associated with intramural touch football injuries. Am J Public Health 59:2144–2156, 1969
26. Lichtor J, Virgin HW, Pisani AJ: On call to the pros. The surgeons of professional football. Int Surg 56:132B–136B, 1971
27. Marks RB, Freed MM: Non-penetrating injuries of the neck and cerebrovascular accident. Arch Neurol 28:412–414, 1973
28. Nedwidek RA: Knee and ankle injuries: articulating opinion with research. Scholastic Coach, pp 18–20, Jan 1969
29. Novich MM: Peroneal nerve syndrome. In Jokl E, Simon E (eds): International Research in Sport and Physical Education. Springfield, Ill., Thomas, 1964, pp 656–659
30. Pearson DE, Mann RJ: Traumatic hip dislocation in children. Clin Orthop 92: 189–194, 1973
31. Rall KL, McElroy GL, Keats TE: A study of the long term effects of football injury to the knee. Mo Med 61:435–438, 1964
32. Rask MR, Lattig GJ: Traumatic fibrosis of the rectus femoris muscle. JAMA 221:268–269, 1972
33. Reid SE, Tarkington JA, Epstein HM, O'Dea TJ: Brain tolerance to impact in football. Surg Gynecol Obstet 133:929–936, 1971
34. Reynolds FC: Injuries of the knee. Clin Orthop 50:137–146, 1967
35. Rogers LF, Jones S, Davis AR, Dietz G: "Clipping injury" fracture of the epiphysis in the adolescent football player: an occult lesion of the knee. Am J Roentgenol 121:69–78, 1974
36. Rose KD, Stone F, Fuenning SI, Williams J: Cardiac contusion resulting from "spearing" in football: a case history. Arch Intern Med 118:129–131, 1966
37. Schneider RC: Serious and fatal neurosurgical football injuries. Clin Neurosurg 12:226–236, 1964
38. Torg JS, Quedenfeld T: Effect of the shoe type and cleat length on incidence and severity of knee injuries among high school football players. Res Q Am Assoc Health Phys Educ 43:203–211, 1971
39. Vincellette P, Laurin CA, LeVesque HP: Footballer's ankle and foot. Can Med Assoc J 107:872–877, 1972
40. Wenger DW: Avulsion of the profundus tendon insertion in football players. Arch Surg 106:145–149, 1973

GOLF

The golf club and the ball may act as weapon and missile, respectively, in producing injuries—especially eye injuries—to golfers and bystanders. Millar reported seven injured patients.[3] Three were hit in the eye by a golf ball and three were struck in the eye by the head of a swinging golf club; global ruptures occurred in two of these patients. The seventh patient sustained a perforating injury of the eye when he struck a piece of glass with a golf club. Burst or explosion injuries to the eye from liquid-center golf balls have been recorded when curious children have cut into the ball to study its contents. Kunkel recorded five such injuries in children during a 13-year period.[2] In such instances the liquid droplets are dense—some contain barium sulfate and zinc sulfide in a compressed center under 2000 to 2400 psi pressure (Fig. 206)—and will be detected on x-rays of the injured face and orbit.

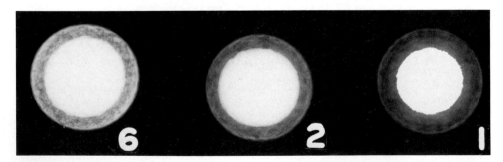

Fig. 206. Three golf balls of the ordinary type were radiographed. The balls were placed next to the numerals designated 6″, 2″, and 1″. The numerals are made of lead and the radiodensity of the numerals can be compared to that of the centers of the golf balls. Note that each ball has a metallic center probably composed of inexpensive suspensions of metals such as barium and zinc. Several varieties of golf balls have been similarly radiographed and each has shown a metallic center. Rarely, explosion injuries to the eye have been reported from golf balls. The injury usually occurs as the pressure-packed center of the ball is cut open by an inquisitive child or adolescent. Radiographs of the injured orbit have shown metallic droplets embedded in the soft tissue.

A forceful swing will occasionally injure the golfer in several ways. First, the golfer may swing with an unimpeded full swing and suddenly experience an injury. The author has seen an example of avulsion of the ischial apophysis that occurred during a swing. Rupture of a branch of the axillary artery due to a golf swing has been reported in a 36-year-old man.[5] In this case, the golfer lost his balance during the swing, immediately had pain, and subsequently noticed a localized pulsatile swelling at the axilla. An arteriogram showed a false aneurysm (a contained leakage of blood) at the origin of the circumflex humeral and subscapular arteries that was repaired surgically.

Second, the golfer may hit the ground near the ball, bury the club in the sand, or strike an object other than the ball. Torisu reported an isolated fracture of a portion of the wrist in a 54-year-old man who felt severe pain at the end of a swing.[6] Oblique x-ray views showed a fracture of the hook of the hamate. A violent contraction of the flexor carpi ulnaris insertion through the pisiform hamate ligament was considered to be the mechanism. Rasad described "golfer's fractures" of the ribs in three patients including himself.[4] Each of the golfers was new to the game and complained of pain and discomfort in the upper back near the shoulder. The fourth, fifth, and sixth, the fourth and fifth, and the sixth and seventh posterior ribs were fractured in these three patients. The right-handed golfers had left-sided rib fractures.

The term "golfer's elbow" has been applied to the painful strain of the origin of the pronator muscles at the medial epicondyle. Curwen notes that strain of the lateral epicondylar area is actually more common in golf than in tennis and that the most common injury in golf is strain of the lower back.[1]

References

1. Curwen IHM: Golf. In Armstrong JR, Tucker WE (eds): Injury in Sport. London, Staples, 1964, pp 200–204
2. Kunkel RE: Exploding golf balls. Rocky Mt Med J 64:82–83, 1967
3. Millar GT: Golfing eye injuries. Am J Ophthalmol 64:741–742, 1967
4. Rasad S: Golfer's fractures of the ribs—report of three cases. Am J Roentgenol 120:901–903, 1974
5. Rosenzweig J, Simon MA: Traumatic aneurysm of the axillary artery: a golf hazard. Can Med Assoc J 93:165–167, 1965
6. Torisu T: Fractures of the hook of the hamate by a golf swing. Clin Orthop 83: 91–94, 1972

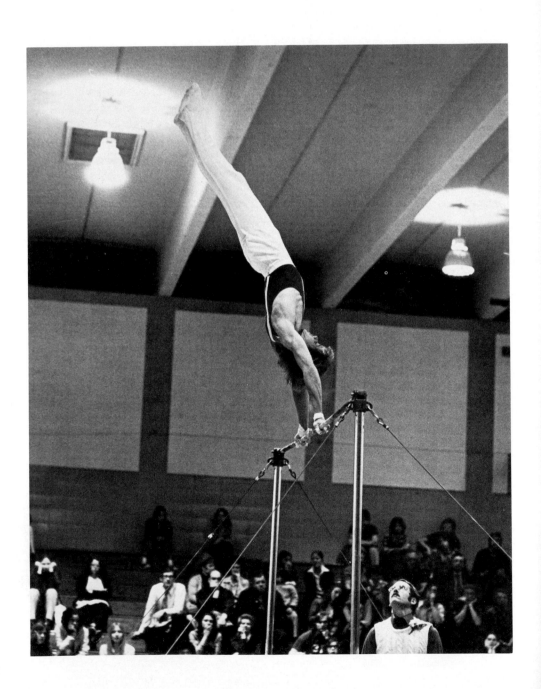

GYMNASTICS

Information on injuries in this sport is sparse. Fractures and dislocations do occur in falls from gymnastic apparatus. A particularly dangerous piece of apparatus is the trampoline. Cervical spine fracture–dislocation with resultant paraplegia is perhaps the most dreaded injury. Fortunately this injury is uncommon if not rare in gymnastics. During 1974 and 1975, the 119 emergency rooms contributing information on injury to the National Electronic Injury Surveillance System pooled data on 1968 gymnastics injuries.[11] These included 107 fractures in 582 injured trampolinists and 383 fractures overall. Only one of the 107 fractures in the trampolinists was a fractured neck.

Potondi et al reported a cervical fracture and dislocation at C5–C6 in a gymnast who was injured when he fell on the nape of the neck while performing a somersault in free exercises without apparatus.[12] The patient was immediately unable to move his limbs. Although the dislocation was reduced and immobilized, the patient died within 2.5 hours of the injury. Autopsy showed rupture of both vertebral arteries, a reddish soft and swollen spinal cord at C5–C6, a lacerated intervertebral disc, and severance of the vertebral column at C5–C6.

Dunn conducted a questionnaire study of the opinions of head gynmnastic coaches of colleges and universities in the United States in 1967 regarding gymnastic safety and rules.[2,3] He reported on 85 questionnaires that satisfied arbitrary requirements that the institution belonged to the National Collegiate Athletic Association, the respondent was the head coach of gymnastics, and a program of intercollegiate competition in gymnastics was being conducted. The number of questionnaires originally distributed was 126 and some form of reply was received from 99 head coaches giving a return of approximately 78 percent. Information on injury was not complete and cannot be conclusively summarized. An average of 37.6 percent of coaches had observed at least one serious injury in trampolining during the past five years. A serious injury was defined as one which required medical evaluation and resulted in two or more weeks of restriction from practice or competition. The two events selected by the coaches as associated with the greatest number of serious injuries were the trampoline and the horizontal bar. In some regions of the country, ie, the Midwest and the Mideast, the horizontal bar was mentioned much more frequently than the trampoline in association with injury. The reverse was true in the western and eastern regions that were polled. A total of 68 serious injuries was reported in all events, including 15 injuries to the neck and back. Five of these injuries were fractured or dislocated vertebrae. No deaths occurred in varsity gymnasts as a result of participating on the trampoline during the five-year period covered by the study.

Bosco edited a study by Rumpf based on questionnaires on trampoline injury that were sent to 246 public secondary schools in California, Florida, Iowa, New Mexico, Pennsylvania, and Washington.[1] The schools were known to have used trampolines in their physical education programs. Adequate responses were obtained from 158 schools. Six divisions of information were requested on the questionnaire including: (1) the length of time the trampoline had been used and the estimated number of students involved per year; (2) the number of accident events; (3) the seriousness of the injuries; (4) the circumstances surrounding the accident; (5) the actual cause of the accident; and (6) the opinion of the respondent regarding the safety of trampolining.

An average of 3078 students used the trampoline at each school. The data cover an average of 7.82 years of trampoline usage at each school. An estimated total of 486,333 students used trampolines in 158 schools. The average number of injured students was 9.93 per school for the 7.82-year period. Abrasions, sprains, and strains accounted for most of the injuries. Less than 6 percent of the injuries were fractures or dislocations. However, one student was killed and two suffered paralysis, emphasizing the severity of some injuries. The exact cause of the fatality is not mentioned nor are the causes of the paralyses discussed.

The majority of the injuries occurred when the trampolinist landed improperly on the bed of the trampoline. The stunt most often associated with injury was a front drop (224 injuries). Other feats linked with injury include the back drop (78 injuries), back somersault (175), and front somersault (127). Approximately 7 percent of all the injuries occurred in the absence of an authorized supervisor or without adequate "spotters." At least four spotters are needed as guardians at the edge of the apparatus to protect the trampolinist from injury off the trampoline or on its frame. Six spotters are needed for trampolines with beds that are larger than 6 × 12 feet. It should be noted that the spotters cannot prevent injury in the middle of the trampoline bed and that most injuries occurred in faulty landings on that bed.

Rumpf concludes that the majority of injuries in trampolining are minor. He emphasizes that the use of safety padding around the springs and frame could prevent some injuries. Trampolines should be folded and locked when not in use and used only with adequate supervision and spotters.

Frederick, as coach of gymnastics at the University of Wisconsin, Superior, Wisc., has observed that those gymnasts who are completely immersed in a special event develop characteristic trauma as a result.[4] He cites the shoulder problems of the ring specialist and the "wrist splints" of the gymnast on the pommel horse. The latter problem is apparently an overuse injury of the forearm and wrist that is analogous to the injury of the soft tissue attachments at the tibia in the runner. Whether this has been studied extensively and whether it has been studied by radiographic means is uncertain. The gymnast with wrist or forearm splints may have pain in the midforearm or at the wrist. Geist believes that most all-around gymnasts are eventually troubled with this problem.[5]

The pattern of injuries in men's gymnastics differs from that in women's gymnastics largely because of the pursuit of different events. Although men perform free exercises or tumbling and vaulting as do women gymnasts, men tend to dominate the activity on the rings, parallel bars, and pommel horse. In participating in and coaching men's gymnastics, Abie Grossfeld has observed lower back injuries as a result of the forces generated in dismounts, tumbling, and vaulting.[6]

A survey of injuries and epidemiologic data related to injuries in girls' and women's gymnastics in America was conducted by Jeffrey and Frankel with the help of Muriel Grossfeld, the coach of the United States Women's Gymnastic Team.[10] Questionnaires were submitted to the 21 coaches of gymnasts competing in the 1974 United States Gymnastic Federation Elite Gymnastics Championships. The coaches were asked to distribute the forms to performers who had reached an arbitrary standard of performance (selected as a score of 32 points or greater in all-around competition on at least one occasion). All but three coaches returned questionnaires. Of 134 gymnasts at risk to injury covered by the 18 coaches, 114 completed questionnaires. The 20 girls who did not respond were unavailable and no longer performing in gymnastics. Only one of these former gymnasts had a disability from injury in gymnastics that prevented further pursuit of the sport. This study then represents a sample of a very cooperative group. Jeffrey et al estimate that the sample represents a significant percentage of the high-level female gymnasts in the United States. Muriel Grossfeld has emphasized that a comprehensive study of women's gymnastics, as in this case, must include information on performers from gymnastic clubs as well as university teams.[7] The majority of high-level women gymnasts in the United States are products of gymnastic clubs.[7]

Of 114 respondents, 76 had been injured and 38 were uninjured. The average age of the entire group was almost 15 years. Some gymnasts had experienced more than one injury, so that 157 injuries were recorded in a 17-month period, ending in May 1974. The major activities in which the injuries occurred were tumbling (51 injuries), uneven bars (35), horse vaulting (19), balance beam (13), general activity involving more than one event (19), and free exercise other than tumbling (10). The ankle, with 39 injuries, was easily the most injured body area; these included 32 ankle sprains, 4 fractures, 1 dislocation, and 2 other injuries. Nearly all the ankle sprains were inversion-type injuries during tumbling and free exercise. Backward tumbling is a dominant maneuver in tumbling and free exercise and was the major activity linked to these injuries. The lower back, with 24 injuries, was the second most injured body area. These injuries are not clearly defined in this group: 12 back injuries were sequelae of general activity, followed unknown activity, or were chronic; 8 were secondary to tumbling and free exercise or vaulting; and 3 followed work on the uneven bars. Other injury sites include the foot (18 injuries) and the knee (12 injuries). Because 21 of the 157 injuries occurred in falls or dismounts from the uneven parallel bars, Jeffrey et al suggest that it may be helpful to examine the effectiveness of spotting and landing mats in preventing these injuries.

Jackson et al have shown that lower back pain in female gymnasts can be a symptom of spondylolysis and spondylolisthesis.[9] In a study of 100 young girl gymnasts, 11 girls had bilateral spondylolysis at the fifth lumbar vertebral level and 6 had spondylolisthesis of L5 on S1. (See the section on the lumbar spine in Part I.)

Hughes has studied the problems of ring-related shoulder injury in college gymnasts on 39 different teams.[8] Some of these athletes were specialists on the rings but others were multievent specialists or all-around gymnasts. Information was obtained by questionnaire and 106 individuals responded. Each respondent had either modified practice techniques or missed gymnastic meets or practices because of shoulder dysfunction or shoulder pain. Ring specialists had more ring-related injuries than the other groups of performers. The weight of the gymnast did not correlate with the frequency of shoulder problems. Only a few respondents indicated that they used rings suspended with rope rather than wire cable. This complicated Hughes' efforts to correlate the frequency of shoulder injury with the type of suspension employed. Rope suspension would logically elongate and provide a cushioning effect on the shoulder; however, no conclusive beneficial result could be shown with rope suspension. Likewise, the author compared ceiling beam suspension (11 examples) and ring frame suspension (52 examples) from the standpoint of associated injuries. Rings mounted on ceiling beam suspensions showed slightly fewer reports of injury. Hughes emphasized that too few examples are recorded in the category of ceiling beam suspension for this comparison to be useful. The specific causes of some injuries are mentioned, ie, swinging moves accounted for 22 injuries and strength moves 11. We can only speculate about the actual anatomic areas damaged in these gymnasts. Hughes indicated that no special radiographic examinations including arthrograms were done. Thus no effort was made to demonstrate rotator cuff tears of the shoulder in these ring specialists.

References

1. Bosco JS: Research and fitness in gymnastics. Mod Gymnast 12:21–22, 1970
2. Dunn JH: A study of the opinions of head gymnastic coaches of colleges and universities concerning recent and proposed rule changes. Unpublished data, 1967
3. _____: The opinions of head coaches of gymnastics in colleges and universities regarding the trampoline. US Gymnast, Dec 1967
4. Frederick AB: Personal communication
5. Geist J: Personal communication
6. Grossfeld A: Personal communication
7. Grossfeld M: Personal communication
8. Hughes E: Report of research on ring related shoulder problems—part I. University of Washington, unpublished data, 1974
9. Jackson DW, Wiltse LL, Cirincione RJ, cited by Martin J: Low back pain may mean spinal defects. Physician and Sports Med 4:15, 1976
10. Jeffrey CC, Frankel V, Grossfeld M: An epidemiological study of injuries in American female gymnasts. Presented at the United States Gymnastics Federation Coaches Congress, Denver Colo, Nov 1975
11. National Electronic Injury Surveillance System Matrix Reports on Trampolines and Gymnastics 7/1/64–6/30/75. U.S. Consumer Product Safety Commission, Washington, DC
12. Potondi A, Rupnik P, Kapusz N: Injuries of the vertebral artery. J Forensic Sci 11:395–403, 1966

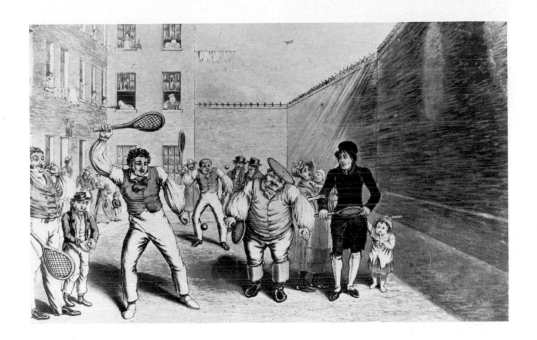

HANDBALL–SQUASH

The American game of handball originated from the English and Irish game of "fives." A ball is struck by a gloved hand against one or more walls of a court. Damage to the hand is usually restricted to minimal soft tissue swelling but rarely periosteal new bone formation has occurred.[4] There are opportunities for injury in collision with opponents or with the walls of the court (Fig. 207). In addition, the arm or hand used in striking the ball may by accident strike an opponent or a barrier. The author has witnessed a metacarpal fracture that occurred when a player struck the wall in an effort to hit the ball and a fibular fracture that occurred as a player landed awkwardly after jumping to reach the ball.

Eye injury and occasional ear injury may occur when the ball strikes a player. The ball is made of black rubber, weighs 2.5 ounces, and measures 4.5 cm in diameter, and, like a squash ball, it can readily injure the eye. Hemorrhage in the anterior chamber of the eye (hyphema) and abrasion of the cornea may result. The only adequate safeguards against "black ball hyphema" are through the use of safety goggles or safety glasses. The author once saw a patient who had been struck on the external auditory meatus by a handball. A fresh but fortunately small perforation of the tympanic membrane was present on examination. The perforation healed without difficulty in several weeks.

The game of squash has obscure origins and is probably derived from a game called "racquets" played in the late Middle Ages.[1] Racquets can be traced to handball and to the French game "jeu de paume" played in the Middle Ages. Thus handball and squash are related historically. The games are also related from the standpoint of injury.

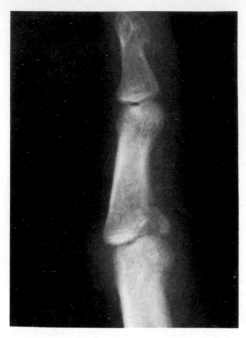

Fig. 207. An enthusiastic handball player hit the left sidewall of the court with his hand in an effort to hit the ball. This view shows an articular margin fracture at the base of the middle phalanx. The fracture healed without surgery.

The squash racquet and the squash ball are linked with eye injury in several reports. North reported 35 cases of ocular injury treated in Melbourne, Australia, between 1968 and 1970:[3] 27 patients were hit in the eye with a squash ball and 8 others were hit by the racquet; 5 patients were wearing glasses (spectacles) that were broken by the injury. Hyphema occurred in 30 patients, corneal damage in 4, retinal damage in 2, and massive vitreous hemorrhage in 1. Two patients required surgery—one for the repair of iris prolapse following a penetrating injury that produced corneal damage from broken glasses and the other to treat a retinal detachment. Ingram and Lewkonia studied 21 players with eye injury in squash in London, England.[2] Details of the 14 more seriously injured patients show that the racquet accounted for as many severe injuries as the ball. Four injuries were of the perforating type in which the globe or cornea and sclera was punctured. Five of the seven most severely injured players were wearing glasses at the time of injury. The squash player that wears glasses during play is advised to use safety lenses or a protective housing around the glasses. North suggests that people with one eye should be advised not to play the game.[3]

References

1. Arlott J (ed): The Oxford Companion to World Sports and Games. London, Oxford, 1975
2. Ingram DV, Lewkonia I: Ocular hazards of playing squash rackets. Br J Ophthalmol 57:434–438, 1973
3. North IM: Ocular hazards of squash. Med J Aust 1:165–166, 1973
4. Wynn-Parry CB: Finger, wrist and hand injuries. In Williams JGP (ed): Sports Medicine. Baltimore, Williams & Wilkins, 1962

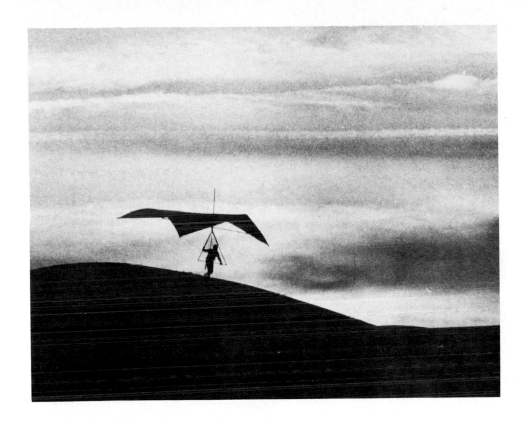

HANG-GLIDING

Injuries and deaths in falls during hang-gliding are described in a report by Krissoff and Eiseman.[1] Four fatalities occurred after flights from mountain cliffs near Denver, Colo. Uncontrolled dives after stall configurations killed two young men. Two others crashed in turbulent wind conditions, with one man falling approximately 90 meters into the chimney and roof of a house. Skull fractures, cerebral and aortic lacerations, and fracture–dislocations of the cervical spine were among the injuries in this group. Eight serious nonfatal injuries in a 12-month period are also described, including tibial, femoral, and vertebral fractures. One unfortunate hang-gliding enthusiast flew into high-tension wires, suffered severe burns of the hands and forearms, and required bilateral amputations of the upper extremity. Lesser injuries, eg, ankle sprains, occur in nearly all participants according to Krissoff and Eiseman. Thus the novice at hang-gliding is exposed to ankle sprain and other minor injury, but the free-wheeling expert who dives from mountain cliffs risks the fate of Icarus.

Reference

1. Krissoff WB, Eiseman B: Injuries associated with hang gliding. JAMA 233:158–160, 1975

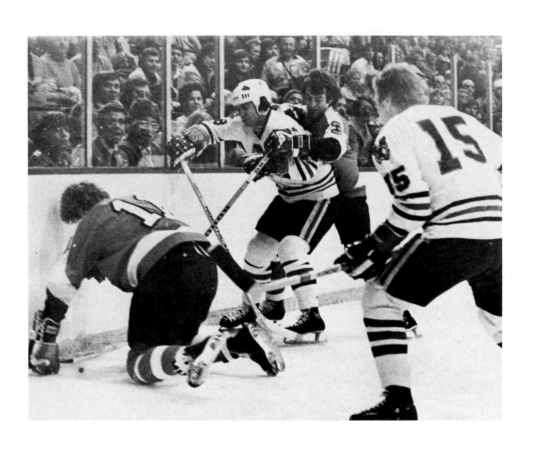

HOCKEY

The potential causes of injury in ice hockey are numerous, including injuries produced by the opponents, puck, stick, skates, ice, boards, and goal posts. The most common injury listed by Michaelson is a laceration.[8] The most common fractures, according to Janes, are those of the nose, cheek, and jaw.[6]

In 1967 there were 3229 teams and 48,435 players registered in the United States Amateur Hockey Association.[8] Juckes estimated the number of Canadian males that play ice hockey to be 500,000, with more than 15,000 active teams.[8] One Canadian insurance plan for players under 18 years of age insured 37,089 players and had 1844 claims for the 1964–1965 season. Therefore, approximately 6 percent of players have injuries significant enough to warrant an insurance claim. Injury rates have apparently decreased following the greater use of mouthguards and helmets. The Canadian Amateur Hockey Association requires use of helmets by all players under the age of 20 years with the exception of players in its Junior "A" classification.

In Czechoslovakia, according to a study by Mathe, less than 1 percent of organized hockey players are injured.[7] This injury rate differs significantly from the aforementioned rate of injury in Canada. It is likely that the freer use of body checking in the North American style of hockey explains this difference. Mathe reported 202 injuries between 1948 and 1951, with an average annual number of players estimated at 35,000. Of these injuries 47 percent were to the head, almost 24 percent inolved the upper extremities, and nearly 20 percent involved the lower extremities. Collisions with opponents were by far the leading method of injury.

Loss of teeth in hockey trauma has been frequent in the past. In 1968, Nadeau estimated that two of every three North American Professional players in the National Hockey League had lost upper teeth in the course of their careers.[8] Extraoral mouth guards are now required in at least one league at the boys' hockey level. In the National Hockey League major injuries of all types occur once in every two games according to Adams.[1] A major injury is defined as one that keeps a player out of play at least three weeks. Three minor injuries occur per game during a season of 70 games.

White has gathered information on injury to Detroit Red Wing players in the National Hockey League in 100 consecutive games.[11] This series spans two seasons. The sample is from a 20-man team and does not include information on injuries in practice. An average of one facial laceration occurred per game. Sprains, strains, and avulsion injuries were the next most common category of injury, totaling 66 injuries. Knee, ankle, wrist, elbow, and hand injuries were the most common in that group. There were 42 fractures, including 15 nasal fractures, 10 at the ribs, and 7 in the hand. Spearing or jabbing with the upper end of the stick produced seven of the rib fractures. Six concussions were recorded, four in players not wearing a helmet and two in those wearing helmets. Nine lacerations of the hand, three acromioclavicular separations and two torn menisci at the knee rounded out the injury picture. Seven of the nasal fractures and approximately 75 percent of the facial lacerations were caused by high sticking, a theoretically controllable infraction of the rules. Fighting within the game, which heretofore has been controlled only partially, accounted for many of the aforementioned injuries, including nine hand lacerations, five nasal, five hand, and one mandibular fractures, and ten hand and four wrist sprains. Fortunately, injuries in this study that were caused by fighting were minor. Nine of the total number of players were hospitalized and seven of these had surgery ranging from a repair of nasal fracture to removal of torn menisci. White believes that the major cause of injury in professional hockey is high sticking and that this could be controlled by strict adherence to the rules of the sport. He estimates that injuries might be reduced by 50 percent if the high sticking rule were rigidly enforced.

Injuries in intercollegiate ice hockey, while frequent, are mostly minor injuries. On the average, slightly more than one injury occurs per game. Hayes collected data from 21 Canadian and 9 American universities participating in 280 games during the 1970–1971 season.[5] There were 328 reported injuries. Craniofacial injuries comprised 45 percent of the total and 88 percent of all injuries involved soft tissue. Body contact produced 38 percent of injuries and 29 percent were produced by blows from a hockey stick. Fractures constituted 4.5 percent and dislocations or subluxations 3 percent. An encouraging note is that 52 percent of the injured were able to return to play within 5 minutes, although 30 percent were sidelined for the remainder of the game. Forwards sustained over 61 percent of the injuries, defensemen over 31 percent, and goaltenders 7 percent. Very few people were injured in striking the goalpost or the boards.

A rare hockey injury, traumatic aneurysm of the temporal artery, has been reported after a puck hit a player's temporal region.[2] As far as the author can determine, this is an isolated event.

A 20-year-old hockey player who sustained a severe knee injury was the subject of a report by Percy in 1971.[10] The player dislocated the patella laterally in a twisting fall after being hit by an opponent. Butt, in describing the findings on x-ray, pointed out a fat–fluid level on the lateral view within the suprapatellar portion of the joint.[10] Fat escaped from a fracture site to produce this finding. An osteochondral fracture of the femur was suspected. When such a fat-fluid level is found every effort must be made to define a fracture. A horizontal x-ray beam is required in order to see the fat–fluid level.

The National Electronic Injury Surveillance System is a system of data collection and analysis following injuries requiring medical care in a selected series of emergency rooms. There are 119 hospital emergency rooms participating in this surveillance system and they comprise a representative sample for the continental United States. Medical reports are submitted only on product-related injuries that require emergency room treatment. Between July 1, 1972, and June 30, 1973, an estimated 30,000 persons received hospital emergency room treatment in the United States for injuries associated with hockey equipment.[3] The surveillance system injury totals include 1607 emergency room treatments for hockey injuries reported in the same fiscal year of 1973. Lacerations, contusions, and abrasions accounted for 75 percent of these injuries, and wounds of the head and face, including the eyes, ears, and mouth, accounted for 64 percent of the total injuries reported, or 1009 injuries. Ten percent (155) of the injuries were fractures. The age span of the injured included primary school and high school players as well as older age groups. The age groups 10 to 14 years and 15 to 19 years each incurred 35 percent of the total injuries. The age group 5 to 9 years incurred 8 percent of the injuries. Of the total 1607 injuries recorded during this period, 91 percent (1457) were to males. There were 40 specific investigations dealing with ice hockey equipment, including 13 that showed that protective equipment was not effective and 11 that showed that normal protective equipment was not used. Ten other injuries were recorded in which no face masks were used. In about half of these accidents, the individual was struck by either the puck or the stick.

Eye injuries account for less than 10 percent of hockey injuries but produce a significant number of handicapped players.[9] A study by the Canadian Ophthalmologic Society shows that 15 percent of those with eye injuries have blindness in one eye.[9] Players in the age group 11 to 15 years group were most often injured. The hockey stick rather than the puck produced most injuries. Eye protectors as visors on helmets are the solution according to the Ophthalmologic Society. Players with preexistent eye damage and those unaware of visual defects are at great risk without eye protection.

The issues of eye and head protection are complex ones and not easily solved. The use of a helmet in ice hockey does not always adequately protect the player from serious head injury and death. Two teenage players in high school hockey in New Brunswick, Canada, died in the 1967–1968 season as a result of head injuries. Both players were wearing "protective" helmets at the time of injury. One player was roughly body checked, and as he fell his left temple struck the ice. He lost consciousness and died within two hours of subarachnoid and subdural hemorrhage. The skull was not fractured. The second player was struck on the right temple by the tip of an opponent's hockey stick. Despite the presence of his helmet he sustained a fractured skull, lost consciousness, and died within six hours of the injury. At autopsy, a depressed fracture of the temporal bone and an epidural hemorrhage were found. Fekete, in reporting these deaths, pointed out the flimsiness of the helmets worn by the teenagers who died.[4] The helmets were made of thin plastic and lined by a layer of plastic foam approximately ⅜ inch in thickness. He called for an improved helmet design with a stronger outer shell and equipped with an inner suspension system similar to those in football.

References

1. Adams RW, cited in: Hockey's hard knocks pose challenge to MD's ingenuity, Med World News, pp 74–79, March 24, 1967
2. Campbell JS, Fournier P, Hill DP: Puck aneurysm. Can Med Assoc J 81: 922–924, 1959
3. Editorial: Accidents associated with hockey equipment. Newslett Nat Electron Injury Surveillance Syst 2:6, Feb 1974
4. Fekete JF: Severe brain injury and death following minor hockey accidents—the effectiveness of the "safety helmets" of amateur hockey players. Can Med Assoc J 99:1234–1239, 1968
5. Hayes D, cited in: College ice hockey injuries frequent but mostly minor. Hosp Trib, p 23, Jan 21, 1974
6. Janes JM: Ice hockey injuries. Clin Orthop 23:67–74, 1962
7. Mathe E: Injuries in ice hockey in sport and health. Proceedings of the International Conference on Sport and Health, Oslo, 1952
8. Michaelson M: Ice hockey safe for your youngster? Today's Health pp 32–37, 80–82, Feb 1968
9. Pashby TJ, Pashby RC, Chisholm LD, et al: Eye injuries in Canadian hockey. Can Med Assoc J 113:663–666, 674, 1975
10. Percy EC (ed): Trauma rounds from Montreal General Hospital. Can Med Assoc J 105:1176–1178, 1971
11. White RT: Unpublished data

HORSEBACK RIDING

Injuries sustained in horseback-riding are among the oldest of all sports injuries. Comprehensive studies of such mishaps are generally lacking despite the number of periodicals dealing with horses and their riders.

Barber surveyed the riding accidents admitted to the Radcliffe Infirmary, Oxford, England, in 1971 and 1972.[1] There were 154 patients admitted to the hospital for such injuries. Lesser trauma not requiring hospitalization is not included in this report. For every patient with an injury due to riding there were 57 with problems unrelated to riding that required admission to the accident unit. Patients with riding injuries ranged in age from less than 10 years of age to more than 70 years of age; however, 90 patients were under 21 years of age. Two-thirds (109) of the patients were female. Thirty-six patients were professionally employed in an occupation involving horses. Except for one instance in which a girl struck her head on a branch, all the injuries were due to falls. In some cases the rider was injured by the horse in addition to having fallen. Concussions numbered 101, skull fractures 14 (4 of these were compound), and facial fractures 4. There were seven pelvic fractures and four spinal fractures, one of which was an odontoid fracture with a Brown-Sequard syndrome in a 71-year-old woman.

Nine patients had rib fractures and four of these had pneumothorax. Two other patients had lung contusions on chest x-ray. There were eight fractures of the clavicle and one fracture of the scapula. One patient died after skull fractures and severe brain injury with a ruptured internal carotid artery and lacerated pharynx. The protective helmet of this unfortunate woman had fallen off before she hit the ground. Incomplete information was collected regarding the wearing of a riding hat but at least 42 patients who had concussions were wearing a hat and 28 were not. The hats were either frontal brimmed hunt caps with flimsy elastic chin straps or strapless formal bowlers or top hats. There was no clear association between the wearing of a hat and the severity of head injury. However, in the fatal case the rider was not protected by a helmet at the time of head injury. This indicates that present-day riding hats of the hunt cap and normal hunt varieties are inadequate protection especially if they can be dislodged before actual impact.

The number of injuries to jockeys in the United States was estimated recently at 600 per year.[2] This was based on records of 1100 jockeys at 97 race-

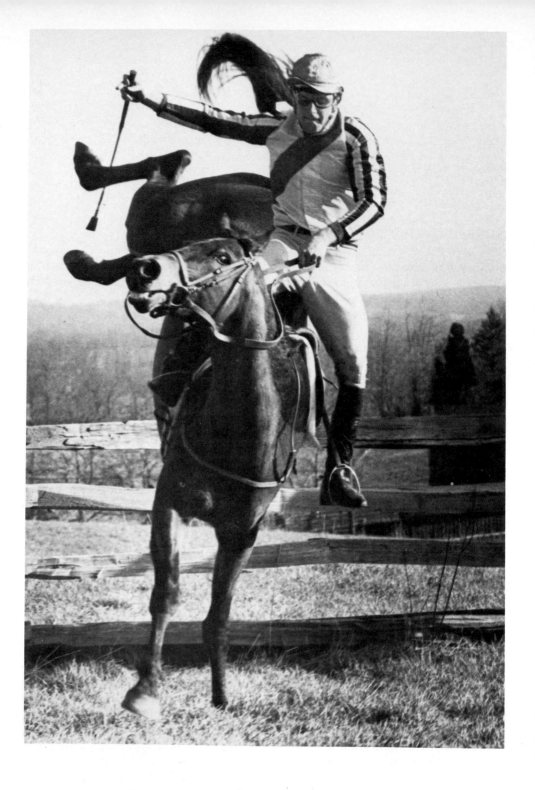

tracks. Kaye pinpointed the clavicle as the jockey's most vulnerable point, followed closely by fractures of the skull, ribs, and extremities.[6] The Jockey Guild, Inc., reported in 1969 that 26 professional jockeys were killed in racing accidents from 1959 to 1969. The average number of professional jockeys riding each year ranges from 1200 to 1500, making a yearly fatality rate of approximately 2 deaths per 1000 riders.

The rodeo rider is one of America's athletes at risk in several ways in rodeo competition. Comprehensive information on injuries to rodeo performers is not available. Some information is available, judging from insurance claim statistics provided by McKnight.[7] In 1975, 150 injuries were considered significant enough to warrant an insurance claim by the injured rodeo performer. This total represents 6 percent of the estimated 2500 contestants of the International Rodeo Association. This group of professional performers is one of the two major associations of rodeo riders in the United States. The most common injuries, according to McKnight, are knee, shoulder, and elbow injuries, in addition to concussions, loss of teeth, and nasal fractures. Rib and lower extremity fractures and concussions occur in falls complicated by compression forces of a horse or bull falling on the rider. Nasal fractures occur from facial impact of the rider with a bucking bull or bronco's back. McKnight emphasizes that bull riding is the most dangerous rodeo event. Many performers retire from competition in their 20s and 30s and only then find time to have injuries fully evaluated and treated. The seven standard events in professional rodeos include bronco and bareback riding, calf roping, barrel racing, steer wrestling, team roping, and bull riding.

Other isolated reports concerning riding injuries include traumatic diastasis of the symphysis pubis in two riders and traumatic femoral artery thrombosis in a man kicked by a horse.[4,5] In all three examples severe forces injured the pelvis. The two riders with rupture and spread of the symphysis pubis were injured as their mounts bucked violently beneath them.

For examples of riding injuries see Figures 60, 63, and 172.

References

1. Barber HM: Horse-play: survey of accidents with horses. Br Med J 3:532–534, 1973
2. Editorial: Trauma at the racetrack. Roche Med Image, pp 24–26, 1968
3. Editorial: Hazardous occupations. Stat Bull Metropol Life Ins Co 50:3–4, 1969
4. Flynn M: Disruption of symphysis pubis while horse riding: a report of two cases. Injury 4:357–359, 1973
5. Hale JE: Traumatic arterial thrombosis, two cases. Proc R Soc Med 67:1024–1025, 1974
6. Kaye A (Editorial), cited in: Trauma at the racetrack. Roche Med Image, pp 24–26, 1968
7. McKnight J: Personal communication, 1976

KARATE–JUDO

Over 50,000 practitioners of karate perform their sport in the United States today.[2] Some karate enthusiasts scarify their hands and feet by striking a straw-covered pliable post (makiwara) over a period of years. Scar tissue accumulates over the injured areas, especially at the index and long finger metacarpophalangeal joints. Gardner reported that entrapment syndromes such as trigger finger and DeQuervain's disease can be recreated in this scar tissue milieu.[2] His report includes the description of a 19-year-old military policeman who, as a devoted karate exponent, practiced with the makiwara. He also pounded his hand into a sack filled with sand and gravel. After several months he developed a dorsal metacarpophalangeal area mass. He could not flex the long finger without severe pain and was unable to salute. Surgical exploration led to the removal of infiltrative scar tissue entrapping the extensor tendon. Gardner has seen many followers of karate with transient swelling and pain at the metacarpophalangeal joints and also notes that fractures of the wrist and hand are common.

Larose and Kim have obtained a number of x-rays of hands abused by this "savage" form of hand conditioning and in those using milder techniques of hand conditioning in karate.[3] In no instances did they find x-ray abnormalities such as soft tissue calcification or damage to the metacarpal heads.

Cantwell and King reported on a 39-year-old woman with abdominal pain, nausea, vomiting, and fainting after a karate lesson six weeks earlier.[1] In that lesson she had received a series of blows to the right upper quadrant of the abdomen in a subcostal location. On physical examination, the edge of the liver was palpable 10 cm below the right costal margin. The liver function tests were abnormal and the hemoglobin and blood pressure were reduced. An upper gastrointestinal series showed displacement of the duodenal bulb to the left. A liver scan showed a large defect in the right lobe of the liver. At laparotomy, the liver was twice normal size and contained a large stellate laceration of the capsule at the dome of the right lobe. An organizing hematoma under the capsule contained approximately 1500 ml of blood. A second laceration was found extending 5 cm and communicated with a subcapsular hematoma. The hematoma was drained and the patient did well. Whether or not she returned to karate lessons is not stated.

Occasionally participants in judo and karate are injured in falls during practice or competition. One unusual response to repeated shoulder injury following falls was described as traumatic osteolysis of the distal clavicle.[5] The outer ends of both clavicles partially resorbed following repeated ligamentous and probable vascular injury.

Sasa et al studied the effects of choking in judo by making cineradiographic recordings of the heart and lungs and electroencephalographic tracings during strangle holds.[4] As choking progressed they observed that the area of the cardiac silhouette decreased and reached a minimum at the time of unconsciousness. Recovery of the normal cardiac silhouette area occurred and was completed within 10 seconds after awakening. Concomitant phlethysmography showed that the blood flow increased in the arm of the person who was strangled. The electroencephalographic tracings showed slow waves during the periods of unconsciousness. The study infers that a decrease in the venous return to the heart is one of the major mechanisms that accounts for the observations during choking.

References

1. Cantwell JD, King JT Jr: Karate chops and liver lacerations, letter. JAMA 224:1424, 1973
2. Gardner RC: Hypertrophic infiltrative tendonitis (HIT syndrome) of the long extensor. The abused karate hand. JAMA 211:1009–1010, 1970
3. Larose JH, Kim DS: Karate hand-conditioning. Med Sci Sports 1:95–98, 1969
4. Sasa T, Ikai M, Ogawa S, Suzuki K, Matsumoto Y: Studies of choking in judo. Physiological and medical aspects. Abstracts of papers presented at the International Congress of Sports Science, Tokyo, Oct 3–8, 1964, p 111
5. Smart MJ: Traumatic osteolysis of the distal ends of the clavicles. J Can Assoc Radiol 23:264–266, 1972

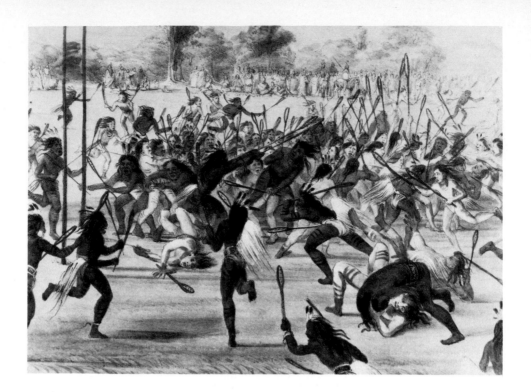

LACROSSE

The warriors of entire Indian nations competed in lacrosse, making the sport one of America's oldest. According to Weyand and Roberts, lacrosse was born of the North American Indian, was christened by the French, and was adopted and raised by the Canadians.[7] Hoffman reported that the game of lacrosse originated without doubt among some of the eastern Algonquian tribes, possibly in the valley of the St. Lawrence River, and was carried among the Huron and Iroquois tribes and later into the country of the Cherokee and other tribes.[5] It was taken west by various tribes of the Algonquian stock. Catlin lived among the Plains Indians for an eight-year period in the mid 1800s and through his noteworthy paintings we have records of the game as it appeared to him.[3]

One account of the origin of the name lacrosse refers to a French word applied to sticks used in a variant of an early form of football.[7] This primitive form of football was called "la soule" in France. In the 1300s a new variety of la soule evolved through the introduction of sticks. The ends of these sticks came to be curved, facilitating striking the ball and, according to Weyand and Roberts, "fanciful persons saw in that curved stick a resemblance to the crosier *(la crosse)* carried at ceremonies by a bishop as a symbol of pastoral office. Thus that crude game of shinny, and varieties of it, became known as la jeu de la crosse."[7] The French settlers in North America conferred the name "la crosse" on the various stick and ball games played by the natives. The city of La Crosse, Wisc., is located on the site of Prairie La Crosse, where the

Winnebago tribes played their matches. Some type of lacrosse was played by at least 48 tribes scattered throughout North America.

The Algonquians called the game *teiontsesiksaheks* and the Iroquois *tehontshik aheks*. The best remembered tribal name is *baggataway* in the Ojibway Chippewa dialect Pagaadowewin. The primitive game was a game played by the masses. Weyand and Roberts cite the account of Nicholas Perrot, a French government agent in Canada who, in 1667, watched a match near Sault Sainte Marie involving more than 2000 Miami warriors.[7] Play lasted for three days in another game recorded between the Senecas and the Mohawks. Thus lacrosse was used not only as a game of recreation but as a game of endurance training of tribal warriors.

Injuries were apparently uncommon among the Indian players, although details of injuries are vague. Beers cites an old Caughnawaga chief as saying that the Indians could play lacrosse all day without an injury.[1] The Iroquois of Caughnawaga had introduced lacrosse to the people of Montreal. Morrill noted that the Montreal Lacrosse Club was formed as early as 1839,[6] serving to bridge the game between the red man and the white man. Rules were soon formulated that prohibited striking, tripping, and throwing the stick or crosse at a player or at the ball.

The most common injuries in lacrosse are contusions, ankle sprains, and muscle tears. These were the most frequent injuries in a survey of the 30-man varsity team of the Johns Hopkins University done in 1975 by Bowerman et al.[2] Records were kept on injury in this study so that the data for an entire season were collected. The intercollegiate lacrosse season spans a three-month period in the United States. Players are protected by helmets and arm padding. The helmets are fitted with face guards that partially protect the player from a thrown ball and from blows from lacrosse sticks. The rules permit a great deal of body contact and allow an opponent to use the stick to hit at the ball carrier in an effort to dislodge the ball. The ball is made of hard rubber, measures between 7.75 and 8 inches in circumference, and weighs between 5 and 5.25 ounces.

There were 13 players injured either once or twice in the Johns Hopkins study, so that a total of 17 injuries were recorded in varsity lacrosse in the 1975 spring season. These included five contusions, three ankle sprains, three muscle tears, two knee injuries, two concussions, one laceration, and one fractured tooth. One of the players with a knee injury missed play for the remainder of the season and underwent surgery for the repair of ligament damage and for the removal of a torn meniscus. Among the injuries to the members of the junior varsity lacrosse team there was one sprained knee, one dislocated knee, and one fracture of the third lumbar vertebral body. The fracture occurred as the player was hit from the side. The two concussions in the varsity players also occurred as players were hit from the side. By way of comparison, there were 50 injuries to 29 players on the 45-member varsity football team at the same university in the 1974 season. The pattern of injuries was generally the same in football as in lacrosse, including 17 contusions, 10 ankle sprains, 4 concussions, and 4 avulsion injuries of muscle.

One myth that can be put to rest is that goalkeepers in lacrosse tend to have serious chest injury from repelling shots with their chest. It has been said, for example, that hemoptysis is common in goalkeepers after normal practice and game conditions. This is not true according to Brandimore, who has cared for players with lacrosse injuries for 30 years.[2] Contusion of the chest wall may occur, but pulmonary contusion or hemorrhage is rare if it occurs at all. Part of the goalkeeper's equipment is a chest protector usually made of a thick rubber pad. This type of protector has been worn for approximately the past ten years. Prior to that time goalkeepers used either an older model padded protector or, for several years, used no chest protector at all.

An unusual injury was reported by Crothers and Johnson in 1973.[4] A 19-year-old boy stepped backward during play and caught his left foot in a hole in the field. He fell on a flexed adducted knee with his foot inverted beneath him. He had immediate pain but was able to walk with moderate discomfort and a limp. Subsequent radiographs showed a dislocation of the proximal fibula. An attempt at nonoperative reduction failed and the fibula was reduced at operation. The fibular head was found displaced to a position anterior to the lateral prominence of the lateral tibial condyle and was held tightly in this location by an intact and taut fibular collateral ligament.

References

1. Beers WG: The National Game of Canada. New York, Townsend, 1869
2. Bowerman JW, Brandimore L, Weiland A, Thompson J, Tolo V: Unpublished data
3. Catlin G: Letters and notes on manners, customs and conditions of the North American Indians, Letter 49. London, Tosswill, 1841
4. Crothers OD, Johnson JTH: Isolated acute dislocation of the proximal tibiofibular joint. J Bone Joint Surg 55A:181–183, 1973
5. Hoffman WJ: The Menomini Indians. In: Fourteenth Annual Report of the Bureau of Ethnology to the Secretary of the Smithsonian Institution; 1892–1893. Washington, DC, Government Printing Office, 1896 (1897)
6. Morrill WK: Lacrosse. New York, Ronald, 1966
7. Weyand AM, Roberts MR: The Lacrosse Story. Baltimore, Herman, 1965

MOTORCYCLING

The use of the motorcycle as a means of transportation and as a vehicle for sport has recently reached new popularity. Similarly, the number of injuries and fatalities have reached new heights. An Associated Press release on July 24, 1974, indicated that sales of motorcycles in 1974 had increased 50 percent over the previous year.[1] In the first four months of 1974 there were 675 deaths of motorcyclists. The rate of death is currently 30 percent ahead of that of 1973 and contrasts with a 24-percent decline in the death rate in all types of accidents involving motor vehicles. At the end of 1973 the Department of Transportation estimated that there were 4,222,000 motorcycles on the road in the United States.

The records of the Maryland State Department of Motor Vehicles show that for 1974 there were 49,771 motorcyles registered in the state.[8] This registration represents an increase of nearly 50 percent over that of 1973, in which there were 34,017 cycles registered. In 1974 there were 48 motorcycle deaths, an increase of almost 40 percent over the 35 deaths in 1973. In addition, there were 1764 injuries to motorcyclists in 2218 accidents in 1973.

Most states require the use of a helmet for all drivers and passengers on motorcycles. Helmet use protects the motorcyclist from severe head injury but affords no protection for the cervical spine and the frequently damaged extremities. Sprains, abrasions, lacerations, fractures, and dislocations of the extremities are the most common injuries in nonfatal motorcycle accidents. Occasionally a rider will fall on the side of the head, damaging the cervical brachial plexus. In this case rupture of the cervical nerve root sheaths can be demonstrated on myelographic examination.

In a survey of motorcycle accidents in Monroe County, N.Y., for the year 1968, Clark and Morton recorded 226 accident victims.[4] There were 5 fatalities, 81 major injuries (those that required hospitalization), and 140 minor injuries. Fifty-three patients suffered 100 fractures. The sites of fracture included the lower extremity (41 percent), the upper extremity (30 percent), and the facial bones (12 percent). There were eight dislocations. Multiple injuries occurred in 39 percent of those injured.

Driver inexperience is one factor to consider regarding the cause of cycle injuries. Bothwell noted that cyclists with less than six months of experience had twice the accident rate of more experienced riders.[3]

Gustilo et al found that 20 percent of a group injured in motorcycle accidents had ridden a cycle less than three times prior to the accident.[6] The age group of the driver is a second factor to consider. In a series reported by Clark and Morton 51 percent of those injured or killed were under the age of 21.[4] Lee reported that a teenage boy has a 2 percent chance of being killed or seriously injured for each year he owns a motorcycle.[7] Ownership of the motorcycle is a third factor related to the causes of accidents. Gustilo et al reported that 70 percent of those injured had either borrowed or rented the motorcycle.[6] A study from staff members of the University of North Carolina showed that 28 percent of the motorcycles were borrowed or rented.[6] The use of alcohol is yet another factor related to the cause of accidents. Graham studied fatal motorcycle accidents and showed that of 193 motorcycle operators surviving less than six hours after injury, 46 percent had a detectable level of blood alcohol.[5] In the same study, 35 percent of the operators had blood alcohol levels greater than 0.1 mg/100 ml at postmortem examinations. Other causative factors include weather conditions—although Clark and Morton note that 90 percent of accidents occur on dry roads—and improper or unsafe driving habits, such as failure to yield the right of way, speeding, and tailgating.[4]

Meyer evaluated and treated injured motorcyclists who performed in national and international races in 1974 and 1975.[9] In his studies of the 1974 and 1975 International Six Day Trials, Meyer refers to those events as the Olympics of motorcycling. The riders race cross country over rugged terrain and travel from 150 to 250 miles in 4 to 6 hours daily for 6 days. At times speeds of 60 to 80 miles per hour are attained, although the average speed is 25 to 30 miles per hour. In the 1975 trials on the Isle of Man, an average of three significant injuries per day were incurred by the American team members. Concussions (3 riders), wounds (2), severe contusions (6), sprains (5), and fractures (8) occurred. Three of the eight contestants with fractures had multiple rib fractures, another fractured his sternum, and another his fibula. One of the Canadian team members was killed in a high-speed fall over the handlebars. Death was attributed to hemorrhage and hemothorax as a result of rupture of the azygous system of veins within the chest.

Meyer examined 276 professional riders in the 1974 International Six Day Trials and obtained information on their prior injuries in practice and in competition.[9] The motorcyclists ranged in age from 17 to 48 years. Two or more fractures had occurred in 45 riders, so that a total of 110 cyclists reported 174 fractures. These included 50 clavicular, 30 ankle, 29 tibial, 16 femoral, and 11 shoulder fractures among several other sites with fewer numbers of fractures. Meyer noted that the femur accounted for only 10 percent of the fractures in trail riding, where Enduro type cycles with relatively low-power engines are used (100 to 250 cc). In contrast, the femur was fractured in 80 percent of street injuries in which higher displacement street cycles were used. Most of the ankle and tibial fractures were produced by torsional forces caused by the rider implanting a foot during a fall or entrapment of the lower extremity under the cycle. His physical examinations of the 276 riders showed that 51 percent had significant knee injury in the past with instability, laxity, or locking as sequelae. Only 9 of these 143 riders had undergone knee surgery.

Bilotta also called attention to the differences in injury patterns in street model motorcycles as compared to Enduro or Motorcross cycles.[2] He studied 34 consecutive hospital admissions in which the patient was injured in a motorcycle crash.[2] The motorcycles included 24 street models (16 of these had an engine displacement of 500 to 750 cc), 6 Enduro models, and 3 Motorcross models. An automobile or truck was involved in 24 injuries and only 4 injuries occurred in the woods or on a track. A total of 66 fractures occurred in only 18 of the 34 patients studied. There were 24 compound fractures. In 60 percent of the cases the accidents were judged to be the fault of the car or truck driver who failed to see the motorcycle or turned in the path of the cycle misgauging its speed. Bilotta made a number of recommendations, including: (1) the institution of a program requiring instruction and licensing in the operation of motorcycles; (2) the maintenance of the present 55-mile-per-hour speed limit; (3) the promotion of cycles with smaller engine displacement rather than those with higher power and speed; (4) the designation of specific secondary routes for motorized and nonmotorized two-wheeled vehicles, separating full-sized automobiles from cycles; (5) the continued support in development of safety devices for the motorcyclist, including crash bars and balloons; and (6) the continued use of the safety helmet and enactment of legislation requiring its use throughout the United States.

Meyer has recommended that all motorcycle road racing apparel be designed to withstand abrasions to body prominences and to permit simple removal once a rider is injured.[9] This would include the use of zippered or latched boots and the abolishment of the unlined, one piece racing suit. These ideas followed observations by Meyer of data on injury to motorcycle racers in Daytona, Fla., in 1974 and 1975. Of 48 riders treated at the track hospital, 30 had abrasions and lacerations on the hands, elbows, hips, or knees that would have been prevented by the use of adequate protective clothing.

References

1. Associated Press Release. Motorcycle sales rise, also deaths. The Baltimore Morning Sun, July 24, 1974
2. Bilotta V: Motorcycle injuries. Paper presented to the Southern Medical Association, Nov 18, 1975
3. Bothwell PW: The problems of motorcycle accidents. Practitioner 188:474–488, 1962
4. Clark DW, Morton JH: The motorcycle accident: a growing problem. J Trauma 2:230–237, 1971
5. Graham JW: Fatal motorcycle accidents. J Forensic Sci 14:79–86, 1969
6. Gustilo RB, Foss DL, Leslie WR, et al: Motorcycle injuries. Minn Med 48: 489–491, 1965
7. Lee JAH: Motorcycle accidents to male teenagers: a contemporary epidemic. Proc R Soc Med 56:365–367, 1963
8. Maryland State Department of Motor Vehicles, Registration Statistics; Maryland State Police Department, Accident Records Division
9. Meyer RD: Injury and treatment report for the 1975 International Six Day Trials, injury to riders in the 1974 International Six Day Trials, and injury reports from Daytona Florida 1974–1975. Unpublished data

MOTOR-RACING

Participants in motor-racing are ever aware of the potential danger to life and limb. The effects of the acute stress in this sport on noradrenaline levels were studied by Taggart and Carruthers in 16 racing drivers at various intervals before and after international competitions.[3] A five- to sixfold increase in plasma noradrenaline levels was observed, with a peak value at 15 minutes after the race.

From the standpoint of fatal injury alone, the Indianapolis 500 Mile Automobile Race is one of the most dangerous sporting events in the world. The death rate among drivers in that race approximates the death rate in the Marine Corps in the Vietnam War at the height of battle.[2] Information compiled by the Statistical Bulletin of the Metropolitan Life Insurance Company based on data from the "500 Mile Record Book" published by the Indianapolis News shows that 36 drivers died between 1955 and 1970 in practice, trial, and final runs.[2] A fatality rate of 35.4 per thousand life-years is given for 500 Mile drivers and is based on a ratio of the number of deaths (36) to the total life-years exposed to the risk of death by the entrants during the same time period (1016). This death rate is extremely high compared to the mortality rate for men of the same age in the United States (approximately 3 per 1000). In addition to the drivers who were killed, 14 mechanics, 9 spectators, and 1 speedway guard have lost their lives during the history of the Indianapolis Race.

By contrast, it is estimated that in 15 years no more than three automobile racing fatalities have occurred at the Bonneville Salt Flats in Utah.[1] Approximately 500 to 700 professional racing drivers use the Salt Flats in Utah or the flat land at Lake Eyre, Australia, for racing, reaching speeds of 600 miles per hour with rocket-propelled cars. Each year nearly 200 permits to use the Salt Flats are issued and about 300 races are run. Simultaneous racing against other drivers is not allowed.

There is evidence that licensed race drivers do not have excellent driving records on the road. Williams and O'Neill compared the on-the-road driving records of 447 race drivers licensed by the Sports Car Club of America with 1053 non-racing drivers who were matched for age, sex, and race as control subjects.[4] Motor vehicle, highway, and public safety departments in Florida, New York, and Texas cooperated in this study. Driving record violations were sorted into three categories: speeding, other moving violations (including reckless driving), and nonmoving violations (including inadequate lights or brakes). The results indicated that in each state the Sports Car Club of America national competition license holders had a greater number of crashes per driver and a greater number of each of the three types of violations per driver than the control group. The biggest difference between race and comparison drivers was in speeding violations, where race drivers greatly exceeded the control group. This study was at least in part performed to shed light on the issue of a Masters Driver's License. The concept of this special license was introduced by the National Highway Traffic Safety Administration. License holders would have to pass a special test proving their expertise in emergency driving procedures such as skid control and off-road recovery. Those who believe that the race driver has fewer crashes, is more law abiding than the average driver, and possibly deserving of a Master Driver's License will have to reevaluate their position in light of the report by Williams and O'Neill.

References

1. Editorial: Championship automobile racing drivers. Stat Bull Metropol Life Ins Co 53:8–9, 1972
2. Editorial: Hazardous occupations and avocations. Stat Bull Metropol Life Ins Co 55:3–5, 1974
3. Taggart P, Carruthers M: Endogenous hyperlipidaemia induced by emotional stress of racing driving. Lancet 1:363–366, 1971
4. Williams AF, O'Neill B: On-the-road driving records of licensed race drivers. Accident Anal Prev 6:263–270, 1974

PARACHUTING

In 1965 there were over 500 sport parachuting clubs in the United States. Kiel reports that although the number of fatalities increased from 3 recorded deaths in 1958 to 35 deaths in 1963 there was an even greater increase in the number of jumps made per year by the estimated 50,000 participants.[2] The total number of jumps made in 1958 was 10,000 (approximately one death per 3300 jumps). In 1963 600,000 jumps were made (one death per 17,000 jumps). Failure to pull the ripcord and pulling the ripcord too late are the leading causes of death in sport parachuting. These faults accounted for 34 of 100 deaths reported by Kiel. Water landings and main chute entanglement or malfunction led to 19 and 16 deaths, respectively. The abrupt deceleration at impact produced lung lacerations (10 deaths), rupture of the heart (9), laceration of the brain (8), rupture of the aorta (7), and spinal fracture–spinal cord injury (6). Over half of these deaths occurred in the periods of preliminary and student training —periods that include 5 static-line jumps and 25 subsequent free falls. Deaths due to electrocution occurred in three jumpers who landed on power lines. Five jumpers died as a result of midair collisions with other parachutists.

Heaton surveyed injures in 50 civilian and 22 military parachute clubs in 1966.[1] The entire membership made 79,573 jumps in that year. One injury occurred in every 372 civilian jumps, compared to one injury in every 468 military jumps. Foot, ankle, leg, and knee injuries accounted for 71 percent of the total of 156 mishaps. Injuries occurred on landing (98.5 percent), at the time of parachute opening (1 percent), and in midair collisions (0.5 percent). Heaton estimated that approximately 12.5 percent or one in eight of the total jumping population in the United States would sustain a doctor-treated injury in the course of a year.

Torp and DeLuca found 10 injuries that required either hospitalization or confinement to quarters in 1966 among military parachutists at Fort Bragg, N. C.[3] In that time period 260 members of the sport parachute clubs at Fort Bragg made 5752 jumps, including 5018 free fall and 734 static-line jumps. The injuries included ankle sprains (2), back sprain (1), vertebral compression fracture (1), shoulder dislocation (1), and lower extremity fracture (5). The last group consisted of two ankle fractures, one foot fracture, and two compound fractures of the tibia and fibula. The injury rate of 1.7 per 1000 jumps occurred without fatality.

226

In a study of 44 fatalities in the United States sports parachuting in 1973 there were 7 (16 percent) due to collisions in free fall or on opening of the parachute.[4] These deaths are a reflection of the increased interest in so-called "relative work," the hand-to-hand contact and aerial formations performed during the free fall phase of jumping. These maneuvers led to death in 23 parachutists between 1968 and 1973. Nevertheless, the great majority of fatalities are attributed to malfunctioning main chutes coupled with reserve chute problems that occurred apart from relative work. This caused 23 of the 44 fatalities in 1973 and 102 of 204 deaths between 1968 and 1973.

References

1. Heaton NE: Review of accident causes: how can they be prevented? Parachutist, pp 9–11, Feb 1968
2. Kiel FW: Parachuting for sport. JAMA 194:264–268, 1965
3. Torp RP, DeLuca SE: Risk of personal injury in sport parachuting. Parachutist, pp 26–27, June 1967
4. Webb AC, Schnimsher J: 1973 fatality study. Parachutist, pp 22–27, Sept 1974

RUGBY

Rugby is generally played without protective equipment and is played enthusiastically in many parts of the world. There are some 1365 rugby clubs in England alone.[2] If there are approximately 40 men per club, then on an average Saturday afternoon in season there are 54,600 players in that country. Rugby easily accounts for the greatest proportion of sports injury in England according to Featherstone.[3] About half of all injuries in rugby occur in tackling.[1,2] Baylis recorded 247 injuries between 1968 and 1972 in a sample of 33 clubs.[2] Ligamentous or joint injuries produced over 28 percent of the injuries, whereas over 20 percent were fractures.

The cost of rugby injuries per year in New Zealand was estimated at more than one million dollars.[4] Dental injuries alone occurred in 26 percent of the players surveyed in Auckland.[5] Another 36 percent had some type of mouth injury. The most detailed account of injuries in rugby is that of O'Connell done in 1954.[6] He reviewed 600 cases in Ireland accumulated over 20 years. Five cases were fatal, including three fracture–dislocations of the cervical spine, one ruptured spleen, and one tetanus infection superimposed on a laceration. All five fatalities were due to charging or collapse of the scrum. These aspects of the game require constant vigilance on the part of the referee. Head and facial injuries accounted for over 21 percent of all injuries, shoulder injuries over 18 percent, and arm injuries over 12 percent. Knee injuries unlike the case in American football, were not frequent and comprised just over 12 percent of the entire group. The forwards and scrum halfbacks received most of their injuries in the head, hands, and face. The three-quarter backs were likely to receive shoulder or leg injuries. The fullback was least likely to be injured of all players on the field.

Archibald surveyed rugby injuries in one season involving 33 teams in Durham County, England.[1] There were 47 injuries serious enough to make the player leave the game permanently on the day of injury. Lacerations (13 players), joint sprains (11 players—4 knee, 4 ankle, 3 shoulder), and fractures (11 players—4 clavicle, 3 wrist, 3 ankle–leg, 1 rib) made up the majority of the injuries.

Roy studied injuries in rugby football in South Africa, where the sport is one of the most popular in that area.[7] There were 300 injuries in the 1973 season. An injury was defined as one requiring private medical treatment. Injuries to the knee (14.5 percent), ankle (13.5 percent), and head–face area (20.5 percent) accounted for almost half the total. There were 15 players with knee injuries and 6 with ankle injuries who required surgery. Other serious injuries included splenic rupture (1 player), concussion (3), transient brachial plexus palsy (1), and compression fracture of the eighth thoracic vertebral body (1). Collisions and falls on the shoulder produced 19 cases of acromioclavicular joint separation. This finding is similar to the incidence of shoulder injury in O'Connell's study. Many of the injuries in Roy's study were "unnecessary," and 34 percent of all the injuries fell into categories of "tackled without the ball," "loose scrum," and "foul play." Stricter control of the game by the official assigned to rule over the players can reduce these unnecessary injuries.

The herpes simplex virus may be inoculated by the close contact and trauma in wrestling and rugby. Scalp, forehead, and neck lesions occurred in two Rugby players reported by Verbov and Lowe.[8] One was admitted to a hospital with unexplained fever. Virus was demonstrated in both patients by electron microscopy of vesicle fluid. In addition, herpes simplex was grown by culture. The editorial staff of *The Lancet* gave this condition the title "herpes rugbeiorum."

References

1. Archibald R McL: An analysis of rugby football injuries in the 1961–62 season. Practitioner 189:333–334, 1962
2. Baylis RG: An analysis of rugby football injuries. Thesis submitted to the Institute of Education, Nottingham University, U.K., 1972
3. Featherstone DF: Sports Injuries—Their Prevention and Treatment. Wright, Bristol, England, 1957, p 1
4. Geiringer E: Sport as a threat to physical and mental health. NZ J Health Phys Educ Recreation 4:5–15, 1971
5. Hawke JE, Nicholas NK: Dental injuries in rugby football. NZ Dent J 65:173–175, 1969
6. O'Connell TCJ: Rugby football injuries and their prevention. A review of 600 cases. J Irish Med Assoc, 1954
7. Roy SP: The nature and frequency of rugby injuries. A pilot study of 300 injuries at Stellenbosch. S Afr Med J 48:2321–2327, 1974
8. Verbov J, Lowe NJ: Herpes rugbeiorum, letter to the editor. Lancet 2:1523–1524, 1974

SKIING

The number of skiers in the United States was estimated at 2.5 million in 1962. The rate of increase of the number of skiers per year has been estimated at 400,000. The number of these per year who cease to be active in the sport is unknown. The estimated average incidence of injury varies from 4 to 7 accidents per 1000 skiers per day in the United States and Sweden.[2,10,11,16,18,19] In 1973 Ellison reported a current injury rate of 4.5 injuries per 1000 skiers per day.[5] He noted that the number of injured had increased from 150,000 in 1961–1962 to 225,000 per year in the United States. Women have a higher incidence of injuries (7.9 per 1000) than do men (greater than 4 per 1000). Cross-country skiing has a lower injury rate than downhill skiing—6.5 per 1000 skiers per day compared to 0.5 per 1000 skiers per day in cross-country skiing.[18]

Teenagers made up the highest proportion of the injured (50 percent) in a review by Clayton.[2] He noted that expert skiers had fewer but generally more severe injuries than the inexperienced skiers. Several professional skiers had ruptures of the Achilles tendon within a two-month period in 1961. Nearly three-fourths of all injuries occur in a situation in which the skier loses control, yet most injuries occur on moderate slopes.

A second comparison of injury patterns in expert and novice skiers was made in an article by Williams.[19] The sites of injury in three groups of recreational skiers in Bavaria, New England, and the Rocky Mountains were compared to those in a unit of British Mountain Troops in Austria. Of 113 injured novice military skiers, almost 48 percent had knee injuries and almost 41 percent had ankle sprains. In the more experienced skiers there was a lower incidence of knee injuries (17 injuries; 22 percent). The percentage of ankle injuries in the recreational skiers ranged from 20 to 55 percent. Ankle fractures were more common in the experienced group at 25 percent (13 injuries), compared to 5 percent in the military group. The most common knee joint injury in this series produced a tear of the medial collateral ligament.

Adequate safety bindings that provide release of the ski in certain stressful positions do reduce injuries. Data suporting this belief that were gathered by Heinkel were cited by Clayton.[2] In 1952, at the American Ski School in Garmisch-Partenkirchen, Germany, 34 fractures of the leg occurred during 500 ski rentals. After changing to a safety release binding and issuing over 100,000 rentals in several seasons, only 60 fractures were recorded. This is a 12-fold reduction in the incidence of fractures. In 1966, Harwood and Strange reported that over 55 types of bindings existed then and that only a dozen were satisfactory from a safety standpoint.[10] They cited work done by Gordon Lipe of Syracuse, N.Y., who designed a system of testing forces needed to effect a toe release in skiers of varying weight and skill. Lipe created a chart relating pressure levels of binding settings with skiers' abilities and needs. Some novice skiers had been setting releases adequate for expert skiers or racers weighing over 200 pounds. Injuries produced by poor release of bindings include knee and ankle sprains and fractures. In a five-year period Harwood and Strange observed 55 fractures of the foot or ankle and 105 fractures of the shaft of the tibia or fibula in skiers in five major ski areas near Syracuse, N.Y. These injuries represented 24 percent of a total of 650 injuries. They found that 30 of these fractures, including 25 tibial or fibular shaft fractures, occurred in skiers whose bindings did not release at the time of injury.

The so-called skier's fracture of the metacarpal is not common. Coventry estimated that such fractures constituted 1.3 percent of all fractures seen in skiing.[3] More than one metacarpal may be fractured.

Sponsel collected injury data on weekend skiers at Mt. Telemark, Cable, Wisc., over a one-year period from 1965 to 1966.[16] Of 215 injured skiers, there were 24 with comminuted tibial fracture and fibular fracture. Seven patients had transverse tibial fractures of the "boot top" variety and several of these were comminuted. One patient fractured the thoracic spine and was paraplegic until recovery after laminectomy. Paraplegia following ski injury has also been reported in skiers who perform stunts or acrobatics on skis. Odom reported two such injuries in a study of spinal cord and head injuries in Denver, Colo., between 1968 and 1972.[15]

The majority of ski injuries are sprains and fractures. Ellison estimated that sprains account for 40 percent of all ski injuries and fractures for 35 percent;[6] 80 percent of all injuries and 89 percent of all fractures occur at the leg;[5] and almost 40 percent of all fractures involve the tibia or fibula or both. Ellison contributed to a film sponsored by the Committee on Sports Medicine of the American Academy of Orthopedic Surgery and by Johnson and Johnson, New Brunswick, N.J., that details the mechanisms in ski injuries.[6]

The problem of the injured athlete who wishes to resume skiing or his chosen sport is discussed by Chrisman and Snook in a report on the problem of refracture of the tibia.[1] Between 1957 and 1964, they treated seven young male athletes with refractures of the lower tibia. Three of the seven refractures occurred in skiing accidents. Since 1964, they have examined the cortex of healing fractures in athletes by tomography. In 18 patients with fracture of the tibia, they found 3 with gaps or defects in the cortex that warranted, in their opinion, continued avoidance of sports for 6 to 12 months until reevaluation with tomography. No instance of refracture occurred in their 18 patients. They thus raise the question, "When is a fracture healed?" and ask, "Healed enough for what?"

The issue of comparison of injury rates between a group of injured athletes with a control group of uninjured athletes at risk in the same activity was investigated by Haddon et al.[9] They reported a controlled study of skiers in action at Mt. Snow, Vt. The control group was composed of every fiftieth person purchasing a ticket to ski on four consecutive weekends in January and February 1961. The entire study group included 438 controls and 130 injured persons. The latter were defined as those persons who were injured while skiing and who reported to the resort's medical facility on the day of injury. Three groups of skiers were created based on turning technique: a snow plow turn group, a stem christie group, and a parallel-wedeln group. Injury rates were higher for the snow plow turn group, which included the highest proportion of beginner and novice skiers. Although this group constituted only 21 percent of those skiing, members of this group contributed 55 percent of the injuries. The injury rate in the snow plow turn group was 16.0 per 1000 ski–man–days compared with rates of 4.1 and 2.9 in the stem christie and parallel-wedeln groups.

The authors noted a significant association between the occurrence of lower extremity musculoskeletal injury and the use of nonrelease bindings among males. Safety or release bindings had a protective effect in male skiers. Among female skiers no significant differences were found between those that used release bindings and those that did not. The forces required to disengage ski boots from the release bindings were felt to exceed the injury thresholds of female skiers but not those of males. Haddon et al proposed four strategies that may be employed to reduce the occurrence and consequence of skiing injuries: (1) provide better training for beginners and have the inexperienced use gentler slopes; (2) develop more effective release bindings; (3) provide the best possible emergency orthopedic and medical care; and (4) provide the best possible follow-up medical care and rehabilitation.

Erskine has observed that the site of leg fractures in skiing has changed from the ankle level to the lower third of the tibia.[7] Although no specific comparative data are cited he suggests that the changes in boot design are responsible for this trend. The rigid molded boots of today protect the malleoli of the ankle but are viselike and permit a leverage of forces to act at the distal tibia. It is essential that release bindings work properly to protect the lower extremity. Erskine believes that the use of silicone spray to lubricate bindings and minimize the hazard of a frozen release system is a vital addition to skiing safety.[7]

The fibula may fracture alone in a boot top injury in a skier. Johnson et al reported 25 examples treated in four Vermont areas between 1969 and 1972.[13] The fracture levels ranged from 7.3 to 12.9 cm above the ankle mortise. In 11 skiers the safety binding did not release, in a like number it did release, and in 3 its function was not known. In 20 skiers, the type of ski boot was known. There were 17 skiers who wore hard plastic boots and 3 who had leather boots. Only 4 of these had new ultrahigh-top boots. Falls produced 23 injuries and collisions led to 2. The fractures were either oblique or, less often, transverse and were a direct result of transverse loading at the upper lateral edge of the boot. The authors estimate that this injury represents 2 percent of all reported injuries in skiers.

It is a consolation to the injured skier to realize that the boot top fracture and other lower tibial fractures of injured skiers have a better prognosis than tibial fractures of a different etiology. Van Der Linden et al studied 600 fractures (including 393 fractures secondary to skiing injury) after admission to the Centrallasarettet, Ostersund, Sweden, between January 1967 and October 1973.[17] The fractures in skiers were more often in the lower third of the tibia and were seldom compound compared to the fractures in nonskiers. Healing was more rapid, the period of hospitalization less, and the incidence of complications lower in the skier group.

Johnson discusses various types of ski bindings in an article that deals practically with the safety of bindings.[12] He reports that his 9-year old daughter suffered a spiral fracture of the femur while skiing with inadequate bindings. He reminds us that bindings must be cleaned and oiled to function safely. The use of silicone spray to reduce friction and ice formation is again recommended.

The ulnar collateral ligament of the thumb can be ruptured in skiing. The usual mechanism of injury is a fall with the leather loop at the handle of the ski pole wrapped around the thumb. Fraser-Moodie suggests that skiers can avoid this injury by gripping the pole very firmly in a fall or by holding the ski stick without using the loop.[8]

It may not be totally safe to go for a fitting for new ski boots. A young woman described by Joynt stood for approximately 12 minutes with her feet in a foam-filled mold inside her new ski boots.[14] She became faint and had a seizure. Fortunately, a fall to the floor was prevented by nearby physical constraints. Ski shop owners have indicated that fainting has occurred infrequently during fittings for foam boots. The prolonged standing with a near motionless body attitude apparently decreased venous return and lowered blood pressure enough to produce the fainting.

Once the skier is past the period of acquiring new boots he faces multiple challenges, including pressure on the first sacral nerve at the boot top. Crelinsten reports that the skier will complain of irritating numbness and tingling of the soles of the feet after a long day on the slopes.[4] He suggests that in some situations the cause will be sensory fiber compression rather than cold injury producing these symptoms. Thus we can add another boot top syndrome to the lower leg injuries at that level.

References

1. Chrisman OD, Snook GA: The problems of refracture of the tibia. Clin Orthop 60:217–218, 1968
2. Clayton M: Ski injuries. Clin Orthop 23:52–66, 1962
3. Coventry MB: Winter sports injuries. Lancet 85:66–70, 1965
4. Crelinsten GL: Ski-boot neuropathy, letter to the editor. N Engl J Med 288:420, 1973
5. Ellison AE: Skiing injuries. JAMA 223:917–919, 1973
6. ⸻, cited in: (Editorial): Ski-mishap novices reveal most common trauma types. Med Trib, p 23, Feb 13, 1974
7. Erskine LA: Recent changes in the pattern of skiing injuries. J Trauma 14:92–93, 1974

8. Fraser-Moodie WA: Gamekeeper's thumb on the ski slopes, letter to the editor. Br Med J 1:640, 1974
9. Haddon W Jr, Ellison AE, Carroll RE: Skiing injuries: epidemiological study. Public Health Rep 77:975–991, 1962
10. Harwood MR, Strange GL: Orthopedic aspects and safety factors in snow skiing. NY State J Med 66:2899–2907, 1966
11. Howorth B: Skiing injuries. Clin Orthop 43:171–181, 1965
12. Johnson HA: Choosing the safest ski binding. Ill Med J 141:288–290, 1973
13. Johnson RJ, Pope MH, Holmes EM: Boot top fractures of the fibula. Clin Orthop 101:198–200, 1974
14. Joynt RJ: Foam fitting faints feigning fits, letter to the editor. N Engl J Med 288:219, 1973
15. Odom JA, cited in: Editorial: Ski-stunts draw fire from doctors. Physician Sports Med 2:19, 1974
16. Sponsel KH: Weekend ski injuries at Mt. Telemark, Cable, Wisconsin, 1965–1966 season. Ind Med Surg 36:35–40, 1967
17. Van Der Linden W, Sunzel H, Larsson K: Fractures of the tibial shaft after skiing and other accidents. J Bone Joint Surg 57A:321–327, 1975
18. Westlin N: Extremity injuries in relation to ski bindings and boots. Lakartidningen 67:3185–3190, 1970
19. Williams JA: Winter sports. In Armstrong JR, Tucker WE (eds): Injury in Sport. London, Staples, 1964, pp 250–258

SNOWMOBILING

The first snowmobiling vehicle was built in 1923 in Valcourt, Quebec, by Joseph-Armand Bombardier.[4] Since that time explosions of injury reports have occurred. Now the severity of snowmobile accidents rivals that of injuries in motorcyclists. Wenzel reported 102 fatalities in snowmobiling in 1970–1971 in the United States.[8] In Wisconsin alone, in 1972–1973, there were 31 deaths and 1000 injuries.[9] Wenzel noted that snowmobiling was nearly nonexistent five years ago, but that 750,000 vehicles were sold in the United States in 1973.[8] Among the 31 deaths in Wisconsin in 1972–1973, 23 occurred at night and one-third of the victims had been drinking. Monge and Reuter at the Duluth Clinic, Duluth, Minn., recorded injures to 267 persons in a study spanning 201 days.[3] Alcohol was a factor in 40 percent of the accidents and figured prominently in the more serious injuries. Soft tissue injury—laceration, contusion, or abrasion—was sustained by 139 patients and ligamentous or cartilaginous tears by 55 patients. There were 7 patients with dislocated joints and 55 patients had fractured a total of 83 bones. There was visceral injury including brain damage in 14 patients and 3 of these died. Leg fractures were found in 40 patients and 16 had skull or facial bone fractures. Five patients had compression fractures of the lumbar vertebrae. Seven patients had concussions, one had an epidural hematoma, and one had an extensive cerebral laceration. There was one complete transection of the spinal cord at the sixth thoracic vertebral level. This occurred when a snowmobiler drove his vehicle over a 50-foot cliff. This patient and the two patients with the most serious brain injuries accounted for the three deaths in this series. The major causes of the accidents were as follows: struck part of the vehicle in riding over rough terrain (56 patients; 20 percent); vehicle capsized (49; 19 percent); struck a fixed object such as a tree, rock, or fence (43; 16 percent); and was thrown from the snowmobile (26; 10 percent).

In a study by Withington and Hall of 59 persons injured in snowmobiles in New Hampshire the disabling nature of many injuries was emphasized.[10] Enough information was provided by 47 victims of collisions or falls in snowmobiles to permit some estimate of disability. Only 22 were disabled temporarily for a period of less than six weeks; 4 of the remaining 25 injured persons were permanently disabled. Facial injury, skull injury, blindness, and fractures of the spine were features of the more severe injuries.

Fractures of the spine were common in a series of 103 patients reported by

Chism and Soule.[1] Fifteen patients had fractures of the spine, most often at T11, T12, or L1. Fractures occurred as high as T4 and as low as L4 in their patients. The second most common injury was a fracture of the tibia or fibula (ten patients). The authors emphasized, apart from the dangers of snowmobile use, that snowmobiles have provided invaluable emergency transportation in many areas of the country where deep snowfall hampers travel.

Few people realize how many snowmobile owners there are in the United States. In Chittenden County, Vt., an area of 99,000 inhabitants, there are approximately 3500 snowmobiles.[7] Slightly more than 2 percent of these vehicles will be involved in accidents each year according to a report by Waller and Lamborn.[7] Information was gathered from questionnaires sent to registered owners and from interviews with injured snowmobilers, uninjured owners, and uninjured neighbors of accident victims. Owners tended to be young (62 percent under age 40) and male (90 percent). Nearly three-fourths of the injured were drivers. The injured drivers over age 18 were twice as likely to report that they had been drinking and drinking heavily before their injury than the uninjured drivers. The higher the speed at the time of injury the greater the likelihood that alcohol had been consumed.

The authors compared the tendency of drivers to feel frustrated in life and in their jobs. Drivers were asked how they responded to frustration and whether they had been involved in fist fights. Almost half of the injured drivers had been involved in at least one fight compared to only one-quarter of the comparison group of uninjured drivers. The injury event was usually a collision with an overhanging object or another fixed barrier. This happened to 33 drivers, or 35 percent of the drivers who were injured. In the immediate postinjury period several noteworthy events occurred. Among those adults who sought care within the first hour after injury, 30 percent had ingested alcohol after the collision or injury event. Of the 115 persons who indicated that time span between the injury and the reception of medical care, 60 percent waited an hour before seeking medical care and 42 percent waited at least six hours.

In reviewing the design features of the snowmobiles the authors suggest that at least half the injuries reported are related to areas of design needing improvement. Some of these problems include inadequate suspension systems, a high center of gravity coupled with a narrow track, inadequate front and rear lights, poor traction on ice, exposed moving parts, and handlebars with poor energy-attenuating characteristics.

Roberts et al tested the seats and suspension systems of the ten best-selling snowmobiles in 1971.[5] An Arctic Cat Panther snowmobile fitted with the test seats and an anthropometric dummy was studied during 2-, 3-, and 4-foot vertical fall and impact situations. The dummy bottomed the seat and was subjected to 20-g forces in the least severe impact and up to 34-g forces in the most severe fall. Such forces are potentially sufficient in all cases to produce compression fractures of the vertebral bodies. It should be noted that asymmetrical loading will produce a concentration of forces in the spine and lead to injuries at a much lower level of impact force than measured. In addition, the vertebral body end-plate will fracture at lower force impact levels than those required to compress the vertebral body. Roberts et al presented seven clinical examples of spinal compression fracture in addition to the test data. They concluded that better seats and better snowmobile suspension systems could be devised to protect the spine from impact forces.

Thomas described the unfortunate example of the snowmobiler who was tuning the motor of his vehicle in his garage when he suddenly fell to the floor and rapidly died.[6] A wound was noted in the upper abdomen. Radiographs showed a metallic foreign body in the right side of the chest and upper abdomen. The metal measured 23.7 × 8.7 cm and matched a defect in the clutch wheel of the snowmobile. No protective shielding was noted on two of the clutch wheels.

Midfacial fractures and lacerations in snowmobilers who were wearing crash helmets at the time of their accidents were reported by Daniel and Midgley in 1972.[2] Four cases were used as examples of poor protection of the face by the helmets worn by the injured. In case one, a 28-year-old driver was struck from behind by another snowmobile. He was thrown forward and hit his face on the handlebars. He sustained facial lacerations, nasal fractures, and a left zygomatic fracture. In other examples, a driver drove off a cliff in unfamiliar terrain, fell from the snowmobile into the path of another vehicle, or drove into an abandoned car in a snow drift. Mandibular and maxillary fractures were commonplace. The authors recommend a different helmet design in which the helmet encircles the nose and mandible, leaving a windscreen visor for vision and eye protection.

References

1. Chism SE, Soule AB: Snowmobile injuries. JAMA 209:1672–1674, 1969
2. Daniel RK, Midgley RD: Facial fractures in snowmobile injuries. Plast Reconstr Surg 49:38–40, 1972
3. Monge JJ, Reuter NF: Snowmobiling injuries. Arch Surg 105:188–191, 1972
4. Percy EC: The snowmobile: friend or foe? J Trauma 12:444–446, 1972
5. Roberts VL, Noyes FR, Hubbard RP, McCabe J: Biomechanics of snowmobile spine injuries. J Biomech 4:569–577, 1971
6. Thomas WC: Snowmobilopathy. N Engl J Med 286:845–846, 1972
7. Waller JA, Lamborn KR: Snowmobiling: characteristics of owners, patterns of use and injury. Proc Am Assoc Automotive Med 383–407, 1973
8. Wenzel FJ, cited in: (Editorial): Strict laws urged to cut down rising snowmobile accidents. Med Trib, p 23, Feb 6, 1974
9. _____, Peters RA, Hintz CS, Olsen TW: Snowmobile accidents in central Wisconsin. Wis Med J 72:89–94, 1973
10. Withington RL, Hall LW: Snowmobile accidents. A review of injuries sustained in the use of snowmobiles in Northern New England during the 1968–1969 season. J Trauma 10:760–763, 1970

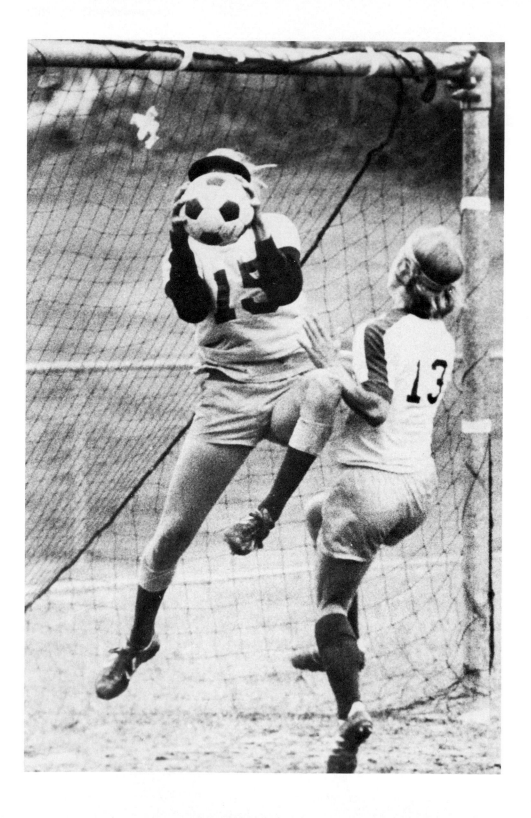

SOCCER

The game of soccer has existed in some form since the earliest records of man. Gardiner[7] and Masterson,[11] in work dealing with the early history of ball-games, suggest that soccer was played in ancient China in the third century BC. The pre-Columbian peoples of the Olmecs, Mayans, and Aztecs, between 500 BC and 300 BC, played games in which a ball was kicked.[11] The Mayan game, known as Pok-ta-Pok, was particularly rigorous, and masks, mitts, and thigh protectors were worn by the participants.[11] Duran has described their play and what must rank among the earliest soccer injuries receiving medical attention.[6] The game was played with a solid rubber ball of four to five inches in diameter. The goals were stone rings set vertically at the sides of the field. Players were allowed to use only their knees, thighs, shoulders, and buttocks to move the ball. Duran[6] relates that

> . . . some of them were carried dead out of the place and the reason was that they ran, tired and out of breath, after the ball from one end of the court to the other. They would see the ball come in the air and in order to reach it first before others, it would strike the pit of the stomach or the groin so that they fell to the ground breathless and some of them died instantly because of their ambition to reach the ball before anyone else. . . They were so quick in that moment to hit the ball with their knees or buttocks that they returned it with extraordinary velocity. With these thrusts, they suffered great damage on the knees or thighs with the result that those, who for dexterity often used them, had their haunches so bruised that they had those places cut with a small knife and extracted the blood which the blows of the ball had gathered.[6]

This gives us an inkling that a trainer or team physician or surgeon was active long before the modern methods of care for the athlete.

That soccer teams of today warrant special medical supervision is scarcely questioned. An idea of the frequency of injury to expert players is given in the three-year injury statistics of the Arsenal Football Club of London cited by Bass.[2] In this time period, 190 injuries were recorded. There were 16 meniscectomies or fractures, comprising 7.5 percent of the injury total. Muscle, tendon, and nonsurgical joint injuries occurred 143 times and accounted for 74 percent of the total injuries. The full-time Arsenal playing staff includes 50 ath-

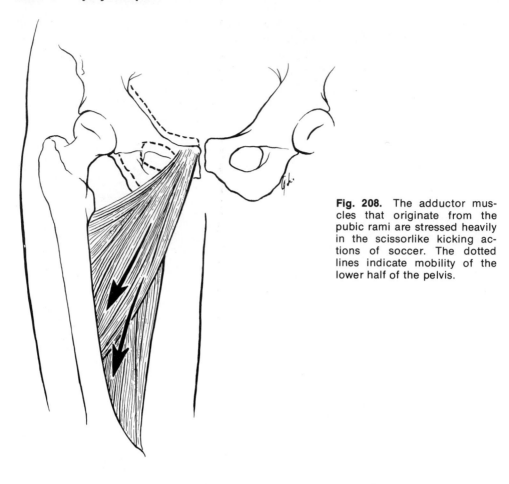

Fig. 208. The adductor muscles that originate from the pubic rami are stressed heavily in the scissorlike kicking actions of soccer. The dotted lines indicate mobility of the lower half of the pelvis.

letes who play or train every day of the week. A portable x-ray unit is available on all match days to provide prompt diagnostic service.

Injury Patterns

The soccer player is one of the most widely studied athletes from the standpoint of injury. Radiographic studies of the ankle and the symphysis pubis are apt to be useful and abnormal. The repeated kicking of a soccer ball has long been suspected to exact a toll from the kicker's foot. Morris described five examples of anterior ankle joint tenderness and swelling in expert kickers of footballs in 1943.[15] New bone formation was found at the dorsal surface of the neck of the talus on x-ray examinations. He felt that a traction force exerted in a position of extreme plantar flexion was responsible for the talus abnormality. McMurray made similar observations in professional soccer players in 1950.[13] He described bony outgrowths from the anterior margins of the tibia as well as the talus in later stages of the disorder. Slight periosteal roughening was found in the early stages of x-ray changes. McMurray joined Morris in attributing the talus abnormality to the effort of kicking with the strain of the blow borne by the dorsal capsule of the ankle joint. The abrupt changes in direction and speed and the jumping required in soccer may cause the observed ankle changes. Only recently x-ray studies of athletes engaged in other sports have shown that the anterior portion of the ankle joint including the dorsal surface of the talus may show degenerative changes.[3,4] Basketball is the sport that perhaps most shares the running and jumping patterns of soccer.

AVULSION INJURY. A most incapacitating injury experienced by soccer players is instability of the symphysis pubis. The ligamentous support of this joint is weakened in association with chronic adductor muscle strain (Fig. 208). Many reports describing these injuries have appeared in the English, German, Italian, and Spanish literature.[5,9,10,19] At present three international players from England are hampered by this injury and more undoubtedly exist. Players often describe no acute episode of injury but have tenderness at the symphysis pubis, especially inferiorly. They complain of groin pain that may be misinterpreted as hip pain or abdominal pain. Symptoms are much worse in full stride, jumping, and in the stretching motion of kicking with power. The actual incidence of this injury is uncertain. Complete radiologic surveys of soccer players with and without symptoms are needed to study its incidence. Luschnitz et al performed serial examinations of 30 soccer players and found 50 percent of the outstanding players to have periosteal reaction at the origin of the adductor muscles.[10] They refer to this particular type of overstrain in soccer players as the gracilis syndrome. In its early stages, semicircular and oval radiolucencies occur at the pubic bone close to the symphysis at the origin of the gracilis muscle and the adductors longus and brevis.

Cochrane lists several things in the x-ray appearance of this disorder in addition to the radiolucencies or erosive avulsion sites: frayed corners of the symphysis pubis, fluffy margins of the symphysis, periosteal reaction at muscle attachments, osteoporosis at the symphysis, a widened symphysis, and, most importantly, an unstable symphysis.[5] This instability can be demonstrated by obtaining two comparison anteroposterior radiographs of the symphysis pubis with the athlete first bearing weight on one leg and then on the other (Fig. 209). This comparison technique will show one side of the symphysis pubis slip to a different position in one weight-bearing view. The uppermost corner of one side of the symphysis will be displaced superiorly as the player bears weight on the corresponding lower extremity. Rest has been the mainstay of treatment although there are some who advocate surgical repair (Fig. 210).

Other conditions can show a similar x-ray appearance, including the relaxation of the symphysis in the childbearing female, the inflammatory changes following supra- and retropubic operations such as prostatectomy, and direct trauma to the pelvis.

Harris and Murray recently surveyed an entire professional soccer club (26 members) for radiographic and clinical evidence of pelvic adductor muscle group avulsion and post-traumatic instability of the symphysis pubis.[9] They also studied a second group of symptomatic athletes (nine soccer players, one

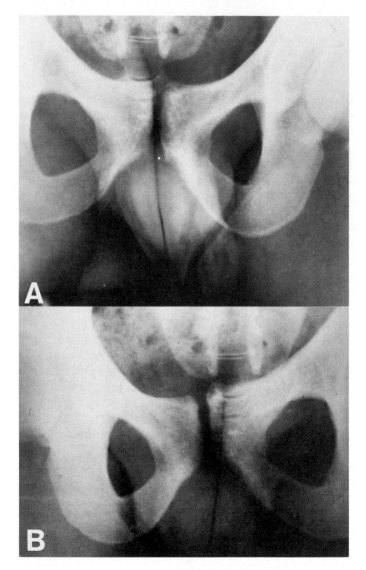

Fig. 209. A painful symphysis pubis was radiographed. **A, B.** Weight-bearing views are shown. What is your diagnosis? **C, D.** Erosive irregularities are present at the lower cortical margin of the inferior pubic rami. The left side of the symphysis is able to slide onto the right side. The diagnosis is instability of the symphysis pubis shown by movement of one side of the symphysis pubis on the other in these weight-bearing views. The comparison views of this symphysis pubis were made with the player first bearing weight on one leg (**C**) and then the other (**D**). This weight-bearing attitude forces one side of the unstable symphysis to slide upon the other (arrows). The views have been informally referred to as "flamingo views" because of the resemblance of the leg position of the patient to that of the great wading bird.

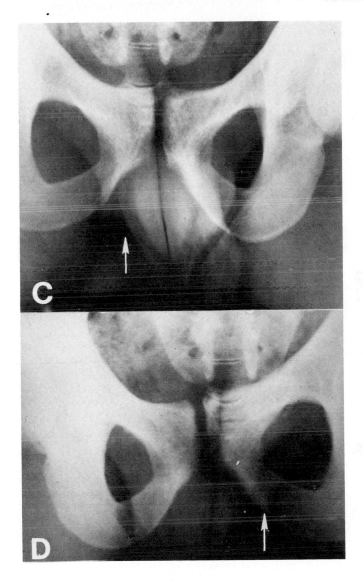

jockey, and one distance runner) in a similar manner. Radiographs of a group of 156 young men provided a comparison and control from the x-ray standpoint. Among the 26 teammates in professional soccer only one had symptoms of groin pain at the time of the study. The two study groups had pelvic radiographs and weight-bearing radiographs of the symphysis pubis, with the player first bearing weight on one leg in one view and then on the other leg for another view (Fig. 209). (Such views have been informally referred to as "flamingo views."[18]) A difference in the height of the superior pubic ramus on each side of more than 2 mm was accepted as abnormal. The width of the

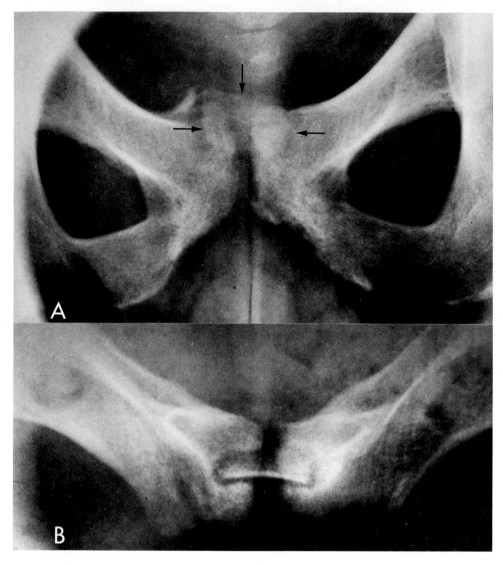

Fig. 210. These views were made postoperatively, with one (**B**) made at a steep angle to the symphysis pubis. A graft of bone (arrows) has been placed across the symphysis in an effort to prevent painful motion at this site in a soccer player.

symphysis was measured using 10 mm as the upper limit of normal. In addition, the margins of the symphysis and the inferior pubic rami were evaluated for marginal irregularity and sclerosis.

Over one-third (9) of the soccer club members had instability of the symphysis, 19 had marginal irregularity, and 17 had reactive sclerosis. There were 14 with stress sclerosis in the iliac portion of one or both sacroiliac joints. In the symptomatic group of 11 athletes there were 7 with instability of the symphysis pubis, 4 with reactive sclerosis, 8 with marginal irregularity, and 2 with an abnormally wide symphyseal cleft. In the control group 70 percent of 156 had some abnormalities at the symphysis pubis. The authors noted that the greater the athletic experience of the control individual the greater the likelihood of an x-ray abnormality.

The clinical features of the symptomatic players include discomfort or pain in one or both groins brought on by physical exertion and relieved by rest. Suprapubic and lower abdominal pain is not uncommon. Tenderness is present over the symphysis and ischiopubic ramus. A rest period of two weeks to three months has been the most reliable method of treatment in this study, although surgical fusion of the symphysis has been used successfully.[9]

Running stresses with attendant falls and tackling in a sliding maneuver to get the ball from an opposing player may lead to avulsion injuries of muscular attachments at the pelvis.[14] (See the section on track and field). Figure 252 is such an injury in an athlete who experienced sudden groin pain. Such appearances may be confused with inflammatory or neoplastic lesions of the pelvis. The adductor muscle group, including the adductor longus and adductor brevis, attach at the inferior pubic ramus.

In a younger player whose skeleton is immature, the cartilaginous growth centers are still visible on radiographs. Separation of the growth center at the ischium is recognized by a gap between the avulsed fragment and the inferior pubic ramus. When an athlete is just beyond the period of skeletal growth and reaches his early twenties, the cartilaginous lines of growth have disappeared radiologically. However, avulsed fragments still occur in the maturing skeletons and the unwary physician may be put off guard by the absence of the lucent bands of cartilage on x-rays. Forgetting that injury alone is the explanation for the radiographic picture he may invoke other diagnoses.

Other less specific injuries occur in this sport and produce a radiologic abnormality (Figs. 211, 212). Occasionally a player will develop chronic leg pain of insidious onset.

STRESS FRACTURE. Radiographs will show a dense, thickened anterior tibial cortex that represents hypertrophy of osseous and periosteal tissue from overuse. A stress fracture may occur in the tibial cortex either unilaterally or bilaterally. Such an occurrence, if unsuspected, may lead to mistaken diagnosis and confusion with osteoid osteoma or other bone lesions. It is a mistake to assume that stress fractures do not occur in accomplished athletes. Figure 213 shows a tibial stress fracture in an expert soccer player. It was initially misdiagnosed as a tumor.

SPINE. Because running and jumping play such an important role in this sport, the spine and pelvis, apart from the symphysis pubis, may show x-ray abnormality. Figure 214 shows a defect in both sides of the fifth lumbar vertebrae at the pars interarticularis in a soccer player. This disorder, known as spondylolysis, can follow heavy lifting and other forms of stress to the spine. It most commonly involves the fifth lumbar vertebral site and is best seen in oblique radiographs of the lumbar spine. The defect is a fracture that rarely unites and is often followed by instability of the spine. The instability may pro-

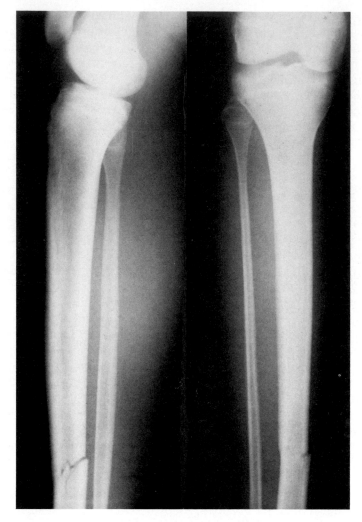

Fig. 211. A soccer player was kicked directly in the lower leg. A tibial fracture resulted.

gress so that one vertebral body at the pars defect and all the vertebral bodies above it slip forward on the vertebral body below the defect. This unstable state is known as spondylolysthesis and is recognized on the lateral radiograph of the lumbar spine by malalignment of the vertical lines of the posterior margins of the vertebral bodies. The intervertebral disc between the slipping vertebrae suffers in this situation and disc degeneration often results.

HIP.   A lifetime of professional soccer, or indeed any extensive athletic participation, can produce the chronic hip pain of osteoarthritis. Murray has observed that the femoral head in many former athletes is not centered in a normal position on the femoral neck, and that extensive osteoarthritis secondary to this situation is not uncommon and is predominantly due to a minimal

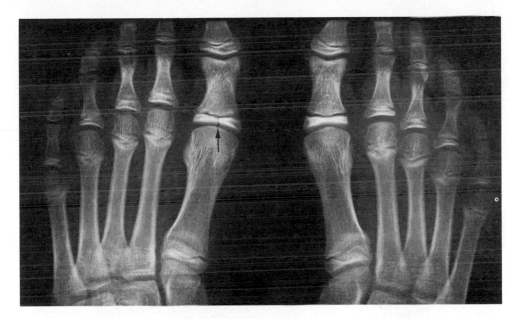

Fig. 212. These foot views were made in a 13-year-old boy who was an active soccer player and trampolinist. He injured his foot in soccer. Both epiphyses of the proximal phalanx of the great toe are dense and an apparent fracture line crosses that of the left great toe. This is a normal variant and not a true fracture line. The line is a cleft between two ossification centers for the epiphysis of the great toe. The increased radiodensity of the proximal epiphyses of the great toes is also a normal variant.

slipped epiphysis of the femoral head at an earlier time in the patient's career.[17] The initial period of slippage may go unnoticed or may be accompanied by mild episodes of pain. The occurrence of slipped femoral capital epiphyses in nonathletic situations—for example, in obese or rangy, lanky adolescent males and in patients with renal disease complicated by metabolic bone disease—is well known.

KNEE. Adams studied the knee joints of 51 professional footballers in a senior club in England.[1] Radiographic examination was performed in all players and assessed by different observers. Both the medial and lateral joint spaces and surfaces were studied in each knee. Only one joint space was abnormal. There was no instance of sclerosis, cysts, angulation, or apparently abnormal patellofemoral joint. Prominence of the tibial spine was a feature of all films.

Adams also conducted a postal survey of injuries in other club members in the English League.[1] He received replies from 61 clubs (66 percent response) including 1490 professional soccer players (70 percent of the entire league). A previous meniscectomy was reported in 159 players (11 percent) and a fracture of the leg in 8 percent. There were 48 players (3 percent) with osteoarthritis of the knee. The players in the radiologic survey included 4 (8 percent) who had had a meniscectomy and 12 (23.5 percent) who had fractured the leg. Adams concludes that osteoarthritis is not common in the knee joints of soccer

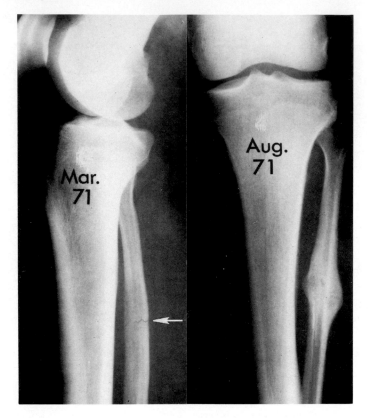

Fig. 213. Occasionally a world class athlete suffers a stress fracture after excessive training. This injury hampered the career of a professional soccer player. There is marked periosteal reaction at the fracture site in the proximal fibula shown after five months. The patient did well with rest for several months and was able to resume play.

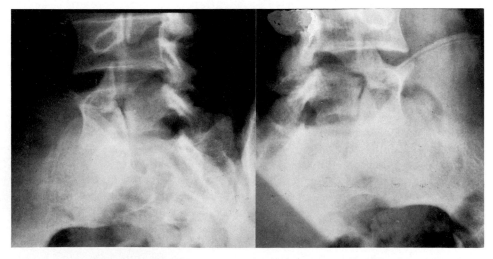

Fig. 214. This 16-year-old male developed back pain while playing soccer. Bilateral pars defects are shown at L5, probably representing stress fracture.

players. It would be of great interest to restudy the same group at various points in time following cessation of active play and to make comparisons with age matched control subjects.

Matthews has reported attacks of migraine triggered by blows to the head by the soccer ball.[12] In such circumstances the player may have visual disturbances and consequently may have to leave the game. The ball weighs approximately 450 grams and reaches speeds of up to 100 km per hour. Matthews states that if a player's head is not positioned to absorb the shock, unskillful heading or accidental blows to the head can initiate the migraine attack.

BLUNT TRAUMA. A report by Morris describes a man who was struck in the epigastrium by a football.[16] He collapsed and complained of epigastric and substernal pain and loss of vision, except when fully recumbent. At immediate hospitalization he was noted to be pale and to have a systolic blood pressure of 50 mm Hg and a pulse rate of 180. A chest x-ray and electrocardiogram were normal, as was the serum amylase level. Laparotomy was performed and all the intra-abdominal viscera were found to be intact. The anesthetist was unable to record the blood pressure and it then seemed likely that a pericardial tamponade was present. A needle was passed through the diaphragm into the pericardium and 300 ml of blood was withdrawn. At this point the blood pressure rose to 150/80 and remained normal. Morris suggests that the important lesson to be learned from this patient's difficulty is that when the degree of cardiovascular collapse in an injured patient is much greater than might be expected from the physical signs, the diagnosis of pericardial tamponade should be excluded by a diagnostic aspiration. The patient did not have extreme dyspnea, pulsus paradoxus, or diminished heart sounds.

Another unusual injury in soccer occurred when a 16-year-old boy was kicked in the upper abdomen.[8] His blood pressure fell to 90/70 mm Hg and his pulse rose to 120 per minute four hours after the injury. At laparotomy blood clots were detected within the left upper quadrant as well as a tear in the mesentery of the small intestine, a one-inch long transverse tear in the jejunum with active bleeding, and a small tear in the serosa of the transverse colon. These areas were repaired; however, four days later the patient vomited bile-stained material. An upper gastrointestinal series showed a sharp cutoff of the second portion of the duodenum. Repeat laparotomy showed a large retroperitoneal hematoma behind and above the convex border of the duodenum. After the hematoma was evacuated, he made a slow but uninterrupted recovery.

References

1. Adams ID: Osteoarthrosis of the knee joint in footballers. J Bone Joint Surg 55B:655, 1973
2. Bass AL: Athletic and soft tissue injuries. Physiotherapy 51:112–114, 1965
3. Blazina ME, Westover JL: Ankle joints of freshman college athletes. Clin Orthop 42:73–80, 1965
4. Bowerman JW, Spence K: Unpublished data
5. Cochrane GM: Osteitis pubis in athletes. Br J Sports Med 5:233–235, 1971

6. Duran D: Historia de Las Indias de Nueva Espana y Islas de Tierra Firme, vol 2. Mexico, Escalante, 1880, p 242
7. Gardiner EN: Athletics of the Ancient World. Oxford, Clarendon, 1930
8. Gue S: Obstruction of the second part of duodenum by retroperitoneal hematoma due to blunt abdominal trauma. Injury 4:65–68, 1972
9. Harris NH, Murray RO: Lesions of the symphysis in athletes. Br Med J 4: 211–214, 1974
10. Luschnitz E, Beyer W, Riedeberger J: Schaden am Knochernen Beckenring bei Fussballspielern. Dtsch Gesund 23:1466–1469, 1968
11. Masterson D: The early history of ball games. Med Biol Illus 15:259–265, 1965
12. Matthews WB: Footballer's migraine. Am Heart J 85:279–280, 1973
13. McMurray TP: Footballer's ankle. J Bone Joint Surg 32B:68–69, 1950
14. Melamed JL, Rabushka SE, Melamed M: Ischial epiphyseolysis: emphasis of the diagnosis of the acute fracture. Clin Radiol 19:465–469, 1968
15. Morris LH: Athlete's ankle. J Bone Joint Surg 25:220, 1943
16. Morris WT: An unusual football injury. Lancet 1:381–382, 1973
17. Murray RO: The aetiology of primary osteoarthritis of the hip. Br J Radiol 38: 810–824, 1965
18. _____: Personal communication
19. Riedeberger J, Luschnitz E, Bauchstiess B: Das Schambein Adduktoren Syndrom bei Fussballspielern. Zentralbl Chir 92:2656–2660, 1967

TENNIS

The reports on injury in tennis include remarks on "tennis elbow," "tennis shoulder," "tennis leg," and "tennis toe." The predominant unilateral use of the upper extremity in this sport accounts for the majority of injuries that are reported. Hypertrophy of both muscle and bone in the dominant arm is an observed sequel to active play by young people. Buskirk et al studied the hands and forearms of seven nationally ranked tennis players in the United States.[3] They found greater muscular and osseous development in the arm that wielded the racquet than in the opposite arm. The length and width of the radius and ulna were increased in the racquet arm. Since these players had participated in tennis during their teenage years, the authors attributed the observed difference to the effects of exercise on bone growth during adolescence.

The term "tennis elbow" generally refers to pain and local tenderness at the lateral epicondyle or, occasionally, at the medial epicondyle. Slapak[16] and Coonrad and Hooper[4] have noted that this diagnostic label is a misnomer, for this condition occurs most commonly in activities unrelated to tennis. Slapak points out that it occurs in badminton, squash, golf, fencing, rowing, violin playing, and manual labor. Of 1000 patients with tennis elbow, or epicondylitis, studied by Coonrad and Hooper fewer than 5 percent played golf or tennis. The lateral epicondyle was involved seven times more frequently than the medial. The syndrome is most likely initiated by macroscopic or microscopic tears in the common origins of the flexor or extensor muscle groups (Fig. 215). These occur in response to stress or trauma at tendon fibers affected by changes of degeneration or aging. In their series the mean age of those affected by such an injury was 42 years. Nirschl and Eberth, in a 1973 study of 81 professional and amateur tennis players, found tennis elbow in 13 percent of the former group and in 50 percent of the latter.[14] They observed that professional players generally avoid strokes with forearm pronation and exert better control of arm power and motion than do amateurs.

Boyd an McLeod, in reporting a series of 871 patients treated for tennis elbow between 1956 and 1972 in Memphis, Tenn., described a subgroup of 37 patients who required elbow surgery.[2] In addition, they referred to the first description of the syndrome given by Runge in 1873.[15] His article was entitled "On the Origin and Treatment of Writer's Cramp." Several authors cite an important review article on the subject by Cyriax.[5]

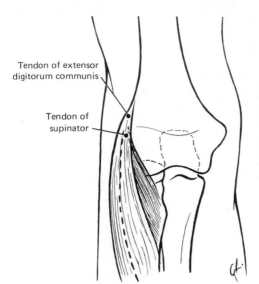

Tendon of extensor
digitorum communis

Tendon of
supinator

Fig. 215. The muscle groups at the lateral epicondyle of the elbow include the supinator and the common extensors of the forearm. Stress leads to soft-tissue injury in the origins of these muscles in many tennis players. The tendon of the supinator muscle takes origin behind the common extensor tendon.

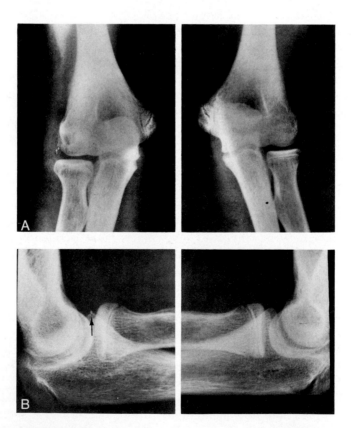

Fig. 216. These views were obtained in a 15-year-old tennis player who complained of chronic elbow pain. The abnormal right elbow on the reader's left is compared to the normal left elbow. **A.** There is faint calcification following tendon injury at the margin of the lateral epicondyle. The capitellar surface is eroded. **B.** The coronoid process has developed a traction spur from chronic stress. The left coronoid process is rounded and is normal.

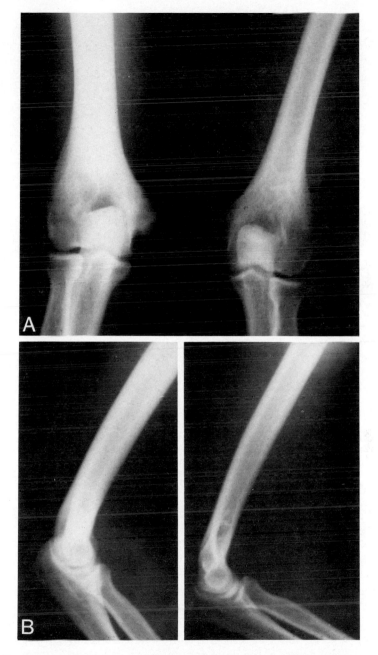

Fig. 217. These views show the bony hypertrophy of the racquet (right) arm (reader's left) of an intercollegiate tennis player compared to the opposite arm. **A.** Anteroposterior view. **B.** Lateral view.

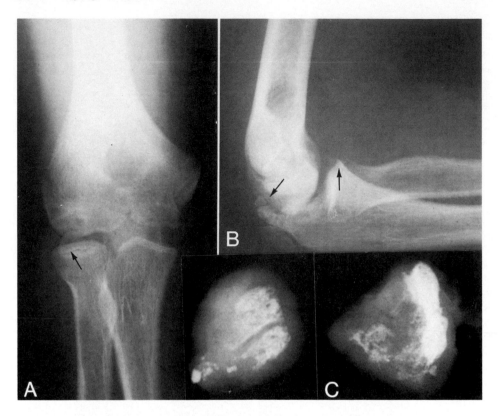

Fig. 218. These views were obtained in the symptomatic elbow of a 13-year-old tennis player. **A.** Loose bodies were suspected on the anteroposterior view adjacent to the capitellar defect. **B.** Loose bodies were suspected on the lateral view in the posterior ulnohumeral area. A traction spur has formed at the coronoid process of the ulna (vertical arrow). **C.** Specimen radiographs of two fragments removed from the elbow of this tennis player show areas of ossification within cartilage. The loose bodies each measured approximately 1 cm in diameter and emanated from the capitellar defect as osteochondral fracture fragments.

Included among the x-ray changes in the tennis player's elbow are erosion and fragmentation of the lateral epicondyle and capitellum, calcification in the soft tissues at the lateral margin of the joint,[12] spur formation at the coronoid process of the ulna, and hypertrophy of the humerus (Figs. 216–218). Nirschl found a medial slope deformity of the lateral condyle of the humerus in 77 (95 percent) of a group of 81 patients with tennis elbow.[13] Calcification was found in the lateral soft tissues in 18 players (22 percent).

Among several kinds of shoulder abnormality in tennis players, including tendon injury and tears of the rotator cuff, is an apparently unusual injury reported by Benton and Nelson.[1] A right-handed 18-year-old tennis player had shoulder pain for four years. The pain was related to activity in tennis and was most severe as he initiated the service with his arm abducted, externally rotated, and hyperextended. Anteroposterior x-ray views of the shoulder were normal. However, on an axillary view giving a vertical profile of the coracoid process and the glenohumeral joint, a transverse avulsion fracture of the distal half of the coracoid process was present. At surgery a loose fragment of bone was found and removed. The fragment was considered too large to represent a secondary ossification center of the coracoid process. This example demonstrates again a message emphasized by F. C. Golding that a number of shoulder abnormalities will be missed unless an axillary view is obtained [10,11]

The lower extremity is occasionally the site of muscle or tendon rupture in tennis.[7] A lead article in the *British Medical Journal* in 1969 referred to a tear of the musculotendinous junction of the medial belly of the gastrocnemius as "tennis leg."[6] Such a rupture may occur in other sports, including squash, cricket, skiing, and track. A gap in the muscle is usually palpable at the site of tenderness. This gap may be demonstrated as an indentation of the soft tissue margins on lateral x-rays of the calf as shown by D. Golding.[9] Xeroradiography of such injuries would also show abnormality.

Finally, Gibbs has noted a number of tennis players who complain of pain in one or more of their toes.[8] In what he refers to as "tennis toe," this pain is associated with hemorrhage beneath the toenails. The toe or toes affected are those that are longest. Gibbs suggests that the injury occurs when the player stops abruptly and the forward motion of the body propels the toes into the box toe and tip of the shoes. The hemorrhage is frequently oriented longitudinally along the nail like the splinter hemorrhages of subacute bacterial endocarditis.

References

1. Benton JN, Nelson C: Avulsion of the coracoid process in an athlete. Report of a case. J Bone Joint Surg 53A:356–358, 1971
2. Boyd HB, McLeod AC: Tennis elbow. J Bone Joint Surg 55A:1183–1187, 1973
3. Buskirk ER, Anderson KL, Brozek J: Unilateral activity and bone and muscle development in the forearm. Res Q Am Assoc Health Phys Educ 27:127–131, 1956
4. Coonrad RW, Hooper WR: Tennis elbow: its course, natural history, conservative and surgical management. J Bone Joint Surg 55A:1177–1182, 1973
5. Cyriax JH: The pathology and treatment of tennis elbow. J Bone Joint Surg 18: 921 940, 1936
6. Editorial, lead article: Tennis leg. Br Med J 3:543–544, 1969
7. Froimson AI: Tennis leg. JAMA 209:415–416, 1969
8. Gibbs RB: Tennis toe. Arch Dermatol 107:918, 1973
9. Golding D: Tennis leg, letter to the editor. Br Med J 4:234, 1969
10. Golding FC: The shoulder—the forgotten joint. Br J Radiol 35:149–158, 1962
11. _____: Radiology and orthopedic surgery. J Bone Joint Surg 48B:320–332, 1966
12. Gondos B: Tennis elbow. A re-evaluation. Am J Roentgenol 79:684–691, 1958
13. Nirschl RP: The etiology and treatment of tennis elbow. In Craig TT (ed): The Medical Aspects of Sports, vol 15. Chicago, AMA, 1973, pp 43–50
14. _____, Eberth E: Etiology and treatment of tennis elbow. J Bone Joint Surg 55A:1305, 1973
15. Runge F: Zur Genese und Behandlung des Schreibekampfes. Berl Klin Wochenschr 10:245–248, 1873
16. Slapak M: Tennis elbow. In Armstrong JR, Tucker WE (eds): Injury in Sport. London, Staples, 1964

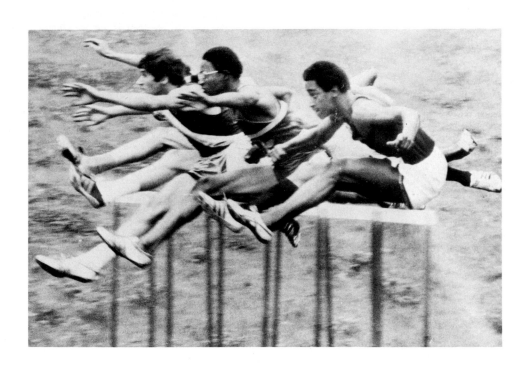

TRACK AND FIELD

The legs, feet, and pelvic musculature are the sites of injury in the sport of running.[1] Acute or chronic injury with bone abnormality such as stress fractures or avulsion fractures are not uncommon in runners or joggers. Bone injuries, however, constitute the minority of a complete survey of injuries in running. Most injuries in running are to muscle, tendon, fascia, and cartilage of the lower extremity. Many injuries will not show an x-ray abnormality. For example, Clancy surveyed the injuries to 310 runners and joggers seen in the Sports Medicine Clinic of St. Luke's Hospital in New York City over a two-year period.[6] Bone injury led to 19 stress fractures and 6 avulsion fractures. Four of the avulsion injuries occurred at the ischial tuberosity, the site of origin for the hamstring muscles; one occurred at the anterior superior iliac spine, the site of origin of the sartorius muscle; and another occurred at the anterior inferior iliac spine, the site of origin of the biceps femoris muscle. He found that 42 runners had muscle strains, 57 had hyaline cartilage damage of the knee (chondromalacia patella), and 21 had shin splints.

Shin splints have been defined by Slocum as a syndrome of pain and discomfort in the lower leg after repetitive overuse in running or walking.[34] He further defines the condition as an aseptic inflammation of the muscle–tendon unit brought about by overexertion. Slocum has most commonly noted tenderness over the posterior tibialis muscle. The second most common site, in his experience, is the anterior tibial muscle with tenderness present at its attachments to the lateral border of the tibia (Fig. 219). The tibia may show no x-ray abnormality in uncomplicated shin splints other than thickening of the bony cortex. However, if pain and local tenderness at the tibia exist a stress fracture must be excluded. Shin splints and other tendon injuries are associated with early season training according to Clancy.[6]

Bill Bowerman, head track coach at the University of Oregon, has observed that injury of the Achilles tendon is a common problem among runners.[5] He also notes from his vast experience that stress fractures are not just occasional events.

Sperryn reported that of 150 consecutive sports injuries treated at Kings College Hospital in London, 32 percent were classified as overuse injuries.[36] If track and field events alone were considered, then 64 percent of new patients had problems due to overuse. Plantar fasciitis (7 runners) and Achilles tendon

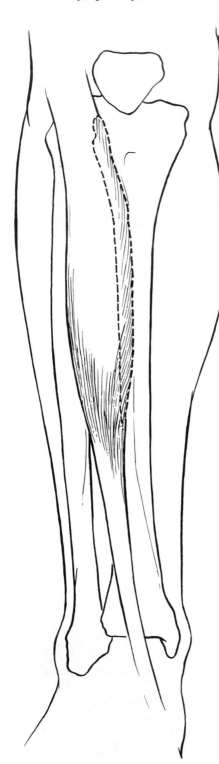

Fig. 219. The medial attachments of the anterior tibialis muscle on the anterior ridge of the tibia are often the site of pain in shin splints. Here the origin of the anterior tibialis is shown in a dotted line posterior to the overlying muscle.

pain (13 runners) occurred in 49 long distance runners studied over a two-year period. In that same time period 23 sprinters had injuries, yet none had plantar fascial or Achilles tendon symptoms. The group of long distance runners with Achilles tendon disorders was further subclassified into those with tendonitis (6 patients), those with paratendonitis or surrounding inflammatory tissue (5), and those with partial rupture of the tendon (2).

Stress fractures are often mistakenly linked only with the novice runner or the athlete in early season form. Murray[23] and Slocum[34] have observed stress fractures in champion athletes, and the latter has observed champion runners in midseason form with stress fractures. Devas describes the stress fracture as one that occurs in the normal bone of a normal person with normal use (for that person) and no injury.[10] He and Sweetnam pinpoint the second metatarsal as the most common site, followed by the fibula.[8-12] The tibia, Devas notes, is the most important site of stress fracture—important because it is common, often overlooked, and occasionally responsible for protracted absence from sport.[8] Other sites include the calcaneus,[45] tarsal navicular,[41] humerus,[10] ribs,[10] and femur[29] (Figs. 220–222). Provost and Morris reported 35 patients with fatigue fractures of the femoral shaft.[29] One was a track athlete and the remainder were military recruits. In Clancy's series of running injuries, there were nine stress fractures of the tibia, six of the second metatarsal, and four of the fibula.[6] Once a stress fracture is suspected, it may take weeks or months to confirm it on x-ray examination. Oblique views may be necessary to detect the fracture line. Liljedahl, in describing common injuries due to conditioning exercises, mentions that the early x-ray may be negative and it is necessary to get follow-up views. He found the fibula to be the most common site of stress fracture.[23]

Slocum notes that the fractures are usually horizontal but can rarely be longitudinal in type.[34] The callus or periosteal new bone formation first appears as a localized haze at the surface of the bone. A line of condensation may appear within the endosteal surface of the bone.[30] Frequently, however, periosteal new bone formation is the only evidence that a stress fracture has occurred. Theros states that the earliest radiographic sign of a stress fracture is minute radiolucent tunneling of the cortex produced by osteoclastic resorption. This is followed by cortical resorption in a fracture line of one cortex and then by periosteal reaction.[40] Rarely, abundant callus may confuse those who interpret the x-ray and a false diagnosis of neoplasm can be the unfortunate result.[21,22,35] Hodson has shown that soft tissue radiography demonstrated stress fractures in 80 percent of cases even when the bone appeared normal in standard views.[19] Rest is the only treatment needed for a stress fracture. Occasionally an extensive stress fracture warrants splinting or casting, especially if the patient is unreliable or unwilling to rest the area of injury.

Man is not the only runner to suffer these injuries. Devas collected examples of five stress fractures in horses from England, Canada, and the United States.[9] The oblique fracture site was at the second metacarpal or shin bone in each animal. Devas commented that another condition described in horses and known as the split pastern may well be the result of a stress fracture comparable to the split tarsal navicular bone in greyhounds.[4]

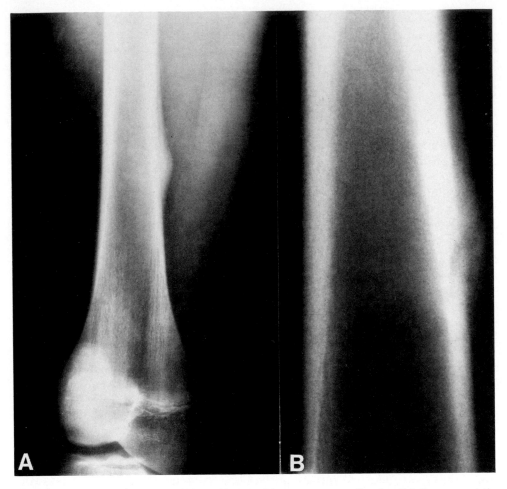

Fig. 220A. Thigh pain developed in a 13-year-old young man active in athletics, especially running. There was no palpable mass on physical examination or fever. What is your diagnosis? **B.** The enlarged view is part of a tomographic series of the lower midshaft of the femur.

Track Injuries

The sprinter and the middle distance track athlete are more prone to injury than are hurdlers, according to James.[20] In a review of 2000 injuries in track and field, he found few injuries in hurdlers. He believes that the hurdlers may be protected by their event and their long-legged body type. The sprinter moves through three phases of running in his event. Watanabe described these as the starting phase, the stride phase, and the finishing phase.[43] He states that most musculotendinous injuries in sprinters occur in the stride phase or during the transition from that phase to that of maximum speed at the finish (Fig. 223). Sudden and severe pain in the buttock or hip region while sprinting oc-

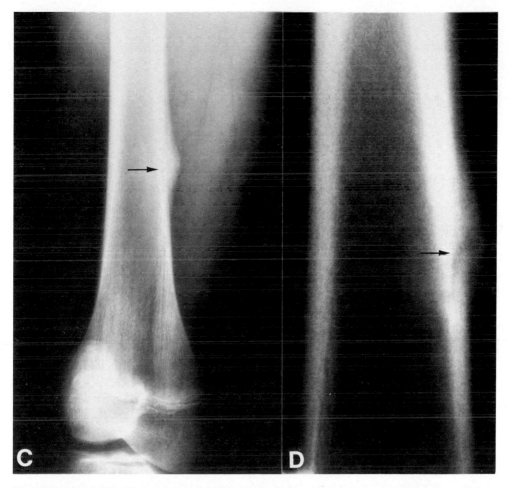

Fig. 220 *(cont.)* **C,D.** These views show periosteal reaction and interruption of the cortex in this patient. Periosteal reaction—actually due to a stress fracture—was attributed to an osteoid osteoma even though such osteomas are usually found in the region of the femoral neck. Surgery was performed and led to a histologic diagnosis of normal callus. This particular site for a stress fracture is slightly unusual. Most stress fractures of the lower extremity are found in the foot, fibula, and tibia.

curred in two teenagers reported by Ellis and Greene.[14] Both boys avulsed the origin of the hamstring musculature at the ischial tuberosity. Radiographs showed large crescent-shaped masses of bone adjacent to the injured ischium. Other avulsion injury sites and other acute injury due to sudden movement at the Achilles tendon are discussed in earlier chapters on those body sites in Part I.

Murray touches upon the concept of the long-term effects of running on the skeleton in his work on hip disease.[26,27] In reviewing a number of hip radiographs in former athletes, mostly former runners, he noticed an increased incidence of osteoarthritis. In addition, there often was a deformity of the nor-

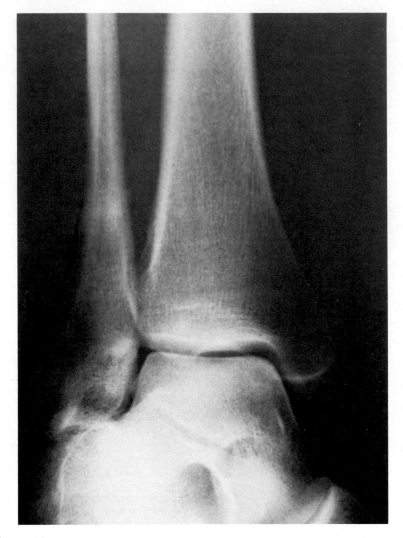

Fig. 221. A young woman complained of lower leg pain after jogging. A stress fracture is present in the distal fibula. The fracture is visible as a focal haze of increased density in the distal shaft.

mal relationship of the femoral head to the femoral neck so that a mild medial and posterior slip of the head was present (Fig. 224). Murray refers to this attitude of the adult hip as the "tilt deformity" and believes that it represents the end result of an earlier juvenile skeletal response to the stress of running. With Duncan, he analyzed radiographs of hips of schoolboys exposed to sports and running in England and compared the findings to those in a similar group of English boys who were not as active in sports.[27] The athletic group showed a higher incidence of slipped capital femoral epiphysis. More controlled studies of this type are needed in order to learn when to limit athletic activity.

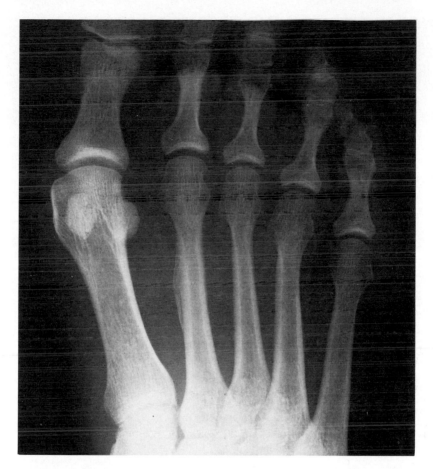

Fig. 222. A long distance runner developed pain in her foot. A stress fracture has produced periosteal reaction of the second metatarsal shaft.

Some runners tolerate heavy training schedules without foot or leg symptoms; however, the symptomatic runner is evidently the most common type of runner. According to a poll conducted by Henderson[18] and Sheehan[32] approximately 60 percent of a sample of 1700 readers of *Runners World* magazine sustained injuries due to overuse in running that required rest for varying periods of time. The injuries involved the entire kinetic chain, including the foot, leg, knee, thigh, pelvis, and lower back. In some of the 1000 injured runners answering the poll there were symptoms in more than one area. The Achilles tendon–ankle–foot complex accounted for 38.6 percent of the injury zones and the knee 23.2 percent.

Assuming that the physical and radiographic examinations of these injury sites are generally within normal limits, where should we look for the cause of the injury? Where should we look for an abnormality? What separates the asymptomatic runner from the runner with symptoms apart from the injury per

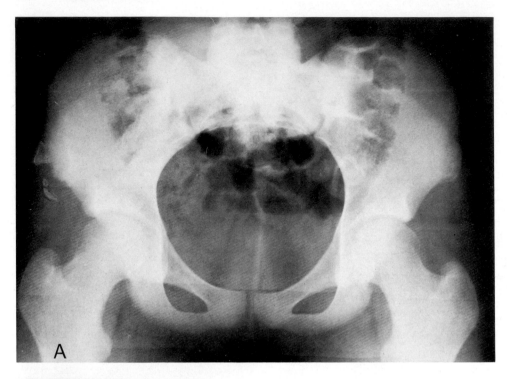

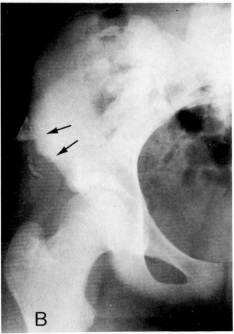

Fig. 223A. A 12-year-old runner twisted her right leg while running. She complained of sudden pain at the right hip. **B.** The displaced bone fragment at the area of the anterior superior iliac spine indicates an avulsion of the sartorius muscle at its origin. Rest alone led to gradual recovery in this patient.

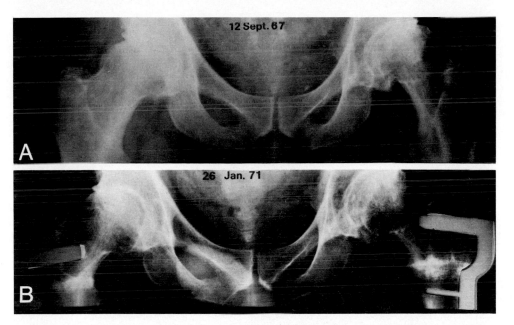

Fig. 224. This 52-year-old man had once been the victor laudorum in his school. He was an exceptionally fast runner, winning most of the shorter distance races. **A.** He now exhibits the tilt deformity of Murray, recognized as a minimal slipped femoral capital epiphysis at both hips. The tilt is more pronounced at the left hip. This deformity leads to incongruity between the femoral head and acetabulum and subsequently to degenerative joint disease. This condition is not a primary osteoarthritis. **B.** Intertrochanteric osteotomies were performed in an effort to aid both hips. (See Murray and Duncan.[27])

se? Schuster,[31] Sheehan,[32] and Subotnick[37–39] would point to the foot, and specifically to variants of normal hind and forefoot structure, as potential causes of symptoms. These variants, including aberrations of metatarsal length and heel tilt, are found in the symptomatic runner too often to be ignored. All would agree that the foot may not be the only problem in each patient. Schuster, according to Sheehan, has treated over 1000 runners and estimates that over 80 percent have a Morton's foot or disproportionately short first metatarsal.[32] Subotnick has studied the overuse syndrome in runners and other athletes as well as methods of control of symptoms using orthotics or foot supports.[39] Those interested in the overuse syndrome and in the biomechanics of subtalar and midtarsal joints are advised to see his papers.[37,38]

Field Injuries

The field events that appear in the literature on injuries are high jumping and javelin throwing. High jumpers have been reported to sustain ruptures of the quadriceps tendon and muscle and cervical spine injury.[28,44] The latter has occurred in devotees of the Fosbury flop, a method of jumping perfected by Dick Fosbury. In his technique the jumper's head and trunk are first over the

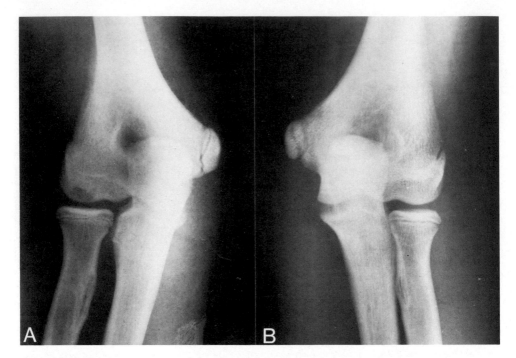

Fig. 225A. The capitellum is eroded after trauma from overuse in javelin throwing in an adolescent. **B.** The normal elbow is shown for comparison.

bar. The jumper lands on his back and often does a backward roll on the landing mat. Enthusiastic but less skillful jumpers have landed on the head and neck instead of the back.[28]

Bateman suggests that in evaluating the patient after injury in the heavy throwing sports such as the hammer throw, javelin, and shotput one should look for tears of the interscapular and scapulocostal muscles as well as rotator cuff tears at the shoulder.[3]

Javelin throwing can produce injury to the throwing arm, as shown in several reports that emphasize elbow abnormalities at the lateral epicondyle and the olecranon.[2,17,24,42] Waris studied elbow injuries in 17 accomplished javelinists in 1946.[42] Each athlete had produced results near or better than the listed world record for that time. Each athlete had elbow pain after the first year of competition. Symptoms were severe enough at certain times such that rest was required in all of those studied. He found that 14 of these men had abnormal elbow x-rays, including one with a complete fracture of the olecranon that had developed a fibrous union in a slightly displaced position. Two men had avulsion fractures of the tip of the olecranon, and the same site showed calcifications or surface irregularity in nine others. In addition, para-articular ossification and intra-articular loose bodies have also been found on elbow x-rays of javelin throwers in studies by Baetzner[2] and by Heiss.[17] Murray[25] and Freiberger[15] have encountered isolated examples of capitellar erosion (Fig.

225) and rupture of the collateral ligaments of the elbow after javelin throwing. The last abnormality was shown by arthrography.

Rarely the javelin injures someone directly as a weapon. An unusual example occurred in 1969 when an Air Force Academy cadet was running toward the intramural playing fields and did not notice a fellow cadet carrying a javelin just ahead of him.[13] The leading end of the javelin suddenly stuck in the ground and the unknowing cadet ran into its elevated opposite end. The wound in the chest was not a minor one. The injured cadet required cardiopulmonary resuscitation and an emergency thoractomy that showed a wound completely through the heart and into the vena cava. Fortunately the injured areas were repaired and the patient was discharged from the hospital two weeks after admission. In addition to the javelin there are other potential injuries in field events in which objects such as the discus, the hammer, and the shot are thrown.

Perhaps the most widespread activity included broadly in the categories of track and field is jogging. Musculoskeletal injury in jogging is common but usually minor. Glick and Katch found 241 such injuries reported by 108 of 120 middle-aged participants in an 11-week jogging program.[16] Nearly half of the injuries were muscle strains, mostly at the calf muscles, 20 percent were joint sprains of the knee and ankle, and 18 percent were foot ailments. One runner sustained bilateral distal fibular stress fractures. Siegal has reported severe heel pain in two joggers, but found no x-ray abnormalities.[33]

The effect of distance running on the heart is discussed briefly in an article by Currens and White.[7] They present some clinical, physiologic, anatomic, and biographic features of Clarence DeMar, a champion marathoner who raced for 49 years. They noted a slightly enlarged left ventricle on chest x-ray at a time when he was still participating in marathon races at age 66. In 1959, DeMar died with peritoneal carcinomatosis following earlier surgery for rectal carcinoma. At autopsy the coronary arteries were estimated to be two or three times the normal diameter. Whether this was always the case with DeMar or represented a response to running is uncertain. Atherosclerosis of the coronary arteries was present but was of mild degree.

References

1. Abrahams A: Injuries to athletes. In Armstrong JR, Tucker WE (eds): Injury in Sport. London, Staples, 1964, pp 143–144
2. Baetzner W, cited by Waris W: Elbow injuries of javelin throwers. Acta Chir Scand 93:563–575, 1946
3. Bateman JE: Athletic injuries about the shoulder in throwing and body-contact sports. Clin Orthop 23:75–83, 1962
4. Bateman JK: Broken hock in the greyhound. Vet Rec 70:621–623, 1958
5. Bowerman WJ: Personal communication
6. Clancy WG Jr: Lower extremity injuries in the jogger and distance runner. Physician Sports Med 2:46–50, 1974
7. Currens JH, White PD: Half a century of running: clinical physiologic and autopsy findings in the case of Clarence DeMar (''Mr. Marathon''). N Engl J Med 265: 988–993, 1961

8. Devas MB: Stress fractures of the tibia in athletes or shin soreness. J Bone Joint Surg 40B:227–239, 1958
9. _____: Shin-splints or stress fractures of the metacarpal bone in horses and shin soreness or stress fractures of the tibia in man. J Bone Joint Surg 49B: 310–313, 1967
10. _____: Stress fractures in athletes. Proc R Soc Med 62:933–937, 1969
11. _____: Stress fractures in athletes. Nurs Times 67:227–232, 1971
12. _____, Sweetnam R: Stress fractures of the fibula: a review of fifty cases in athletes. J Bone Joint Surg 38B:818–829, 1956
13. Editorial: An Air Force cadet survives javelin puncture of the heart. Hosp Trib, p 23, Nov 3, 1969
14. Ellis R, Greene A G: Ischial apophyseolysis. Radiology 87:646–648, 1966
15. Freiberger R: Personal communication
16. Glick JM, Katch VL: Musculoskeletal injuries in jogging. Arch Phys Med 51: 123–126, 1970
17. Heiss F, cited by Waris W: Elbow injuries of javelin throwers. Acta Chir Scand 93:563–575, 1946
18. Henderson J: Personal communication
19. Hodson CT, cited in: Panel discussion on sports injuries. Proc R Soc Med 62:943, 1969
20. James SL, cited in: Editorial: Tribune sports report. Hosp Trib, p 21, Feb 23, 1970
21. Kahn LB, Wood FW, Ackerman LV: Fracture callus associated with benign and malignant bone lesions and mimicking osteosarcoma. Am J Clin Pathol 52:14–24, 1969
22. Levin DC, Blazina ME, Levine E: Fatigue fractures of the shaft of the femur: simulation of malignant tumor. Radiology 89:883–885, 1967
23. Liljedahl SO: Common injuries in connection with conditioning exercise. Scand J Rehabil Med 3:1–15, 1971
24. Miller JE: Javelin thrower's elbow. J Bone Joint Surg 42B:788–792, 1960
25. Murray RO: Personal communication
26. _____: The aetiology of primary osteoarthritis of the hip. Br J Radiol 38: 810–824, 1965
27. _____, Duncan C: Athletic activity in adolescence as etiologic factor in degenerative hip disease. J Bone Joint Surg 53B:406–419, 1971
28. O'Hanlon JT: The Fosbury flop. Va Med Mon 95:717–719, 1968
29. Provost RA, Morris JM: Fatigue fracture of the femoral shaft. J Bone Joint Surg 51A:487–498, 1969
30. Savoca CJ: Stress fractures: a classification of the earliest radiographic signs. Radiology 100:519–524, 1971
31. Schuster R, cited in personal communication from Sheehan GA
32. Sheehan GA: Personal communication
33. Siegel IM: Jogger's heel. JAMA 206:2899, 1968
34. Slocum DB: The shin-splint syndrome: medical aspects in differential diagnosis. Am J Surg 114:875–881, 1967
35. Solomon L: Stress fractures of the femur and tibia simulating malignant bone tumors. S Afr J Surg 12:19–25, 1974
36. Sperryn PN: Runner's heel. Br J Sports Med 5:236–238, 1971
37. Subotnick SI: Orthotic foot control and the overuse syndrome. Physician Sports Med 3:75–79, Jan 1975
38. _____: The abuses of orthotics in sports medicine. Physician Sports Med 3: 73–75, July 1975
39. _____: Podiatric Sports Medicine. Mt Kisco, NY, Futura, 1975
40. Theros E: Personal communication
41. Towne LC, Blazina ME, Cosen LN: Fatigue fracture of the tarsal navicular. J Bone Joint Surg 52A:376–378, 1970

42. Waris W: Elbow injuries of javelin throwers. Acta Chir Scand 93:563–575, 1946
43. Watanabe RS, cited in: Editorial: Tribune sports report. Hosp Trib, p 21, Jan 12, 1970
44. Weigert M: Spontaneous rupture of patellar tendon during high jump. Z Orthop 104:429–431, 1968
45. Winfield AC, Dennis JM: Stress fractures of the calcaneus. Radiology 72:415–418, 1959

WATER SPORTS

Activity in water sports encompasses many pursuits, including swimming, boating, fishing, water skiing, surfing, diving, and underwater events such as snorkeling or scuba diving. Swimming and its hazard of drowning are pertinent to all these activities. Approximately 6500 people drown in the United States each year according to a report by Dietz and Baker in 1974.[10] Drowning is the second leading cause of accidental death in the age group 5 to 24, while death due to motor vehicles is first.[10]

Dietz and Baker studied the epidemiology of drowning in Maryland in order to determine the areas of need for water safety instruction, the prevalence of alcohol intoxication in relation to drowning, and the possibilities of injury control.[10] In 1972 there were 133 accidental drownings in Maryland, which has 3.9 million inhabitants. Of these deaths 16 occurred during tropical storm Agnes and are not sports related. However, 61 persons (52 percent) drowned in creeks or rivers while swimming and wading. Immediately before drowning most persons were swimming (40 persons; 34 percent) or boating (34 persons; 29 percent). In this study drowning was rarely associated with ocean swimming or with sailing despite their popularity in Maryland.

In order to study the relationship of alcohol to immersion death, the authors reviewed the drownings in Baltimore City from 1968 to 1971. Records of blood alcohol determinations in these deaths were complete. There were 45 deaths in the group they studied, selected so that all victims were age 15 or older, were not immersed during a truck or car collision, and were submerged less than 12 hours. Of these victims 21 (47 percent) had elevated blood alcohol concentrations. Alcohol use was especially common in swimming deaths, being present in 11 of 14 deaths (78 percent). This linkage of alcohol to drowning is not unique to the geographic area studied, as the authors cite other studies from California, Finland, and Australia in which alcohol was also implicated in death by drowning.

Radiographs of the lungs in fatal and near fatal drownings show the pattern of pulmonary edema (Fig. 226). Patients who recover have a rapid disappearance of the pulmonary infiltrates within days. Apart from this, the morbidity of swimming is restricted largely to occasional complaints of shoulder pain in competitive swimmers. Kennedy and Hawkins found 81 athletes with shoulder symptoms in a survey of 2496 Canadian swimmers.[13] The freestyle and but-

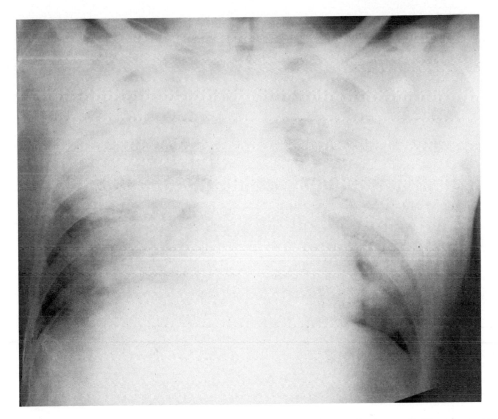

Fig. 226. This chest x-ray was obtained in a young man who nearly drowned. The view was made in the first 24 hours after he was pulled from a mountain lake. The diffuse pulmonary infiltrate and edema pattern follows cerebral hypoxia as well as transudation of fluid and aspiration of water. He recovered after a stormy hospital course. An electrode with its attached wire overlies the upper part of the chest.

terfly strokes were most commonly involved. The swimmers usually had discomfort or pain after swimming, a painful arc of motion of the shoulder, tenderness over the supraspinatus or biceps tendons, and restricted motion of the shoulder. The authors have also encountered shoulder joint subluxation in backstrokers. The stress of a turn in the water with the arm fully abducted and externally rotated and immediately followed by sudden push off on the wall with the swimmer's hand can produce shoulder complaints. Kennedy and Hawkins have done cineradiography to show subluxation of the shoulder in such athletes.[13]

Diving

Fracture and dislocation of the mid and lower cervical spine with resultant spinal cord injury is the most common serious mishap associated with diving. The unfortunate victim nearly always overestimates the depth of the water or

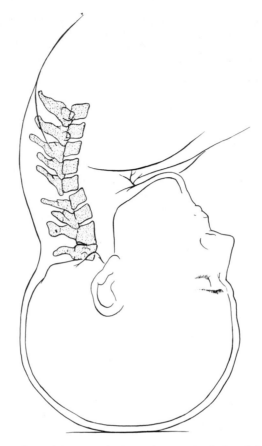

Fig. 227. The careless diver risks paraplegia and even death by diving into shallow water. Here the diver has sustained a fracture dislocation of the cervical spine.

neglects to consider the actual or possible variance of the depth of the water when diving (Fig. 227). Laursen treated 11 such patients in one summer in Odense, Denmark.[15] Burke reported 52 patients with spinal cord injury due to aquatic sporting accidents in Victoria, Australia, over an eight-summer period.[4] All but four patients were injured in diving into shallow water. Of the 52 patients, 51 had cervical injuries and nearly 90 percent of these were compression fracture or "burst" fractures. The fifth cervical vertebra was fractured in 25 patients, the sixth vertebra in 12 patients, and the fourth, seventh, and third cervical vertebra less frequently, in that order of decreasing incidence. In Burke's series, 28 patients had complete paralysis of all extremities and 23 had incomplete tetraplegia. Nine patients with incomplete paralysis made a full recovery.

In some diving injuries the odontoid process is fractured at the second cervical vertebra. Such fractures are often difficult to detect, as mentioned earlier, in the chapter concerning the evaluation of x-rays of the cervical spine in Part I. A burst fracture or compression fracture of the ring of the first cervical vertebra is a potential injury in diving. This fracture, known as the Jefferson fracture, was described by Jefferson in a victim of an aircraft accident.[11] The fracture is detected on the anteroposterior view of the C1–C2 region. (See Figures 50 and 65.)

Diving injuries occurred in a variety of bodies of water in a study of 23 patients in Central California.[14] Rivers, an irrigation reservoir, creeks, streams, lakes, and swimming pools all claimed victims. One patient macerated his spinal cord at the C4 level and died two days after injury. There were 13 patients who had complete tetraplegia without recovery and the remainder had lesser neurologic injury ranging to no neurologic loss at all. The majority of the victims were males (91 percent) and tended to be young (between 15 and 47 years of age). Several patients admitted that they had been drinking alcoholic beverages immediately before the injury. The fact that 43 percent of the patients were under the legal age for drinking weighs against an even larger proportion of the study group having an alcohol content at the time of injury. There were 22 patients with 29 cervical vertebral fractures, associated with 29 subluxations (especially at C4–C5 and C5–C6) and 2 frank dislocations. None of the patients had x-ray evidence of thoracic or lumbar injury.

Both Burke[4] and Laursen[15] emphasize the need to provide continued public information about the dangers of diving into shallow water. Bohlman[3] and others[2,8,18,20,25] have directed attention to the anterior portion of the spinal cord where compression can occur from bone or disc material following trauma. Consideration of anterior factors and anterior surgical approaches to the cervical spine is important in the evaluation and treatment of cervical injury.

Occasionally, the diver is unfortunate enough to hit the diving board or some adjacent immovable object. Aach and Kissane reported an example of splenic rupture associated with subsequent ischemic renal failure and death in a 16-year-old who slipped while attempting to dive and fell on nearby rocks.[1]

Water Skiing

Moore outlined four causes of injury in waterskiing: falling in the water, striking a solid object, entangling in rope, and striking the boat or being run over by the boat.[16] The most common injuries are sprains, muscle tears, and dislocations from falling in the water. The higher the boat speed, the harder the water surface to the falling skier and the more likely the injury. Moore cites torsional fracture of the femur, knee and hip dislocation, and cervical spine fracture dislocation following falls in the water.[16] A hazard to both men and women is perineal laceration from forced entry of water after falling. This is most dangerous to women. Vaginal and vulvar lacerations, abortion, and bowel perforation have occurred in female skiers.[17] Tweedale strongly recommends protection through the use of rubber wet suits or rubber pants in place of or in addition to the swimming suit.[24]

A typical example of the problems of perineal injury in waterskiers who persist in wearing bathing suits instead of waterskiing suits is described in a report by Ramey.[17] A 23-year-old woman fell while waterskiing in the Miami,

Fla., area. As she hit the water her bikini bathing suit pulled to one side of the perineum. She felt sudden pressure in the lower abdominal and rectal area followed by some crampy pain in the left lower quadrant. Bleeding was noticed from a rectal source. At a nearby hospital, anoscopic and proctoscopic examinations were performed showing an apparently superficial tear in the anterior wall of the rectum. The rectum was packed with two-inch vaginal packing; however, the bleeding continued. The patient was taken to surgery, where a 6-cm tear was repaired at the anterior rectal wall beginning about 4 cm above the anal verge. The tear extended through all layers of the rectum to the vaginal submucosa. The patient did well and was discharged on the fifth postoperative day.

Powerboat propeller injuries may compound the hazards of waterskiing. Such trauma is remarkable for its sudden severity. Compound fractures, deep multiple wounds, and lacerations of peripheral nerves and arteries may occur. Sand and debris contaminate the wounds and the injured may lose limb and life.

Waterski federations are explicit in ruling that swimming and waterskiing must be separate activities. The towing boat must contain two capable persons—one to drive and one to watch the skier. Consider the case history described by Sleight involving two people who ignored the two-in-the-boat rule.[21] A 27-year-old woman fell while water skiing in the late afternoon. The driver, apparently alone in the boat, circled back to pick her up but was dazzled by the sunlight reflected on the water and ran over her. Her injuries included a comminuted subtrochanteric fracture of the right femur through a deep buttock wound. She also had left thigh, calf, and popliteal fossa lacerations that required a through-knee amputation. She was discharged walking on a prosthesis after spending more than six months in hospital and rehabilitation units.

An unusual waterskiing injury occurred when an 11-year-old girl was struck while sitting on a ramp used for waterski jumping.[6] She was injured by a tow rope pulling a waterskiier behind an inboard power boat. The tow rope hit the front of her neck, knocking her unconscious and into the water. She was immediately pulled from the water but was apneic and cyanotic. At a hospital an emergency tracheostomy was performed. X-rays of the neck showed upward displacement of the hyoid bone, soft tissue swelling, subcutaneous emphysema, and a large mass of extravasated air between the trachea and the base of the tongue. At surgery, the larynx was found to be avulsed between the cricoid cartilage and the thyroid cartilage. The lower third of the thyroid cartilage had been crushed and disorganized. In addition, the pharynx had been avulsed and distracted from the esophagus. The injured structures were reapproximated at surgery. After a difficult postoperative course of fever and aspiration pneumonia, the patient survived and had residual dysphonia.

Underwater Diving

Snorkeling and scuba diving share drowning as the most common hazard. In a study of 21 deaths from scuba diving over a seven-year period in

Michigan, Denney and Read found that 10 divers drowned.[9] Of the 21 divers, 15 were new to the sport, but 6 had two or more years of experience and formal training in diving. The ages of the divers ranged from 12 to 42 years. The water depth was 25 feet or less in 18 of the 21 deaths. A few divers were trapped beneath ice or by weeds. There were 11 divers who showed signs of barotrauma with air embolism as a probable mechanism of injury. They were stunned or unresponsive on surfacing. Four autopsies in these 11 examples showed acute pulmonary emphysema with edema, hemorrhage, and rupture of alveolar walls as well as severe cerebral congestion. Butterfield et al, in a two-part review article on the hazards of skin diving, cited the work of Comeau.[5] Comeau reported that 9 of 15 diving deaths in Massachusetts occurred at the surface after a face mask filled with water or was lost.[7] Of the 15 victims, 12 were inexperienced divers and 10 had received no formal instruction in diving techniques.

Weeth has categorized diving hazards into five categories: suction and blast injuries, gas expansion injuries, decompression sickness, gas poisoning, and emotional reactions.[26] To these we can add hazards of fishing spears and those of contact with marine organisms and animals. Approximately 1000 species of marine organisms are toxic to man according to Johnston and Burger.[12] They cite a comprehensive review of these dangers by Russell.[19] Tanton and Elliott describe an eye injury from a fishing spear.[23] The mechanism of injury was most unusual. A young man placed one of his 48-inch-long spears in the ground with the barbed end pointing upward. He bent over quickly, ignoring or forgetting the spear, and drove it deeply into his right orbit. X-rays later showed the tip of the spear extending along the orbital floor to the temporal bone. The spear was removed at an operation and the patient had no residual abnormality when examined six months postoperatively.

Surfing

Surfing injuries include head injuries and blunt abdominal trauma from collisions with surf boards—an average board weighs between 25 and 45 pounds —as well as fractures and dislocations from falls in shallow water. At Maryland's nearby ocean resorts cervical spine fracture–dislocations, identical to those mentioned in diving mishaps, and shoulder dislocations are seasonal surfing events. Less worrisome are the hyperkeratotic skin nodules of the legs and feet known as "surfers knots." Swift described southern California surfers with these nodules at the anterior tibial surface, over the tibial tubercles, and at the dorsum of the feet over the metatarsophalangeal joints.[22] In addition, he described swelling of a bursa at the proximal aspect of the dorsum of the foot that forms in the synovial sheath of the tendon of the extensor digitorum longus. The lesions are related to kneeling on the surfboards and are a minor nuisance and a major status symbol among surfers.

References

1. Aach R, Kissane J: Renal failure following blunt trauma: clinicopathologic conference. Am J Med 50:368–379, 1971
2. Bailey RW: Observations of cervical disc lesions in fractures and dislocations. J Bone Joint Surg 45A:461–470, 1963.
3. Bohlman HH: Pathology and current treatment concepts of cervical spine injuries. In: Instructional Course Lectures. American Academy of Orthopedic Surgeons, St. Louis, Mosby, 21:108–115, 1972
4. Burke DC: Spinal cord injuries from water sports. Med Aust 2:1190–1194, 1972
5. Butterfield DE, Mack JD, Majno G: Hazards to health: skin diving—parts I and II. N Engl J Med 269:147–149, 255–259, 1963
6. Chandler JR: Avulsion of the larynx and pharynx as the result of a water ski rope injury. Arch Otolaryngol 96:365–367, 1972
7. Comeau GF: Report on skin diving fatalities. Prepared by Division of Accident Research, Underwater Society of America, Stoneham, Mass, 1962
8. Davis D, Bohlman H, Walker AE, Fisher R, Robinson R: The pathological findings in fatal craniospinal injuries. J Neurosurg 34:603–613, 1971
9. Denney MK, Read RC: Scuba-diving deaths in Michigan. JAMA 192:120–122, 1965
10. Dietz PE, Baker SP: Drowning, epidemiology and prevention. Am J Public Health 64:303–312, 1974
11. Jefferson G: Fracture of the atlas vertebra. Br J Surg 7:407–422, 1920
12. Johnston DG, Burger W: Injury and disease of scuba and skin divers. Postgrad Med 49:134–139, 1971
13. Kennedy JC, Hawkins RJ: Swimmer's shoulder. Physician Sports Med 2:35–38, 1974
14. Kewalramani LS, Laxman S, Taylor RG: Injuries to the cervical spine from diving accidents. J Trauma 15:130–142, 1975
15. Laursen B: Diving accidents: cervical spine fracture from diving into too shallow water. Ugeskr Laeger 131:1121–1122, 1969
16. Moore AT: Waterskiing. In Armstrong JR, Tucker WE (eds): Injury in Sport. London, Staples, 1964, chap 19
17. Ramey JR: Intrarectal tear with bleeding from water skiing accident. J Fla Med Assoc 61:162, 1974
18. Robinson RA: Anterior and posterior cervical spine fusions. Clin Orthop 35:34–62, 1964
19. Russell FE: Marine toxins and venomous and poisonous marine mammals. Adv Marine Biol 3:255–384, 1965
20. Schneider RC: The syndrome of acute anterior spinal cord injury. J Neurosurg 12:95–122, 1955
21. Sleight MW: Speedboat propeller injuries. Br Med J 2:427–429, 1974
22. Swift S: Surfer's "knots." JAMA 192:123–124, 1965
23. Tanton JH, Elliott DC: Fishing spear injury of the orbit. Am J Ophthalmol 64:973–974, 1967
24. Tweedale PG: Gynecological hazards of water skiing. Can Med Assoc J 108:20–22, 1973
25. Verbiest H: Anterolateral operations for fractures and dislocations in the middle and lower parts of the cervical spine. J Bone Joint Surg 51A:1489–1530, 1969
26. Weeth JB: Management of underwater accidents. JAMA 192:115–119, 1965

WEIGHT LIFTING

Only a few injuries or hazards are recorded in weight lifters. Occasionally muscle, bone, and joint injuries occur. Fractures of the epiphyseal cartilage of the distal radius can occur in adolescents lifting excessive weight. Bakalim reported an acute rupture of a muscle tendon unit in a 24-year-old man.[1] The victim felt a sudden pain while lifting 190 kg while supine on a bench. An audible dull snap occurred at the moment of injury. He was unable to move the right arm across the chest toward the left arm. A large hematoma developed by the next day and extended to the medial forearm and elbow. At operation a total rupture of the pectoralis major tendon was found at the posterior bicipital ridge of the humerus. The tendon was sutured to the humerous through a drill hole into the bicipital ridge. The patient resumed weight lifting eight weeks post operation.

Weight lifter's "blackout" or syncope was studied by Compton et al in New Zealand.[2] Two champion weight lifters were studied in an effort to explain the loss of consciousness observed occasionally during competition. Respiratory carbon dioxide levels, heart, rates, and intraesophageal pressures were obtained in each man. The subjects lifted weights of 90 to 150 kg in the clean and jerk method. Both men lowered their expired carbon dioxide levels through hyperventilation. Both developed tachycardia, not bradycardia, and extremely high intrathoracic pressures during the lifts. The maximum intrathoracic pressures recorded were 257 and 161 mm Hg. These levels compare with maximum values recorded in observations of coughing reported by Sharpey-Schafer.[6] A cineradiographic recording was made during another lift. The cardiac size was greatly reduced and pulsations of the heart, pulmonary artery, and aorta were barely visible. After the release of pressure, pulsations returned immediately to the pulmonary artery but were delayed at the aorta until the third or fourth beat. The authors believe that syncope probably results from cerebral ischemia produced by a large transient fall in arterial pressure when the elevated intrathoracic pressure is released. They recommend that weight lifters avoid hyperventilation and prolonged squatting prior to a lift. Squatting reduces the venous return to the heart. The weight should be lifted as rapidly as possible so that normal breathing is resumed.

As in many sports in which the lumbar spine is stressed, weight lifting is associated with an increased incidence of spondylolysis (Figs. 228, 229). Kotani

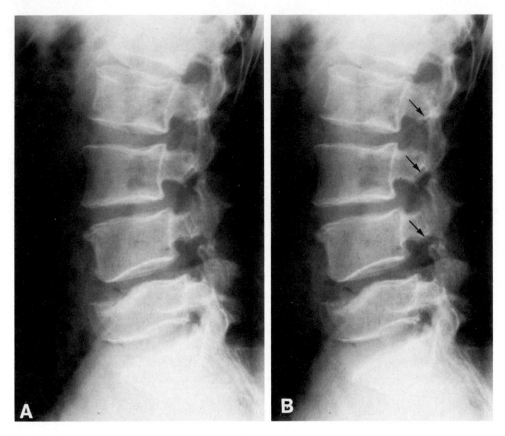

Fig. 228A. In his teenage years and his early twenties this man was a dedicated weight lifter and wrestler. He is now 35 years of age and has severe pain in the lower back. What is your diagnosis on the lateral view of the lumbar spine? **B.** The lateral view of the lumbar spine shows an old compression fracture deformity of the L5 vertebral body. Of greater interest is the series of spondylolyses (stress fractures) at the pars interarticularis area of L2, L3, and L4. (See also Figure 229.)

et al studied the lumbar spine x-rays of 26 weight lifters in Japan.[5] Eight of the 26 had spondylolysis. Six of these eight men gave a history of episodes of low back pain. D. W. Jackson and Wiltse reported spondylolysis in 20 young athletes over a five-year period.[3] Several sports were involved in producing these injuries, including weight lifting. (See the section on the lumbar spine in Part I.)

F. E. Jackson et al described an example of acute rupture of two lumbar intervertebral discs in a 17-year-old weight lifter.[4] This young man was attempting a "clean and press" lift without prior instruction in lifting techniques when he experienced one episode of severe back pain. Subsequent lifting led to continued back pain and to left leg pain. Myelographic examination showed extradural defects at L3–L4 and L4–L5. At surgery a completely extruded disc was found at L3–L4 and a herniated disc was found at L4–L5. In a similar manner, fracture of a lumbar vertebral body can occur during lifting. This must

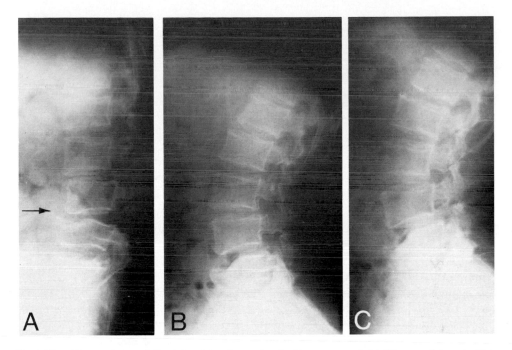

Fig. 229. Stress views of the lateral lumbar spine in the same weight lifter as shown in Figure 228 were taken with the patient in the standing position. **A.** Limit of flexion. **B.** Normal position. **C.** Limit of extension. The anterior part of the L4–L5 intervertebral disc space narrows in flexion (arrow) and a spondylolisthesis is demonstrated at the same level. The patient faces either nonoperative treatment or a major posterior lower lumbar operation.

be a rare event, although the author has observed it in a medical student who developed sudden back pain while lifting.

Jackson et al also recorded an example of injury to a 30-year-old weight lifter who was lifting a barbell from the supine position. The weight slipped from his grasp and fell on his face, producing fractures of the mandible and teeth and a through-and-through oral facial laceration. The lifter in the supine position should be protected by a support for the weight that will serve to catch the weight if it should fall.

References

1. Bakalim G: Rupture of the pectoralis major muscle. Acta Orthop Scand 36: 274–279, 1965
2. Compton D, Hill PM, Sinclair JD: Weight-lifters' blackout. Lancet 2:1234–1237, 1973
3. Jackson DW, Wiltse LL: Low back pain in young athletes. Physician Sports Med 2:53–60, Nov 1974
4. Jackson FE, Sazima HJ, Pratt RA, Back JB: Weight lifting injuries. J Am Coll Health Assoc 19:187–189, 1971
5. Kotani PT, Ichikawa N, Wakabayashi W, et al: Studies of spondylolysis found among weight lifters. Med Sport 25:154–160, 1972
6. Sharpey-Schafer EP, cited by Compton D, et al: Weight-lifters' blackout. Lancet 2: 1234–1237, 1973

WRESTLING

Wrestling produces numerous injuries, but few with radiologic findings. Grant reported that wrestling leads in injury rates among physical education activities in the United States.[1] Wrestling accounted for 16 injuries per 1000 participants compared to 9.7 per 1000 for boxing, 8.6 per 1000 for swimming, 5.1 per 1000 for gymnastics, and 5.3 per 1000 for fencing. He also lists a study of 448 injuries to 920 wrestlers over a five-year period. Approximately 10 percent of the injuries were fractures, most commonly of the ribs and fingers. The acromioclavicular and finger joints were the most common sites of dislocations. Roeser and Gentaz reported that bone spurs were a common finding in the cervical spines of 14 male wrestlers ranging in age from 31 to 68 years old.[3] The adjacent intervertebral disc spaces were normal. Five of these men had spurs or degenerative changes at the C1–C2 joint. Only 6 of 50 nonwrestlers in the 50-year-old age group had similar atlantoaxial changes. Limitation of motion of the neck was the chief difficulty in the wrestler group.

Wrestling led to a rupture of the left pectoralis major in a 28-year-old man who complained of pain in his left shoulder after a match.[2] Four weeks earlier his left arm had been caught under a training mat in a practice match. On physical examination there was tenderness over the belly of the left pectoralis major muscle with thinning of the axillary fold. Surgical repair was not attempted. The patient was able to resume training despite this injury.

References

1. Grant R: Wrestlers' problems with injuries. Br J Sports Med 5:161–166, 1970
2. Gudmundsson B: A case of agenesis and a case of rupture of the pectoralis major muscle. Acta Orthop Scand 44:213–218, 1973
3. Roeser J, Gentaz R: Lesions of the cervical column in wrestlers. J Radiol Electrol Med Nucl 50:699–702, 1969

PART III
RADIOGRAPHIC EXAMPLES OF INJURY

In most of these examples an athlete was injured while participating in sport. Many of the cases that follow are arranged so that two identical radiographic views are displayed side by side or as an upper and a lower figure on the same page. Instructions will be given in the legends when this double presentation occurs so that the reader can cover the second figure while surveying the first figure as an unknown. The second figure will be marked with arrows indicating the site or sites of injury.

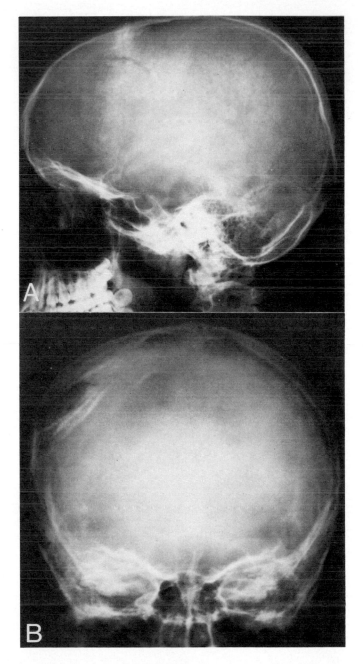

Fig. 230. Blunt trauma to the skull led to a suspicion of a skull fracture. What is your diagnosis based on the selected lateral and anteroposterior views? *(Examine A and B and make your decision before turning to C and D.)*

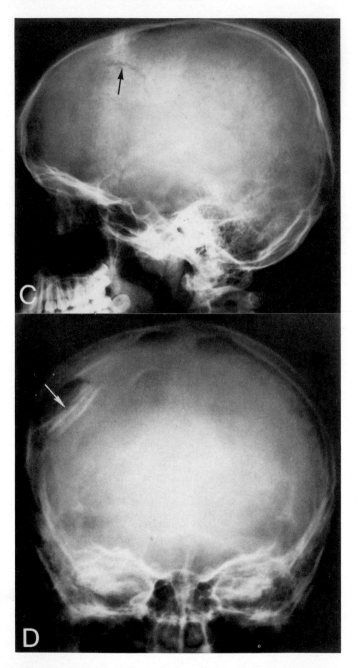

Fig. 230 (cont.).   The lateral view of the skull (**A** and **C**) shows an unusual radiolucent line at the frontoparietal area (arrow). A gauze dressing overlies this site (arrow). The frontal view (**B** and **D**) shows an area of increased density associated with radiolucency at its lateral margin. This area corresponds with the abnormal radiolucent zone noted on the lateral view and represents a depressed skull fracture. Not all skull fractures produce sharp, long radiolucent lines crossing a part of the skull. Depressed skull fractures do not produce areas of increased radiodensity on all views.

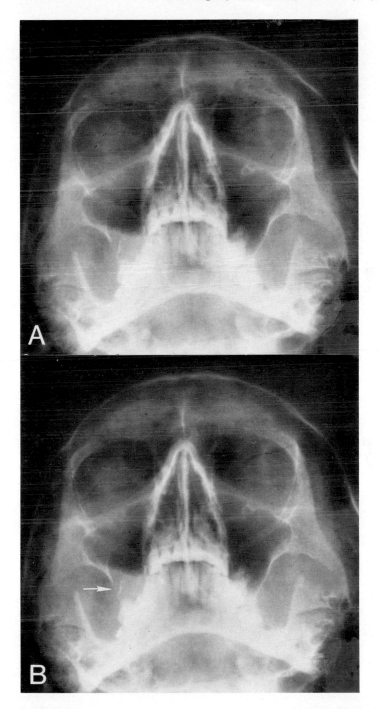

Fig. 231A. This view was obtained after facial injury. What is your diagnosis? *(Cover B before making your decision.)* **B.** The lateral wall of the right maxillary antrum is fractured (arrow) and soft-tissue swelling or hemorrhage has developed at the base of the injured sinus. The remaining facial areas are unremarkable.

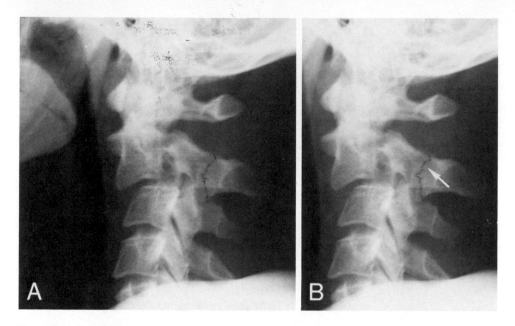

Fig. 232A. A young man injured his neck by diving into shallow water. What are your findings based on the lateral view of the upper portion of the cervical spine? *(Cover B.)* **B.** A fracture is present through the neural arch of the second cervical vertebrae and is associated with a dislocation of C2 and C3. A fracture of this type is referred to as a hangman's fracture because similar injuries have been produced by that form of capital punishment. Fortunately this patient escaped neurologic damage by a very narrow margin.

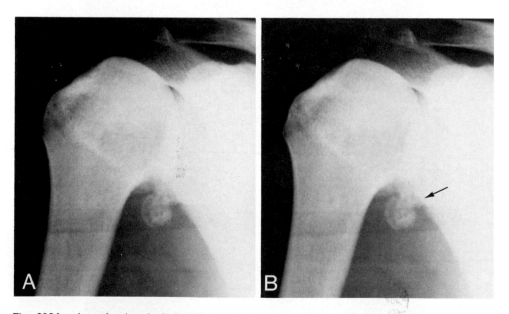

Fig. 233A. A professional pitcher in baseball complained of pain in the shoulder. How do you interpret these findings? *(Cover B.)* **B.** A rounded fragment of bone with irregular ossification is present adjacent to the infraglenoid margin. The fragment has been avulsed from the scapular margin in a chronic injury of the long head of the triceps muscle of the type described by Bennett. (See the section on baseball in Part II.) The size of the fragment suggests that it has enlarged since it separated from the scapula. The superolateral slope of the humeral head is slightly sclerotic and steep, suggesting degenerative or post-traumatic changes at the cortex. There was no history of shoulder dislocation in this patient.

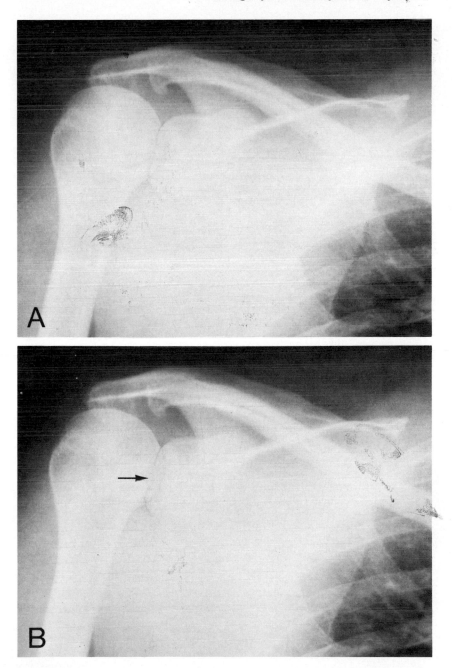

Fig. 234A. Is this a normal anteroposterior view of the shoulder? *(Cover B.)* **B.** The margins of the glenohumeral joint overlap with no intervening cartilage or joint space. This should lead you to a presumptive diagnosis of a posterior dislocation of the shoulder that was present in this patient.

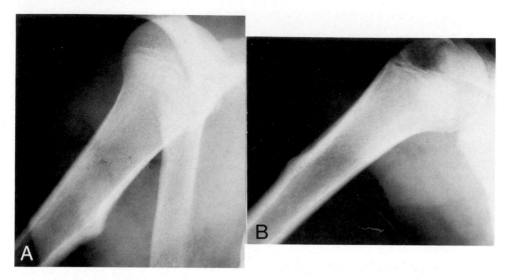

Fig. 235. Two views of the same humerus are shown in different positions of humeral rotation. The promontory on this humeral shaft was detected several months after injury in a wrestler. The position is correct for the promontory to be a deltoid tubercle. The author knows of no other variant of normal at this site. An osteochondroma could account for the cortical enlargement, but so could an avulsion injury at the deltoid muscle insertion. This promontory did not change on subsequent radiographs made six months after the injury.

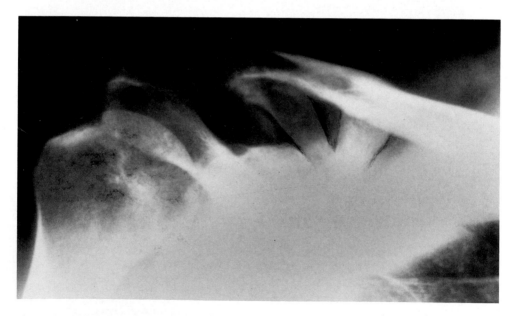

Fig. 236. The lateral and medial portions of the coracoclavicular ligaments are ossified following prior ligament rupture that separated both the acromioclavicular and coracoclavicular joints.

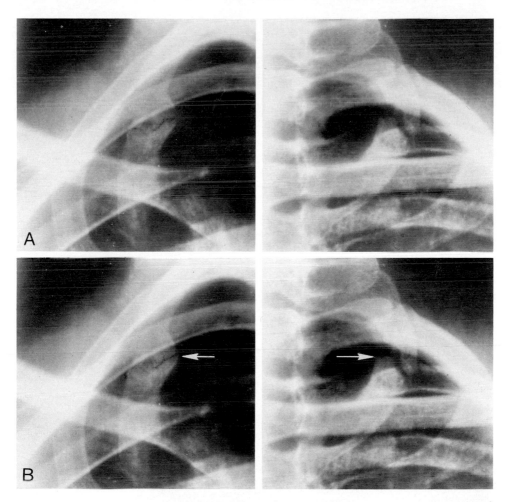

Fig. 237A. Heavy use of the shoulder girdle in throwing and lifting can produce this injury. What is your diagnosis? *(Cover B.)* **B.** Stress fractures of the first ribs are present (arrows). The defects show little or no periosteal reaction. Identical fractures have been observed in baseball pitchers on rare occasion and in individuals carrying heavy loads in knapsacks. (See Figure 186.)

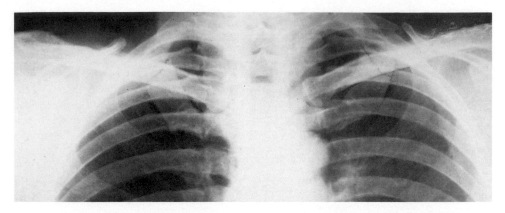

Fig. 238. Heavy use of the shoulders in another patient led to bilateral stress fractures of the first rib that were discovered incidentally when the patient was struck in the left upper chest, receiving a fracture to the left second rib.

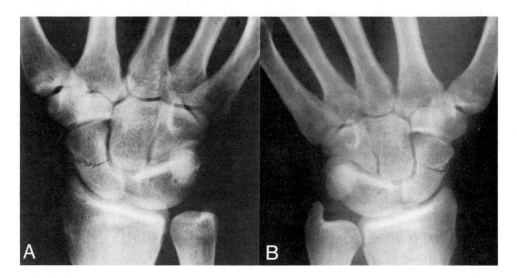

Fig. 239A. An ice skater fell on the ice and injured both wrists in that fall. What is your diagnosis based on these views of both wrists? **B.** The x-ray diagnosis is identical for each side—fracture of the waist of the carpal navicular or scaphoid bone. Both wrists also show congenital fusion or failure of segmentation between the lunate and the triquetrum. Whether or not this normal variant of carpal structure contributed to the injury on each side is uncertain.

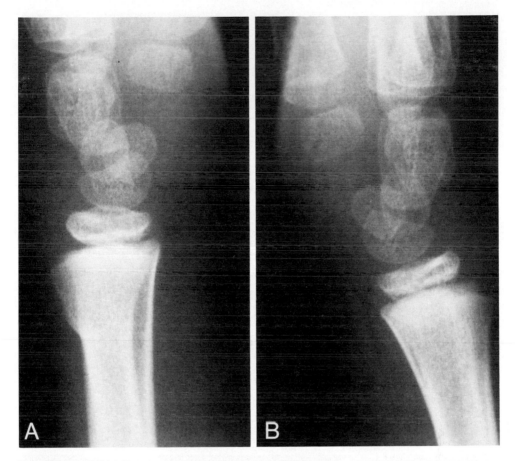

Fig. 240. A child fell while running. **A.** The lateral view of the injured forearm. **B.** The uninjured side. Study the views carefully before you come to any conclusion. The posterior cortex of the injured radius is indented in a torus fracture. The torus fracture is one that buckles the cortex of the long bone. The cortical bump resembles the foot or torus of the end of an ancient architectural column—hence its name. The examiner must study the cortical areas carefully to detect a torus fracture.

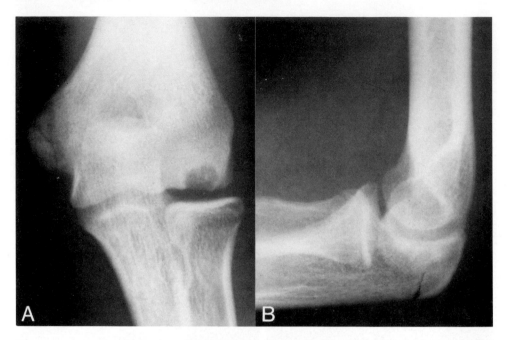

Fig. 241. A 14-year-old quarterback in football complained of sudden pain in the elbow after throwing a pass. He was unable to extend his elbow fully and was admitted for further evaluation. **A.** This view shows a radiolucent defect in the capitellar surface due to chronic injury to the articular surface. A loose fragment was suspected but was not found at operation. **B.** The lateral view shows displacement of the anterior fat pad indicating an effusion. A residual epiphyseal growth plate is present in the olecranon.

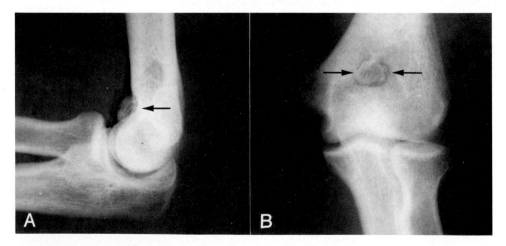

Fig. 242. At age 14 this teenage wrestler fell on his elbow. The original lateral view is not displayed here, but showed a small density in the antecubital fossa, suggesting a fracture fragment. These follow-up views, made two years later, showed enlargement of this loose body in the interim.

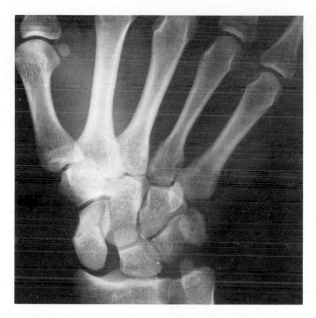

Fig. 243. A rugby player injured his wrist in a fall during a rugby match. What is your diagnosis based on this view? (See Figure 244.)

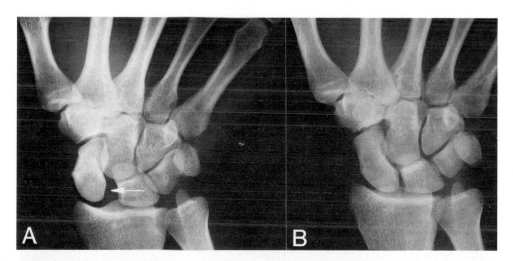

Fig. 244. Comparison views of the left and right wrists were made in the same rugby player as shown in Figure 233. **A.** The navicular (scaphoid)–lunate ligaments have been ruptured in the left wrist, leading to a widened navicular (scaphoid)–lunate intercarpal joint space. The right wrist is normal. **B.** The patient had tenderness at the anatomic snuff box and the pre-radiographic diagnosis was fracture of the carpal navicular (scaphoid).

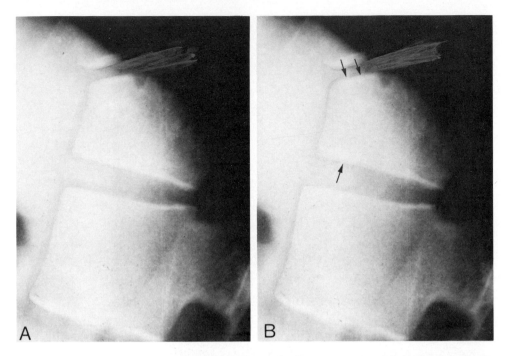

Fig. 245A. A medical student interested in weight lifting developed sudden back pain during a lift. This enlargement shows the junction of the thoracolumbar spine in the lateral projection. **B.** A compression fracture of the first lumbar vertebral body is present.

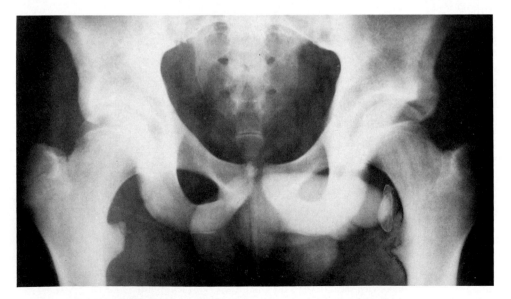

Fig. 246. This view was taken several weeks after a sprinter experienced sudden pain at the left hip while running. What is your diagnosis? Ossification is present in the soft tissues adjacent to the left lesser trochanter. The trochanter has been displaced superiorly following an avulsion injury to the insertion of the left iliopsoas muscle.

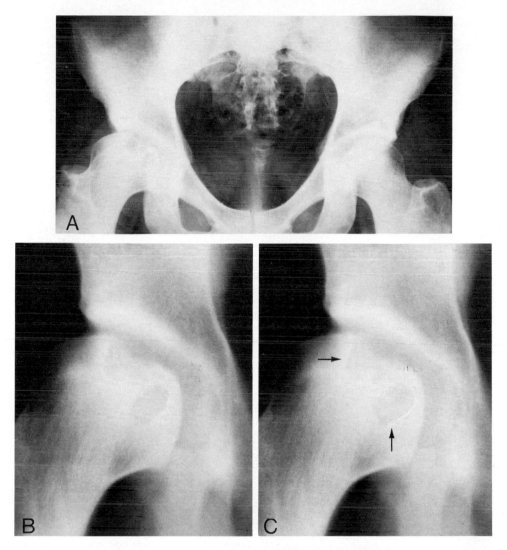

Fig. 247. A rugby player complained of right hip pain after persistent play and running. **A.** The right hip is abnormal on this x-ray. What is your diagnosis? *(Cover B and C)* **B.** A tomographic view was also obtained. **C.** A radiolucent area (vertical arrow) has formed in the femoral head adjacent to a widened fovea capitus (horizontal arrow). This radiolucent and cystic area shown on tomography represents a post-traumatic cyst of the type more commonly found in the ankle or knee.

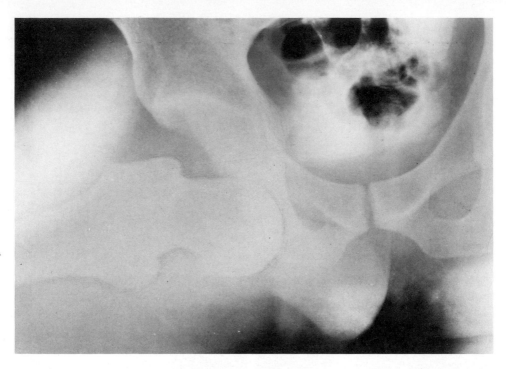

Fig. 248. A young man attempted to throw his opponent in judo. He lay on his back with his foot aimed at his opponent's body as a throwing platform or fulcrum. The opponent, without cooperating in this maneuver, fell on the patient's leg and injured the hip. What is your diagnosis? The right hip is dislocated. The patient was anesthetized and the hip was relocated from a position of anterior dislocation.

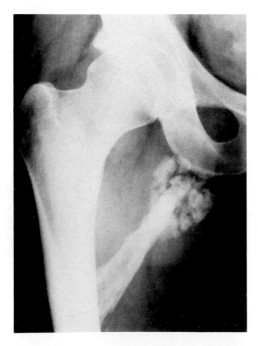

Fig. 249. A strutlike mass of bone has developed following an adductor muscle avulsion injury in a gymnast. The inferior two-thirds of the lesion shows trabeculation and a poorly delimited cortex, indicating a mature organization that has evolved many months after the day of the injury. (From Murray, Jacobson: The Radiology of Skeletal Disorders, 1971. Courtesy of Churchill Livingstone).

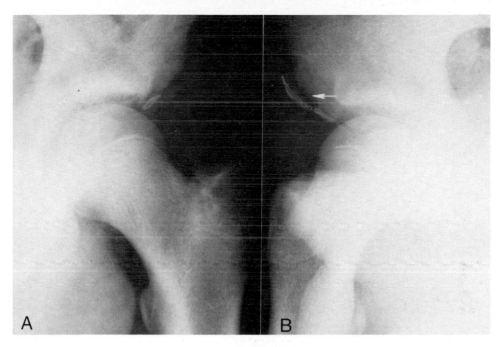

Fig. 250. Sudden hip pain while running led to this demonstration of an avulsion of the origin of the biceps femoris at the anterior inferior iliac spine. **A.** A normal ossification center is present at the edge of the acetabular margin in both the injured and uninjured hips. (Shown here is the uninjured hip.) **B.** The injured hip shows a large flake of bone superior to the rim of the acetabulum (arrow).

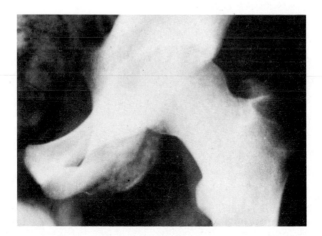

Fig. 251. Ossification is present at the margin of the ischial tuberosity. The bone developed following a sudden avulsion injury during delivery of the ball by a bowler in cricket.

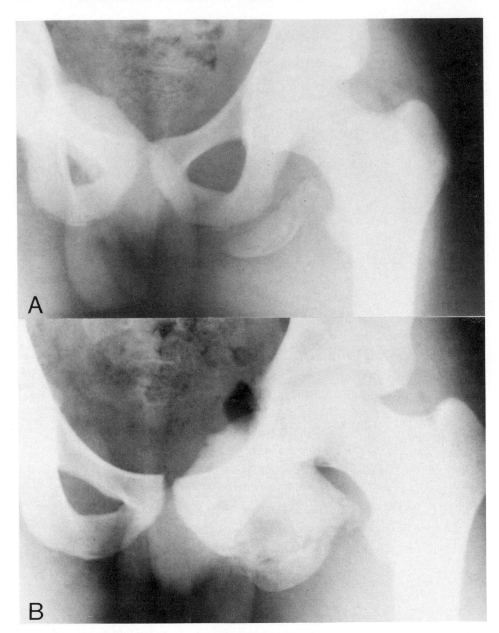

Fig. 252A. A football player experienced severe groin pain suddenly while running. What is your diagnosis? The entire ischial tuberosity has been avulsed on the left side of the pelvis. This is the origin of the hamstring muscles, which have pulled violently, producing this injury. **B.** A subsequent radiograph made two months later shows the mass of bone that has developed at the injury site. This particular appearance of the large area of bone has on occasion been mistaken for a neoplasm involving the skeleton.

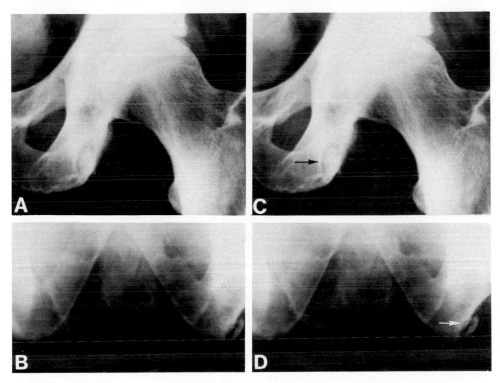

Fig. 253. Cover C and D of this figure. A golfer experienced sudden pain at his left groin during a forceful swing at a golf ball. **A.** The frontal view of the ischial tuberosities. **B.** A steeply angled view. **C, D.** A small avulsion fragment is present at the margins of the ischium, indicating an injury of the origin of the hamstring muscles.

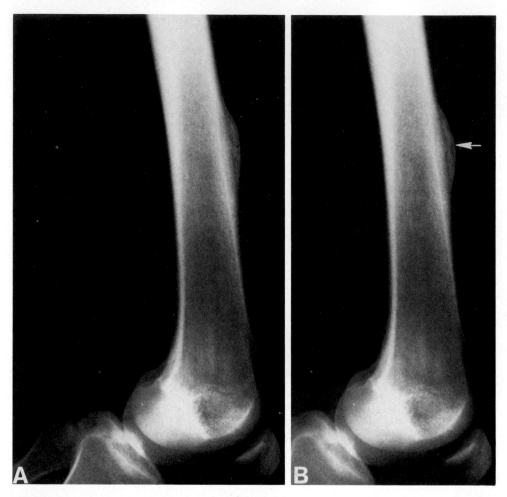

Fig. 254A. A collision in basketball produced an injury months before this x-ray was obtained. What is your diagnosis? *(Cover B.)* **B.** A periosteal-based mass of bone is present on the surface of the femur. This is a form of myositis ossificans of the post-traumatic type that occasionally shows periosteal attachment. The lesion is too regular and too orderly to represent a bone tumor.

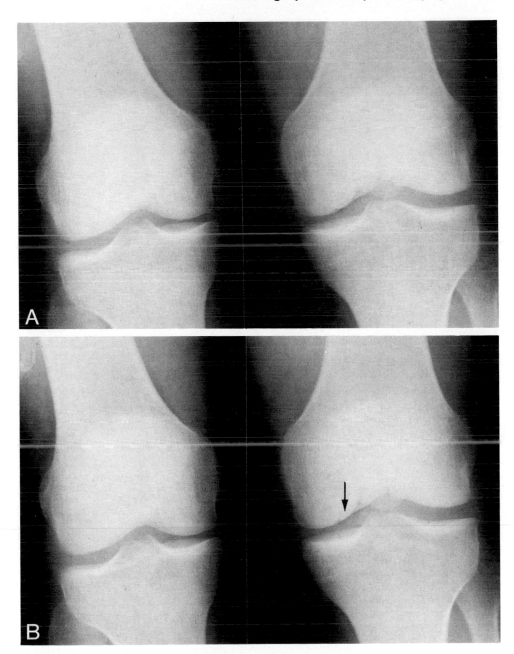

Fig. 255A. A runner complained of left knee pain. The right knee (reader's left) is normal but the left knee is not. What is your diagnosis? *(Cover B.)* **B.** The irregularity in the left knee of the cortical surface of the medial femoral condyle at its lateral aspect is diagnostic of osteochondritis dissecans. This finding is usually attributed to surface injury of the condyle or to injury of underlying vessels affecting surface bone. Although asymptomatic examples of this finding are occasionally noted, the lesion is usually associated with pain and knee discomfort. The right knee is normal.

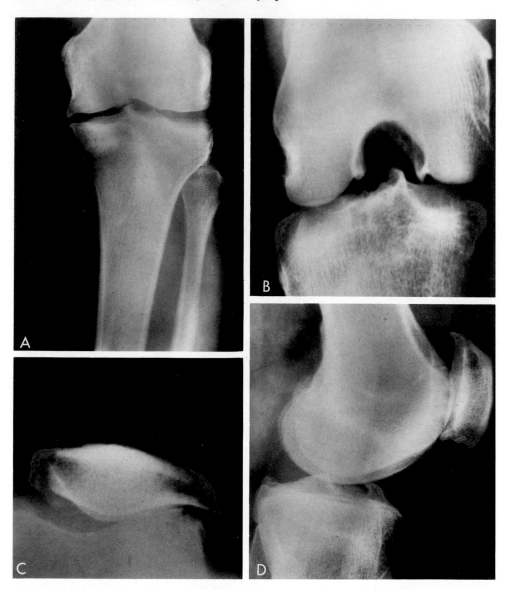

Fig. 256A. A professional squash player in his early thirties complained of knee pain. The anteroposterior view of the knee shows degenerative disease with spur formation at the tibial intercondylar eminence and at the medial margin of the femorotibial joint. **B.** The notch or intercondylar notch view shows additional degenerative spurs at the inner margins of the femoral condyles. **C.** The axial view of the patella shows narrowing of the patellofemoral joint, lateral subluxation of the patella, and spur formation. **D.** The lateral view shows patellar articular spurs and posterior joint margin spurs.

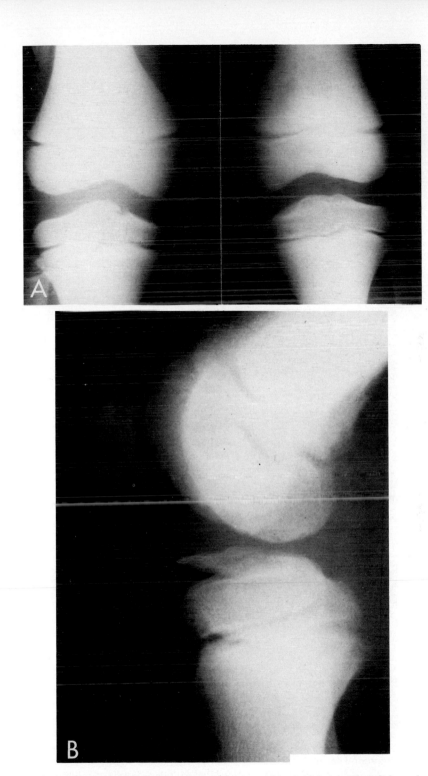

Fig. 257. A young boy fell while bicycling and injured his right knee. His left knee is normal. **A.** The anteroposterior view of both knees. **B.** The lateral view of the right knee. What is your diagnosis?

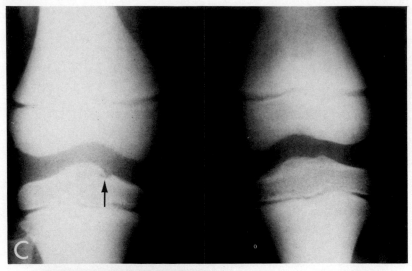

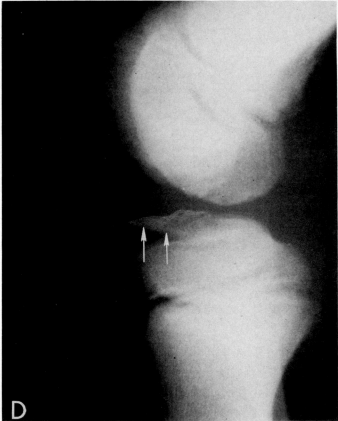

Fig. 257 *(cont.)* **C.** The comparison anteroposterior view of both knees shows slight irregularity of the right intercondylar eminence of the tibia. **D.** The lateral view of the right knee shows the displaced avulsion fragment of bone at the tibial articular margin. At operation this fragment was attached to the anterior cruciate ligament. In similar cases meniscal attachments may also be found.

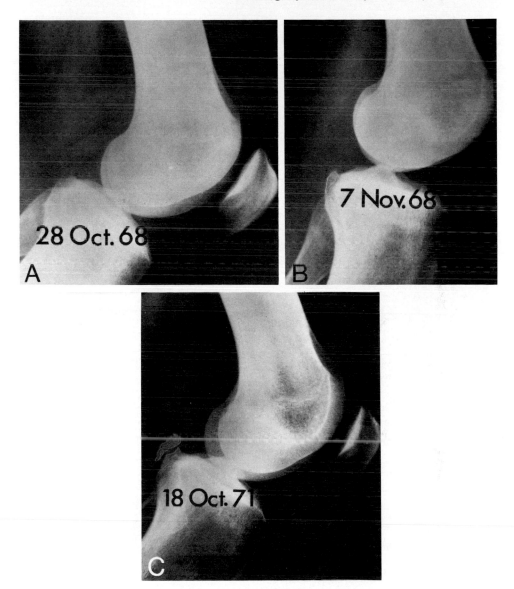

Fig. 258. A 26-year-old athlete injured his left knee in a fall in sport. **A.** The lateral view made on October 28, 1968, is normal. **B.** A post-traumatic exostosis has developed at the posterior margin of the tibia in the view made on November 7, 1968. This is a hamstring insertion site and represents an avulsion injury with hemorrhage and subsequent ossification. **C.** The ossification increased in size in the years following injury and is shown in a view made on October 18, 1971.

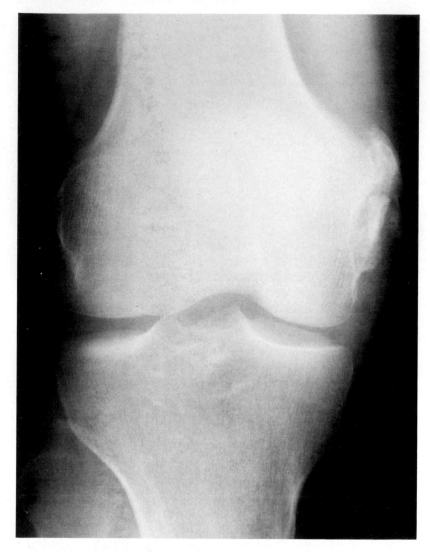

Fig. 259. This anteroposterior view of the knee shows marked ossification at the origin of the medial collateral ligament, demonstrating the Pelligrini-Stieda type lesion following ligament injury in the past.

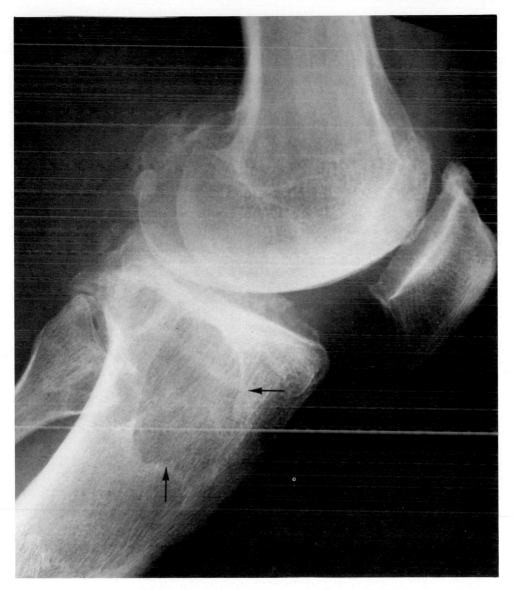

Fig. 260. Marked degenerative changes in exathletes and in nonathletes can be associated with large subchondral cysts. Here a subchondral or post-traumatic cyst (arrow) occupies most of the proximal end of the tibia.

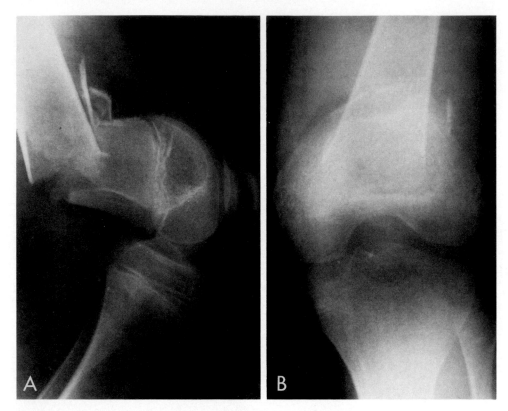

Fig. 261A. A motorbike accident produced this injury in a teenager. The displacement of this comminuted femur threatens the popliteal artery. Fortunately no permanent vascular damage occurred. **B.** The frontal view of the femur again shows the comminuted fracture fragments.

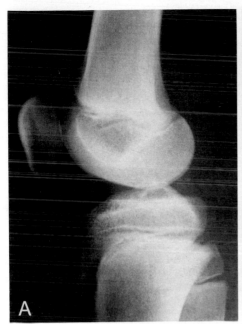

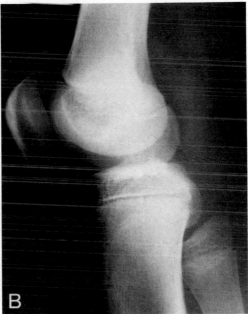

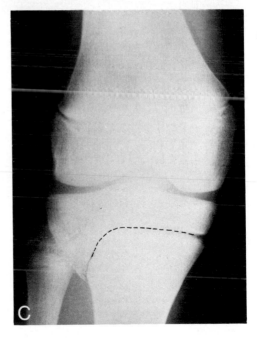

Fig. 262. A 12-year-old injured his knee while motorcycling. **A.** The lateral view of the injured knee. **B.** The normal knee. Compare the positions of the proximal tibial epiphyseal and epiphyseal plate areas in the two knees. The bony epiphysis is displaced forward in the injured knee, giving a widened posterior epiphyseal cartilage compared to the normal knee. **C.** The anteroposterior view shows that the transepiphyseal cartilage fracture has extended across the metaphysis of the tibia.

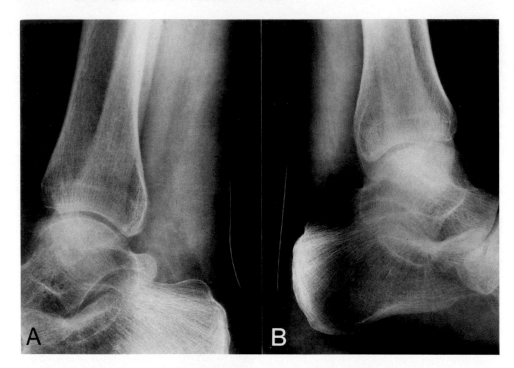

Fig. 263. This R.A.F. officer was unfortunate on two occasions. While diving he ruptured one Achilles tendon and while playing tennis he ruptured the other. The radiographs of the ankles show the soft-tissue swelling that obliterates the normal radiolucent space above the calcaneus. The space is normally triangular in shape and is bound by the calcaneus, Achilles tendon, and posterior tibial muscles and soft tissues. Do not forget that other conditions, including inflammatory diseases of the tendon and its surrounding tissue, can obliterate this triangle. (See Goldman et al: Disruptions of the tendo Achilles. Mayo Clin Proc 44:28–35, 1969.)

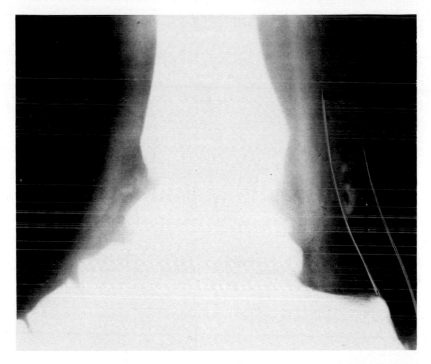

Fig. 264. This lateral view was obtained after partial rupture of the Achilles tendon in a tennis player. The player is a former National Junior Champion. Edema obliterates the normal margins of the tendon and the posterior radiolucent triangle. In addition, calcification is present in the tendon from an earlier injury. Occasionally, xanthomata form within the tendon and produce similar calcification in the Achilles tendon or elsewhere. Some examples of tendon xanthomata are secondary to hyperlipidemia. The lower portions of the Achilles tendon have been outlined on the photograph although these lines appeared on the original x-ray.

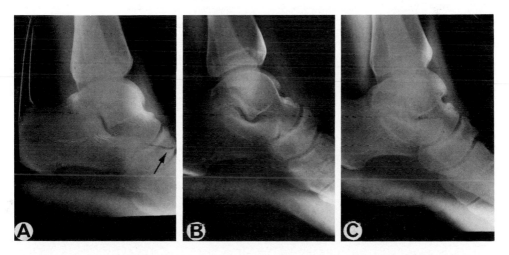

Fig. 265. A young woman injured her foot while practicing judo. **A.** The fracture line in the tarsal navicular (scaphoid) is obvious. Of incidental importance is the beautiful example of the normal radiolucent triangle above the calcaneus on this lateral projection. The Achilles tendon has been outlined as in Figure 264. **B, C.** The subsequent views show the healing process and irregularity of the dorsal surface of the talus over a period of months.

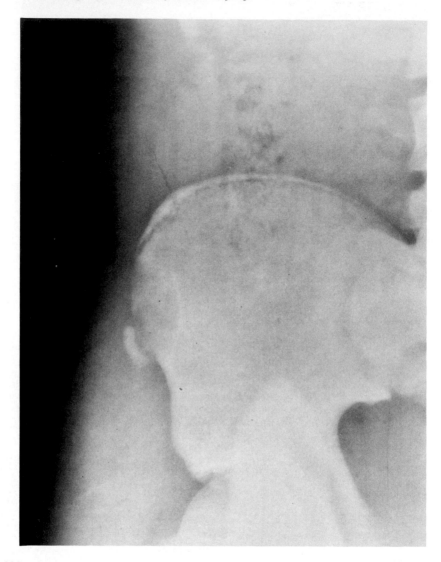

Fig. 266. An 18-year-old boy reached for a pass while running at full speed in football. As he stretched to reach the ball he experienced a sudden pain at the pelvic margin near the right hip. At the emergency room an x-ray of the pelvis showed an avulsion fragment of bone at the origin of the sartorius muscle at the anterior superior iliac spine. His treatment consisted solely of ice packs and pain medication. He recovered uneventfully.

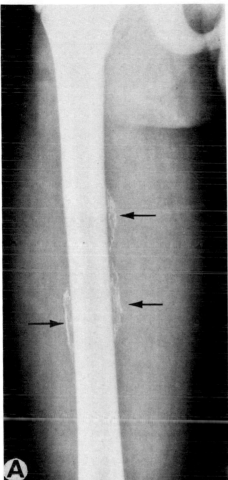

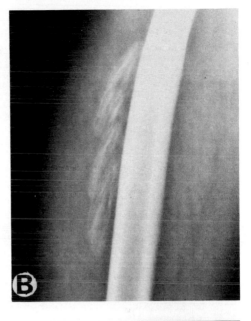

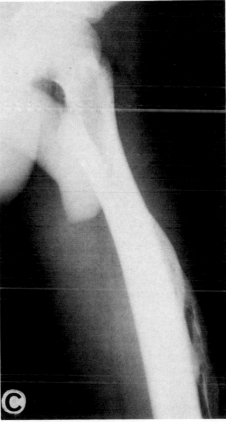

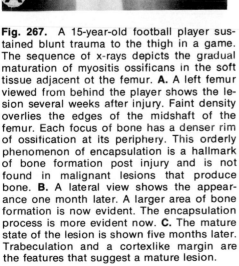

Fig. 267. A 15-year-old football player sustained blunt trauma to the thigh in a game. The sequence of x-rays depicts the gradual maturation of myositis ossificans in the soft tissue adjacent ot the femur. **A.** A left femur viewed from behind the player shows the lesion several weeks after injury. Faint density overlies the edges of the midshaft of the femur. Each focus of bone has a denser rim of ossification at its periphery. This orderly phenomenon of encapsulation is a hallmark of bone formation post injury and is not found in malignant lesions that produce bone. **B.** A lateral view shows the appearance one month later. A larger area of bone formation is now evident. The encapsulation process is more evident now. **C.** The mature state of the lesion is shown five months later. Trabeculation and a cortexlike margin are the features that suggest a mature lesion.

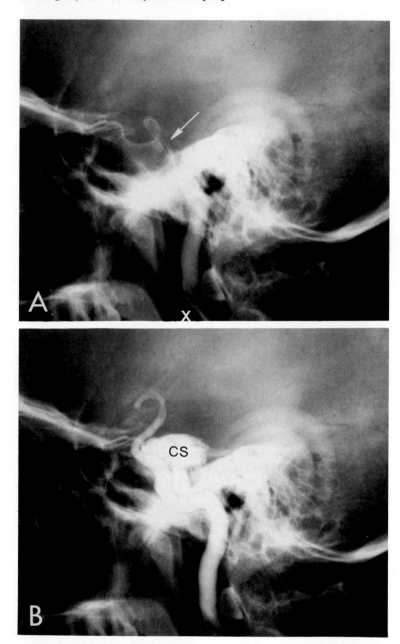

Fig. 268. A jockey fell from his mount and injured his head. He complained of headache and a persistent pulsating noise in his head. A bruit was present on auscultation. **A.** This enlargement shows the area of the sella turcica from the lateral viewpoint. A fracture is present at the clivus Blumenbachi (arrow). A catheter (×) has been placed in the common carotid artery and threaded into the internal carotid system. Contrast material appears in the internal carotid artery in this early view at arteriography. **B.** Just fractions of a second later the contrast material has outlined the intracranial portion of the internal carotid artery and the adjacent cavernous sinus (CS). The sinus has filled via a traumatic arteriovenous fistula produced by the shearing forces of the fall.

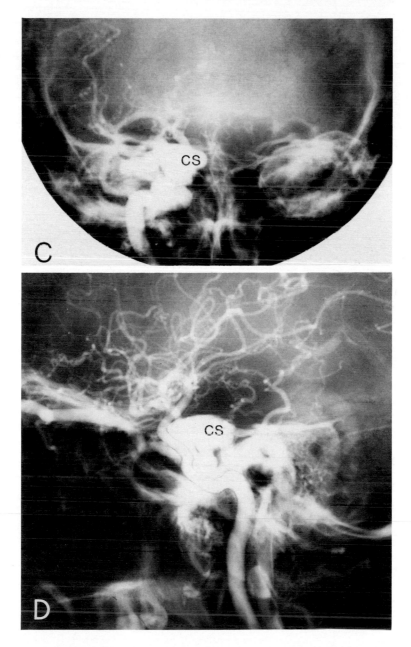

Fig. 268C. An anteroposterior view made a few seconds later shows the intimate relationship of the internal carotid artery and the cavernous sinus from the frontal plane. **D.** The lateral view made at the same time as C shows filling of intracerebral branches of the anterior and middle cerebral arteries despite the short circuit through the cavernous sinus.

INDEX

(Page numbers within parentheses indicate illustrations)